DALLAS AREA (Including Grand Prairie, Garland, and Irving)

1 Bachman Lake Trail (p. 18)
2 Boulder Park Trail (p. 22)
3 Campion Trail (p. 26)
4 Downtown Dallas Urban Trail (p. 30)
5 Duck Creek Greenbelt (p. 35)
6 Fair Park Loop (p. 39)
7 Fish Creek Linear Trail (p. 43)
8 Katy Trail (p. 47)
9 L. B. Houston Nature Trail (p. 52)
10 Rowlett Creek Nature Trail (p. 56)
11 Spring Creek Park Nature Trail (p. 60)
12 Trinity River Audubon Trail (p. 64)
13 Turtle Creek Leisure Trail (p. 69)
14 White Rock Lake Trail (p. 73)

FORT WORTH AREA (Including Grapevine Lake, Colleyville, and Euless)

15 Bear Creek–Bob Eden Trail (p. 80)
16 Benbrook Dam Trail (p. 84)
17 Benbrook Lake Trail (p. 88)
18 Colleyville Nature Trail (p. 92)
19 Fort Worth Nature Center: Canyon Ridge Trail (p. 96)
20 Fort Worth Nature Center: Prairie Trail (p. 100)
21 Horseshoe Trail (p. 104)
22 Knob Hill Trail (p. 108)
23 Northshore Trail (p. 112)
24 River Legacy Trail (p. 116)
25 Rocky Point Trail (p. 120)
26 Sansom Park Trail (p. 124)
27 Trinity River Trail (Northside) (p. 128)
28 Trinity River Trail (Oakmont Park) (p. 132)

NORTH OF DALLAS–FORT WORTH (Including Plano, McKinney, Lake Ray Roberts, and Lake Lewisville)

29 Arbor Hills Loop (p. 139)
30 Black Creek–Cottonwood Hiking Trail (p. 143)
31 Breckenridge Park Trail (p. 147)

32 Cicada–Cottonwood Loop (p. 151)
33 Elm Fork Trail (p. 155)
34 Erwin Park Loop (p. 159)
35 Lavon Lake: Trinity Trail (p. 163)
36 Parkhill Prairie Trail (p. 167)
37 Pilot Knoll Trail (p. 171)
38 Ray Roberts Greenbelt (p. 175)
39 Ray Roberts Lake State Park, Isle du Bois Unit: Lost Pines Trail (p. 179)
40 Ray Roberts Lake State Park, Johnson Branch Unit: Johnson Branch Trail (p. 183)
41 Sister Grove Loop (p. 187)
42 Walnut Grove Trail (p. 191)

SOUTH OF DALLAS–FORT WORTH (Including Cedar Hill, Glen Rose, and Cleburne)

43 Bardwell Lake Multiuse Trail (p. 198)
44 Cedar Hill State Park: Talala–Duck Pond Loop (p. 202)
45 Cedar Mountain Trail (p. 206)
46 Cedar Ridge Preserve Trail (p. 210)
47 Cleburne State Park Loop Trail (p. 215)
48 Cottonwood Creek Trail (p. 220)
49 Dinosaur Valley Trail (p. 224)
50 Purtis Creek Trail (p. 229)
51 Visitor's Overlook: Joe Pool Lake Dam Trail (p. 233)
52 Walnut Creek Trail (p. 237)
53 Waxahachie Creek Hike & Bike Trail (p. 241)
54 Windmill Hill Preserve Trail (p. 245)

WEST OF FORT WORTH

55 Lake Mineral Wells State Park: Cross Timbers Trail (p. 252)
56 Lake Mineral Wells State Trailway (p. 257)
57 Lost Creek Reservoir State Trailway (p. 261)

EAST OF DALLAS

58 Lake Tawakoni Nature Trail (p. 268)
59 Post Oak Trail (p. 272)
60 Samuell Farm Trail (p. 276)

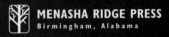

MENASHA RIDGE PRESS
Birmingham, Alabama

60 HIKES WITHIN 60 MILES

DALLAS– FORT WORTH

INCLUDING TARRANT, COLLIN, AND DENTON COUNTIES

SECOND EDITION

JOANIE SÁNCHEZ

60 HIKES WITHIN 60 MILES: DALLAS–FORT WORTH

Copyright © 2012 by Joanie Sánchez
All rights reserved
Printed in the United States of America
Published by Menasha Ridge Press
Distributed by Publishers Group West
Second edition, third printing 2016

Library of Congress Cataloging-in-Publication Data

Sánchez, Joanie
   60 hikes within 60 miles, Dallas, Fort Worth: includes Tarrant, Collin, and Denton counties / Joanie
Sánchez. — 2nd ed.
      p. cm.
   ISBN-13: 978-0-89732-606-3 (pbk.)
   ISBN-10: 0-89732-606-7
   1. Hiking—Texas—Dallas Region—Guidebooks. 2. Hiking—Texas—Fort Worth Region—Guidebooks.
   3. Trails—Texas—Dallas Region—Guidebooks. 4. Trails—Texas—Fort Worth Region—Guidebooks.
   5. Dallas Region (Tex.)—Guidebooks. 6. Fort Worth Region (Tex.)—Guidebooks. I. Title. II. Title:
   Sixty hikes within sixty miles.
   GV199.42.T492D35 2011
   917.64'28—dc23
                                    2011041180

Cover and text design by Steveco International
Cover photo by Andrew Sánchez
Author photo by Andrew Sánchez
Cartography and elevation profiles by Scott McGrew, Lohnes+Wright, and Joanie Sánchez
Indexing by Ann Cassar/Cassar Technical Services

Menasha Ridge Press
AdventureKEEN
2204 Fist Avenue South, Suite 102
Birmingham, AL 35233
menasharidge.com

DISCLAIMER

**TO MY MOTHER AND FATHER, FOR TEACHING ME MY FIRST FEW STEPS
AND GUIDING ME ON EACH ONE THEREAFTER.**

— JOANIE SÁNCHEZ

TABLE OF CONTENTS

OVERVIEW MAP . . . . inside front cover

ACKNOWLEDGMENTS. vii

FOREWORD viii

ABOUT THE AUTHOR. ix

PREFACE x

HIKING RECOMMENDATIONS xiii

INTRODUCTION 1

DALLAS AREA (including Grand Prairie, Garland, and Irving) 16
1	Bachman Lake Trail 18
2	Boulder Park Trail 22
3	Campion Trail. 26
4	Downtown Dallas Urban Trail .30
5	Duck Creek Greenbelt. 35
6	Fair Park Loop. 39
7	Fish Creek Linear Trail. 43
8	Katy Trail 47
9	L. B. Houston Nature Trail 52
10	Rowlett Creek Nature Trail. 56
11	Spring Creek Park Nature Trail 60
12	Trinity River Audubon Trail. .64
13	Turtle Creek Leisure Trail 69
14	White Rock Lake Trail 73

FORT WORTH AREA (Including Grapevine Lake, Colleyville, and Euless) 78
15	Bear Creek–Bob Eden Trail 80
16	Benbrook Dam Trail 84
17	Benbrook Lake Trail. 88
18	Colleyville Nature Trail 92
19	Fort Worth Nature Center: Canyon Ridge Trail 96
20	Fort Worth Nature Center: Prairie Trail. 100
21	Horseshoe Trail 104
22	Knob Hill Trail 108
23	Northshore Trail 112
24	River Legacy Trail. 116
25	Rocky Point Trail 120
26	Sansom Park Trail. 124
27	Trinity River Trail (Northside). 128
28	Trinity River Trail (Oakmont Park) 132

NORTH OF DALLAS–FORT WORTH (Including Plano, McKinney, Lake Ray Roberts, and Lake Lewisville) 136

29 Arbor Hills Loop 139
30 Black Creek–Cottonwood Hiking Trail 143
31 Breckenridge Park Trail 147
32 Cicada–Cottonwood Loop 151
33 Elm Fork Trail 155
34 Erwin Park Loop 159
35 Lavon Lake: Trinity Trail 163
36 Parkhill Prairie Trail 167
37 Pilot Knoll Trail 171
38 Ray Roberts Greenbelt 175
39 Ray Roberts Lake State Park, Isle du Bois Unit: Lost Pines Trail 179
40 Ray Roberts Lake State Park, Johnson Branch Unit: Johnson Branch Trail 183
41 Sister Grove Loop 187
42 Walnut Grove Trail 191

SOUTH OF DALLAS–FORT WORTH (Including Cedar Hill, Glen Rose, and Cleburne) 196

43 Bardwell Lake Multiuse Trail 198
44 Cedar Hill State Park: Talala–Duck Pond Loop 202
45 Cedar Mountain Trail 206
46 Cedar Ridge Preserve Trail 210
47 Cleburne State Park Loop Trail 215
48 Cottonwood Creek Trail 220
49 Dinosaur Valley Trail 224
50 Purtis Creek Trail 229
51 Visitor's Overlook: Joe Pool Lake Dam Trail 233
52 Walnut Creek Trail 237
53 Waxahachie Creek Hike & Bike Trail 241
54 Windmill Hill Preserve Trail 245

WEST OF FORT WORTH 250

55 Lake Mineral Wells State Park: Cross Timbers Trail 252
56 Lake Mineral Wells State Trailway 257
57 Lost Creek Reservoir State Trailway 261

EAST OF DALLAS 266

58 Lake Tawakoni Nature Trail 268
59 Post Oak Trail 272
60 Samuell Farm Trail 276

APPENDIXES AND INDEX 281
APPENDIX A: Outdoor Shops 283
APPENDIX B: Places to Buy Maps 285
APPENDIX C: Hiking Clubs 287
INDEX 289
MAP LEGEND ....inside back cover

ACKNOWLEDGMENTS

Without question, it would have been impossible for me to have written either edition of this book without the enthusiasm of the park rangers, office staff, and volunteers who promote and stand guard over the trails in their domain. On my first visits, they had me eagerly lacing up my boots and seeking out their trailheads. Since then, their passion has kept me eager to revisit and explore more. I cannot thank these watchful custodians enough for their tips, insights, recommendations, and knowledge which help and inspire all who pass through their doors.

I would also like to thank others without whose help the first edition of this book truly would never have been written, much less updated: my father, Orlando Sánchez, whose enthusiasm and excitement motivate me; Bob Shauchunas, who always seems to have the right tip at the right time; my mother, Joan Shauchunas, who inspires me with her company and impresses me with her own adventures; and my brother, Andrew Sánchez, who has never—regardless of weather, insects, or logistics—turned me down on an adventure. These hikes would not have been nearly as easy or as fun to execute without his assistance, advice, and companionship.

—JOANIE SÁNCHEZ

FOREWORD

Welcome to Menasha Ridge Press's *60 Hikes within 60 Miles*. Our strategy was simple: First, find a hiker who knows the area and loves to hike. Second, ask that person to spend a year researching the most popular and very best trails around. And third, have that person describe each trail in terms of difficulty, scenery, condition, elevation change, and all other categories of information that are important to hikers. "Pretend you've just completed a hike and met up with other hikers at the trailhead," we told each author. "Imagine their questions, and be clear in your answers." An experienced hiker and writer, author Joanie Sánchez has selected 60 of the best hikes in and around the Dallas–Fort Worth metropolitan area. From the greenways and urban hikes that make use of parklands to flora- and fauna-rich treks along the cliffs and hills in the hinterlands, Sánchez provides hikers (and walkers) with a great variety of hikes—and all within roughly 60 miles of Dallas–Fort Worth.

You'll get more out of this book if you take a moment to read the Introduction explaining how to read the trail listings. The "Topographic Maps" section will help you understand how useful topos will be on a hike and will also tell you where to get them. And though this is a where-to rather than a how-to guide, those of you who have hiked extensively will find the Introduction of particular value. As much for the opportunity to free the spirit as well as to free the body, let these hikes elevate you above the urban hurry.

**All the best,
The Editors at Menasha Ridge Press**

ABOUT THE AUTHOR

An avid hiker, camper, and traveler, **JOANIE SÁNCHEZ** first fell in love with the outdoors when an opportunity came to work one summer with the Youth Conservation Corps in Yosemite National Park. That summer led to her serving as a leader of the group the following year, teaching and mentoring as she shared her passion for nature. Since then her adventures have taken her backpacking across Europe, on a state-to-state bike tour across New England, and hiking through the Caribbean

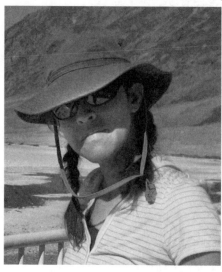

islands. She has traveled extensively throughout Mexico and has written an adventure guidebook to Mexico's Gulf Coast. A graduate of Yale University, Sánchez grew up and lives in the Dallas area. She spends her free time showing fellow hikers the beauty that Texas trails have to offer.

PREFACE

In the few years since the last edition of this book was published, the Dallas–Fort Worth–Arlington Metroplex has seen tremendous growth—in fact, 2010 Census figures show that this is one of the fastest-growing metropolitan areas in the country. Enticed by a low cost of living, excellent job opportunities, and warm Texas weather, people from all around the country are moving in.

But what does this population growth mean for the outdoors enthusiast, adventure seeker, and hiker? Will the trails that we love be reclaimed by their creators for necessities like housing, roads, and new developments? When I set out to update *60 Hikes within 60 Miles: Dallas–Fort Worth,* it was with these questions in mind. And while there is certainly evidence of expansion everywhere you look, what I found for the hiker and outdoorsperson was wonderfully surprising.

Recognizing the needs of their growing populations, cities and towns have gone out of their way not only to preserve and expand existing areas but also develop new green spaces. In south Dallas, for example, a former eyesore and landfill has been reclaimed and transformed into a beautiful and unforgettable nature preserve. In your own community you may have noticed miles of expansion to local greenbelts and linear parks as local leaders attempt to create outside opportunities for their citizens. And North Texas now has more than just trails for hikers: new trails have been developed . . . on water! The Metroplex now boasts an impressive 57 miles of paddling trails for those who want to explore the area's rivers and lakes.

In the last edition of this book, I tried to select trails from all corners of the Metroplex so that no matter where you lived, you could find something close to home. For this edition I've taken out a few trails and replaced them with new ones that have impressed me in different ways. Happily, however, I've kept most of your favorites—and many of these are now better than ever in terms of length and amenities.

As I mentioned in the last edition, I've done my best to describe the trails in this book, but don't be surprised if, on your own explorations, you discover things that differ slightly from what I've found. A trail you've been on before (or heard about) can be an entirely new experience in another season. Don't like a trail in the winter? Go back in the spring, when the flowers are in bloom and the trees are budding. Conversely, a hot prairie path can be a delight on a sunny winter day, but probably not as pleasant at the peak of summer.

Regardless of when you go or where you go, just make sure that you *go*. If you know of a hike I haven't included here, that doesn't mean it's not worthy— some hikes didn't make my list because of weather or logistics; nevertheless, don't be afraid to check them out. If you've thumbed through this book and found a hike that interests you but that seems too short or too long, try it anyway: any hike can be shortened, and many of these can be lengthened.

And when you're done trying the hikes in this book . . . keep going! So many more trails out there await your discovery. I hope you enjoy them as much as I have.

—Joanie Sánchez

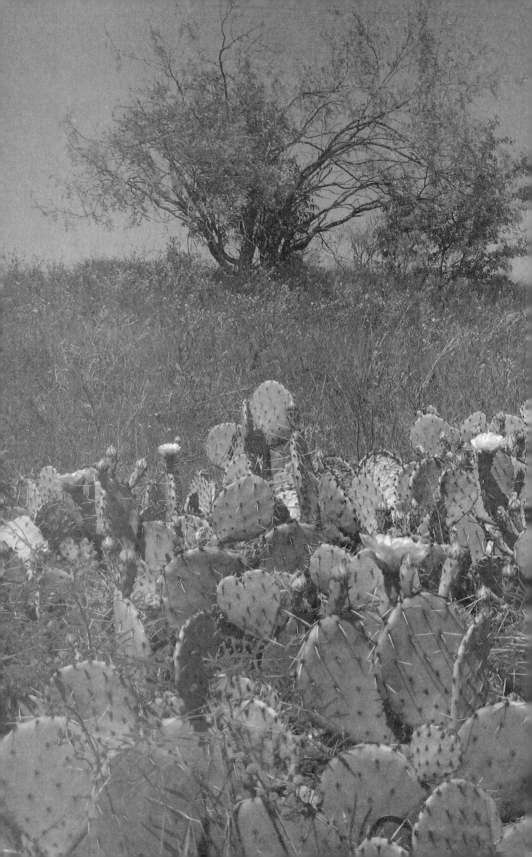

HIKING RECOMMENDATIONS

HIKES 1–2.9 MILES

2 Boulder Park Trail (page 22)

5 Duck Creek Greenbelt (page 35)

6 Fair Park Loop (page 39)

9 L. B. Houston Nature Trail (page 52)

11 Spring Creek Park Nature Trail (page 60)

12 Trinity River Audubon Trail (page 64)

18 Colleyville Nature Trail (page 92)

20 Fort Worth Nature Center: Prairie Trail (page 100)

26 Sansom Park Trail (page 124)

29 Arbor Hills Loop (page 139)

32 Cicada–Cottonwood Loop (page 151)

34 Erwin Park Loop (page 159)

36 Parkhill Prairie Trail (page 167)

37 Pilot Knoll Trail (page 171)

39 Ray Roberts Lake State Park, Isle du Bois Unit: Lost Pines Trail (page 179)

41 Sister Grove Loop (page 187)

43 Bardwell Lake Multiuse Trail (page 198)

45 Cedar Mountain Trail (page 206)

48 Cottonwood Creek Trail (page 220)

50 Purtis Creek Trail (page 229)

52 Walnut Creek Trail (page 237)

54 Windmill Hill Preserve Trail (page 245)

58 Lake Tawakoni Nature Trail (page 268)

59 Post Oak Trail (page 272)

60 Samuell Farm Trail (page 276)

HIKES 3–5 MILES

1 Bachman Lake Trail (page 18)

3 Campion Trail (page 26)

4 Downtown Dallas Urban Trail (page 30)

7 Fish Creek Linear Trail (page 43)

10 Rowlett Creek Nature Trail (page 56)

13 Turtle Creek Leisure Trail (page 69)

14 White Rock Lake Trail (page 73)

16 Benbrook Dam Trail (page 84)

17 Benbrook Lake Trail (page 88)

19 Fort Worth Nature Center: Canyon Ridge Trail (page 96)

21 Horseshoe Trail (page 104)

25 Rocky Point Trail (page 120)

27 Trinity River Trail (Northside) (page 128)

28 Trinity River Trail (Oakmont Park) (page 132)

31 Breckenridge Park Trail (page 147)

33 Elm Fork Trail (page 155)

35 Lavon Lake: Trinity Trail (page 163)

38 Ray Roberts Greenbelt (page 175)

40 Ray Roberts Lake State Park, Johnson Branch Unit:
    Johnson Branch Trail (page 183)

42 Walnut Grove Trail (page 191)

44 Cedar Hill State Park: Talala–Duck Pond Loop (page 202)

46 Cedar Ridge Preserve Trail (page 210)

49 Dinosaur Valley Trail (page 224)

51 Visitor's Overlook: Joe Pool Lake Dam Trail (page 233)

55 Lake Mineral Wells State Park: Cross Timbers Trail (page 252)

56 Lake Mineral Wells State Trailway (page 257)

HIKES > 5 MILES

 8 Katy Trail (page 47)

15 Bear Creek–Bob Eden Trail (page 80)

22 Knob Hill Trail (page 108)

23 Northshore Trail (page 112)

24 River Legacy Trail (page 116)

30 Black Creek–Cottonwood Hiking Trail (page 143)

47 Cleburne State Park Loop Trail (page 215)

53 Waxahachie Creek Hike & Bike Trail (page 241)

57 Lost Creek Reservoir State Trailway (page 261)

BEST HIKES FOR CHILDREN

11 Spring Creek Park Nature Trail (page 60)

18 Colleyville Nature Trail (page 92)

20 Fort Worth Nature Center: Prairie Trail (page 100)

29 Arbor Hills Loop (page 139)

31 Breckenridge Park Trail (page 147)

32 Cicada–Cottonwood Loop (page 151)

39 Ray Roberts Lake State Park, Isle du Bois Unit: Lost Pines Trail (page 179)

59 Post Oak Trail (page 272)
60 Samuell Farm Trail (page 276)

BEST HIKES FOR SOLITUDE
27 Trinity River Trail (Northside) (page 128)
42 Walnut Grove Trail (page 191)
55 Lake Mineral Wells State Park: Cross Timbers Trail (page 252)
57 Lost Creek Reservoir State Trailway (page 261)
58 Lake Tawakoni Nature Trail (page 268)

BEST-MAINTAINED TRAILS
11 Spring Creek Park Nature Trail (page 60)
12 Trinity River Audubon Trail (page 64)
15 Bear Creek–Bob Eden Trail (page 80)
31 Breckenridge Park Trail (page 147)
32 Cicada–Cottonwood Loop (page 151)
53 Waxahachie Creek Hike & Bike Trail (page 241)
59 Post Oak Trail (page 272)

BUSIEST TRAILS
1 Bachman Lake Trail (page 18)
 3 Campion Trail (page 26)
 8 Katy Trail (page 47)
 9 L. B. Houston Nature Trail (page 52)
10 Rowlett Creek Nature Trail (page 56)
14 White Rock Lake Trail (page 73)
21 Horseshoe Trail (page 104)
23 Northshore Trail (page 112)
29 Arbor Hills Loop (page 139)

EASIEST HIKES
5 Duck Creek Greenbelt (page 35)
 7 Fish Creek Linear Trail (page 43)
16 Benbrook Dam Trail (page 84)
20 Fort Worth Nature Center: Prairie Trail (page 100)
24 River Legacy Trail (page 116)
32 Cicada–Cottonwood Loop (page 151)
38 Ray Roberts Greenbelt (page 175)
39 Ray Roberts Lake State Park, Isle du Bois Unit: Lost Pines Trail (page 179)
40 Ray Roberts Lake State Park, Johnson Branch Unit:
       Johnson Branch Trail (page 183)
52 Walnut Creek Trail (page 237)

FLAT HIKES

1 Bachman Lake Trail (page 18)

3 Campion Trail (page 26)

7 Fish Creek Linear Trail (page 43)

8 Katy Trail (page 47)

15 Bear Creek–Bob Eden Trail (page 80)

16 Benbrook Dam Trail (page 84)

20 Fort Worth Nature Center: Prairie Trail (page 100)

24 River Legacy Trail (page 116)

32 Cicada–Cottonwood Loop (page 151)

38 Ray Roberts Greenbelt (page 175)

52 Walnut Creek Trail (page 237)

53 Waxahachie Creek Hike & Bike Trail (page 241)

57 Lost Creek Reservoir State Trailway (page 261)

HIKES ALONG CREEKS AND RIVERS

3 Campion Trail (page 26)

5 Duck Creek Greenbelt (page 35)

7 Fish Creek Linear Trail (page 43)

11 Spring Creek Park Nature Trail (page 60)

13 Turtle Creek Leisure Trail (page 69)

15 Bear Creek–Bob Eden Trail (page 80)

24 River Legacy Trail (page 116)

27 Trinity River Trail (Northside) (page 128)

28 Trinity River Trail (Oakmont Park) (page 132)

52 Walnut Creek Trail (page 237)

53 Waxahachie Creek Hike & Bike Trail (page 241)

HIKES FOR RUNNERS

1 Bachman Lake Trail (page 18)

3 Campion Trail (page 26)

7 Fish Creek Linear Trail (page 43)

8 Katy Trail (page 47)

14 White Rock Lake Trail (page 73)

16 Benbrook Dam Trail (page 84)

21 Horseshoe Trail (page 104)

23 Northshore Trail (page 112)

24 River Legacy Trail (page 116)

31 Breckenridge Park Trail (page 147)

38 Ray Roberts Greenbelt (page 175)

53 Waxahachie Creek Hike & Bike Trail (page 241)

56 Lake Mineral Wells State Trailway (page 257)
57 Lost Creek Reservoir State Trailway (page 261)

BEST HIKES FOR DOGS

3 Campion Trail (page 26)
 5 Duck Creek Greenbelt (page 35)
 8 Katy Trail (page 47)
11 Spring Creek Park Nature Trail (page 60)
15 Bear Creek–Bob Eden Trail (page 80)
18 Colleyville Nature Trail (page 92)
21 Horseshoe Trail (page 104)
24 River Legacy Trail (page 116)
29 Arbor Hills Loop (page 139)
31 Breckenridge Park Trail (page 147)
38 Ray Roberts Greenbelt (page 175)
40 Ray Roberts Lake State Park, Johnson Branch Unit:
      Johnson Branch Trail (page 183)
43 Bardwell Lake Multiuse Trail (page 198)
54 Windmill Hill Preserve Trail (page 245)

LAKE HIKES

1 Bachman Lake Trail (page 18)
14 White Rock Lake Trail (page 73)
16 Benbrook Dam Trail (page 84)
17 Benbrook Lake Trail (page 88)
18 Colleyville Nature Trail (page 92)
21 Horseshoe Trail (page 104)
23 Northshore Trail (page 112)
25 Rocky Point Trail (page 120)
26 Sansom Park Trail (page 124)
30 Black Creek–Cottonwood Hiking Trail (page 143)
31 Breckenridge Park Trail (page 147)
33 Elm Fork Trail (page 155)
35 Lavon Lake: Trinity Trail (page 163)
37 Pilot Knoll Trail (page 171)
39 Ray Roberts Lake State Park, Isle du Bois Unit: Lost Pines Trail (page 179)
40 Ray Roberts Lake State Park, Johnson Branch Unit:
      Johnson Branch Trail (page 183)
42 Walnut Grove Trail (page 191)
50 Purtis Creek Trail (page 229)
51 Visitor's Overlook: Joe Pool Lake Dam Trail (page 233)
57 Lost Creek Reservoir State Trailway (page 261)

MOST DIFFICULT HIKES

19 Fort Worth Nature Center: Canyon Ridge Trail (page 96)
26 Sansom Park Trail (page 124)
47 Cleburne State Park Loop Trail (page 215)
49 Dinosaur Valley Trail (page 224)

MOST SCENIC HIKES

11 Spring Creek Park Nature Trail (page 60)
13 Turtle Creek Leisure Trail (page 69)
12 Trinity River Audubon Trail (page 64)
14 White Rock Lake Trail (page 73)
15 Bear Creek–Bob Eden Trail (page 80)
21 Horseshoe Trail (page 104)
23 Northshore Trail (page 112)
31 Breckenridge Park Trail (page 147)
36 Parkhill Prairie Trail (page 167)
39 Ray Roberts Lake State Park, Isle du Bois Unit: Lost Pines Trail (page 179)
42 Walnut Grove Trail (page 191)
46 Cedar Ridge Preserve Trail (page 210)
48 Cottonwood Creek Trail (page 220)
49 Dinosaur Valley Trail (page 224)
59 Post Oak Trail (page 272)

STEEPEST HIKES

19 Fort Worth Nature Center: Canyon Ridge Trail (page 96)
23 Northshore Trail (page 112)
26 Sansom Park Trail (page 124)
46 Cedar Ridge Preserve Trail (page 210)
47 Cleburne State Park Loop Trail (page 215)
49 Dinosaur Valley Trail (page 224)

URBAN HIKES

1 Bachman Lake Trail (page 18)
3 Campion Trail (page 26)
4 Downtown Dallas Urban Trail (page 30)
5 Duck Creek Greenbelt (page 35)
6 Fair Park Loop (page 39)
7 Fish Creek Linear Trail (page 43)
8 Katy Trail (page 47)
13 Turtle Creek Leisure Trail (page 69)
14 White Rock Lake Trail (page 73)
15 Bear Creek–Bob Eden Trail (page 80)
21 Horseshoe Trail (page 104)

24 River Legacy Trail (page 116)
27 Trinity River Trail (Northside) (page 128)
31 Breckenridge Park Trail (page 147)
53 Waxahachie Creek Hike & Bike Trail (page 241)

WHEELCHAIR-ACCESSIBLE TRAILS

1 Bachman Lake Trail (page 18)
 5 Duck Creek Greenbelt (page 35)
 7 Fish Creek Linear Trail (page 43)
14 White Rock Lake Trail (page 73)
15 Bear Creek–Bob Eden Trail (page 80)
21 Horseshoe Trail (page 104)
24 River Legacy Trail (page 116)
27 Trinity River Trail (Northside) (page 128)
29 Arbor Hills Loop (page 139)
31 Breckenridge Park Trail (page 147)

WILDFLOWER HIKES

22 Knob Hill Trail (page 108)
29 Arbor Hills Loop (page 139)
31 Breckenridge Park Trail (page 147)
34 Erwin Park Loop (page 159)
36 Parkhill Prairie Trail (page 167)
41 Sister Grove Loop (page 187)
43 Bardwell Lake Multiuse Trail (page 198)
44 Cedar Hill State Park: Talala–Duck Pond Loop (page 202)
56 Lake Mineral Wells State Trailway (page 257)
60 Samuell Farm Trail (page 276)

WILDLIFE HIKES

17 Benbrook Lake Trail (page 88)
19 Fort Worth Nature Center: Canyon Ridge Trail (page 96)
20 Fort Worth Nature Center: Prairie Trail (page 100)
22 Knob Hill Trail (page 108)
30 Black Creek–Cottonwood Hiking Trail (page 143)
37 Pilot Knoll Trail (page 171)
42 Walnut Grove Trail (page 191)
44 Cedar Hill State Park: Talala–Duck Pond Loop (page 202)
46 Cedar Ridge Preserve Trail (page 210)
49 Dinosaur Valley Trail (page 224)
57 Lost Creek Reservoir State Trailway (page 261)
58 Lake Tawakoni Nature Trail (page 268)

BIRDING HIKES

 7 Fish Creek Linear Trail (page 43)
11 Spring Creek Park Nature Trail (page 60)
12 Trinity River Audubon Trail (page 64)
19 Fort Worth Nature Center: Canyon Ridge Trail (page 96)
30 Black Creek–Cottonwood Hiking Trail (page 143)
31 Breckenridge Park Trail (page 147)
32 Cicada–Cottonwood Loop (page 151)
38 Ray Roberts Greenbelt (page 175)
44 Cedar Hill State Park: Talala–Duck Pond Loop (page 202)
46 Cedar Ridge Preserve Trail (page 210)
49 Dinosaur Valley Trail (page 224)
53 Waxahachie Creek Hike & Bike Trail (page 241)
58 Lake Tawakoni Nature Trail (page 268)
60 Samuell Farm Trail (page 276)

HIKES OF HISTORICAL INTEREST

 4 Downtown Dallas Urban Trail (page 30)
 6 Fair Park Loop (page 39)
32 Cicada–Cottonwood Loop (page 151)
33 Elm Fork Trail (page 155)
49 Dinosaur Valley Trail (page 224)
53 Waxahachie Creek Hike & Bike Trail (page 241)
60 Samuell Farm Trail (page 276)

60 HIKES
WITHIN 60 MILES

DALLAS–FORT WORTH
INCLUDES
TARRANT, COLLIN, AND DENTON COUNTIES

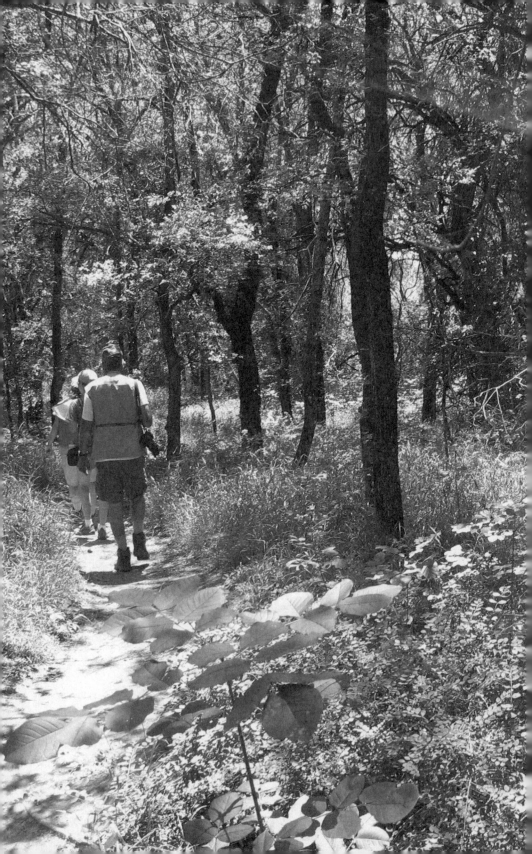

INTRODUCTION

Welcome to *60 Hikes within 60 Miles: Dallas–Fort Worth.* Whether you're new to hiking or a seasoned trekker, take a few minutes to read the following introduction. We explain how this book is organized and how to use it.

HOW TO USE THIS GUIDEBOOK

THE OVERVIEW MAP AND OVERVIEW-MAP KEY

Use the overview map on the inside front cover to assess the exact locations of each hike's primary trailhead. Each hike's number appears on the overview map, on the map key facing the overview map, and in the table of contents. As you flip through the book, a hike's full profile is easy to locate by watching for the hike number at the top of each right-hand page. A map legend of the symbols found on trail maps appears on the inside back cover.

REGIONAL MAPS

The book is divided into regions, and prefacing each regional section is an overview map of that region. The regional map provides more detail than the overview map, bringing you closer to the hike.

TRAIL MAPS

Each hike contains a detailed map that shows the trailhead, the route, significant features, facilities, and topographic landmarks such as creeks, overlooks, and peaks. The author gathered map data by carrying a Garmin eTrex Legend GPS unit while hiking. This data was downloaded into the Topo! State Series digital mapping program and processed by expert cartographers to produce the highly accurate maps found in this book. Each trailhead's GPS coordinates are included with each profile.

ELEVATION PROFILES

Corresponding directly to the trail map is a detailed elevation profile for each hike. The elevation profile provides a quick look at the trail from the side, enabling you to visualize how the trail rises and falls. Key points along the way are labeled. Note the number of feet between each tick mark on the vertical axis (the height scale). To avoid making flat hikes look steep and steep hikes appear flat, height scales are used throughout the book to give an accurate image of the hike's climbing difficulty.

GPS TRAILHEAD COORDINATES

To collect accurate map data, the author hiked each trail with a handheld GPS unit (Garmin eTrex series). Data collected was then downloaded and plotted onto a digital United States Geological Survey (USGS) topo map. In addition to providing a highly specific trail outline, this book also includes the GPS coordinates for each trailhead in latitude–longitude format. These coordinates tell you where you are by locating a point west (latitude) of the 0° meridian line that passes through Greenwich, England, and north or south of the 0° longitude line that belts the Earth, aka the equator.

For readers who own a GPS unit, whether handheld or aboard a vehicle, the latitude–longitude coordinates provided on the first page of each hike may be entered into the GPS unit. Just make sure your GPS unit is set to navigate using WGS84 datum. Now you can navigate directly to the trailhead.

Most trailheads, which begin in parking areas, can be reached by car, but some hikes still require a short walk to reach the trailhead from a parking area. In those cases, a handheld unit is necessary to continue the GPS navigation process. Still, readers can easily access all trailheads in this book by using the directions given, the overview map, and the trail map, which shows at least one major road leading into the area. But for those who enjoy using the latest GPS technology to navigate, the necessary data has been provided.

To learn more about how to enhance your outdoor experiences with GPS technology, refer to *GPS Outdoors: A Practical Guide for Outdoor Enthusiasts* (Menasha Ridge Press).

HIKE DESCRIPTIONS

Each hike contains eight key items: an In Brief summary of the trail, a Key At-a-Glance Information box, directions to the trail, GPS trailhead coordinates, a trail map, an elevation profile, the trail description, and notes on nearby activities. Combined, the maps and information let you assess each trail from the comfort of your favorite reading chair.

IN BRIEF

This section gives you a taste of the trail. Think of this as a snapshot focused on the historical landmarks, beautiful vistas, and other sights you may encounter on the hike.

KEY AT-A-GLANCE INFORMATION

The following information gives you a quick idea of the statistics and specifics of each hike:

LENGTH This indicates the length of the trail from start to finish. There may be options to shorten or extend the hikes, but the mileage corresponds to the described hike. Consult the hike description to help you decide how to customize the hike for your ability or time constraints.

CONFIGURATION This information tells you what the trail might look like from overhead. Trails can be loops, out-and-backs (trails on which one enters and leaves along the same path), figure-eights, or a combination of shapes.

DIFFICULTY The degree of effort an average hiker should expect on a given hike is provided here. For simplicity, the trails are rated as easy, moderate, hard, or sometimes a combination of different ratings.

SCENERY This short summary gives an overview of the attractions offered by the hike and what to expect in terms of plant life, wildlife, natural wonders, and historic features.

EXPOSURE A quick check of how much sun you can expect on your shoulders during the hike helps you plan when to go and what to wear.

TRAIL TRAFFIC How busy is the trail on an average day? Traffic, of course, varies from day to day and season to season. Weekend days typically see the most visitors. This part tells you what kinds of other trail users may be encountered on the way.

TRAIL SURFACE The path may be paved, rocky, gravel, dirt, boardwalk, or a mixture of elements.

HIKING TIME You'll want to know how long it takes to hike the trail. A slow but steady hiker will average 2–3 miles an hour, depending on the terrain.

ACCESS A notation of any fees or permits that you may need to access the trail or park at the trailhead is given here, along with daily/seasonal operating times.

If you plan to do a lot of hiking, consider buying a Texas State Parks Pass, which waives the daily entrance fee to the state parks and historic sites within the state, allowing pass-holders unlimited free access. The annual pass costs $60 for a one-card membership or $75 for a two-card membership (with the stipulation that both pass-holders live at the same residence), and allows everyone in the vehicle admittance. If you don't have a State Parks Pass, you'll need to pay the daily entrance fee, which varies from park to park (most within 60 miles of Dallas–Fort Worth cost $5). Passes can be purchased at the visitor centers at most state parks. Seniors and veterans, may be eligible for reduced or free admission. For more information, visit **tpwd.state.tx.us/spdest/parkinfo/passes.**

Most of the parks I've listed that are operated by the U.S. Army Corps of Engineers require no admission or parking fees, but most city parks offering recreation areas, such as camping, boating, and picnicking, typically charge a small entrance fee.

FACILITIES Indicates whether restrooms and water are available at the trailhead or nearby.

WHEELCHAIR TRAVERSABLE Indicates whether or not the trail offers accommodations for persons with disabilities.

SPECIAL COMMENTS Helpful information that doesn't fit any other category.

SUPPLEMENTAL MAPS Included for a number of hikes are online sources for trail maps from public and private entities.

DRIVING DISTANCE FROM MAJOR INTERSECTION Shows how far you can expect to travel from a familiar highway reference point.

DIRECTIONS

Used in conjunction with the overview map, the driving directions will help you locate each trailhead. Once at the trailhead, park only in designated areas.

GPS TRAILHEAD COORDINATES

The trailhead coordinates can be used in addition to the driving directions if you enter the coordinates into your GPS unit before you set out. See page 2 for more information.

DESCRIPTION

The trail description is the heart of each hike. Here, the author summarizes the trail's essence and highlights any special traits the hike has to offer. The route is clearly outlined, including landmarks, side trips, and possible alternate routes. Ultimately, the hike description will help you choose which hikes are best for you.

NEARBY ACTIVITIES

Look here for information on things to do or points of interest in the area. Sites might include nearby parks, museums, restaurants, or places to shop.

WEATHER

There's an old saying—"If you don't like the weather, wait 5 minutes and it'll change"—and nowhere is that more true than in North Texas. You can find yourself wearing a winter jacket one day and shorts the next, or be dismayed by severe thunderstorms wreaking havoc on your day, only to find the sun shining brightly an hour later.

Winters are usually mild, with average daily temperatures in the 50s during December and January. Occasionally, much colder weather sets in, and you'll have a few days of below-freezing temperatures. Although winter storms rarely bring snow, a few times each year storms combine with overnight freezing temperatures to cause "black ice" to form on roads and bridges, temporarily immobilizing the city. The coldest month is January, with temperatures rising around 7–8 degrees each subsequent month before finally peaking in July.

Spring peaks around mid-April, when Texas's favorite wildflower—the bluebonnet—blankets highway medians, parks, and undeveloped fields. Daytime temperatures during this time are typically in the high 70s, and it's not uncommon for showers and severe thunderstorms to threaten at least a couple of days a week. In conjunction with the storms, threats of tornados also increase in the spring.

Summers are typically hot, with temperatures in the 90s, and include an average of two weeks when readings are above 100—typically during July and August.

AVERAGE DAILY TEMPERATURES BY MONTH (°F): DALLAS						
	JAN	FEB	MAR	APR	MAY	JUN
HIGH	55°	61°	69°	77°	84°	92°
LOW	36°	41°	49°	56°	65°	73°
	JUL	AUG	SEP	OCT	NOV	DEC
HIGH	96°	96°	89°	79°	66°	57°
LOW	77°	76°	69°	58°	47°	39°

WATER

How much is enough? Well, one simple physiological fact should convince you to err on the side of excess when deciding how much water to pack: a hiker working hard in 90-degree heat needs about 10 quarts of fluid per day. That's 2.5 gallons—12 large water bottles, or 16 small ones. In other words, pack along one or two bottles, even for short hikes.

Some hikers and backpackers hit the trail prepared to purify water they find along the route. This method, while less dangerous than drinking it untreated, comes with risks. Purifiers with ceramic filters are the safest. Many hikers pack the slightly distasteful tetraglycine–hydroperiodide tablets (sold under the names Potable Aqua, Coughlan's, and others) to debug water.

Probably the most common waterborne bug hikers face is giardia, which may not hit until one to four weeks after ingestion. It will have you living in the bathroom, passing noxious rotten-egg gas, vomiting, and shivering with chills. Other parasites to worry about include E. coli and cryptosporidium, both of which are harder to kill than giardia.

For most people, the pleasures of hiking make carrying water a relatively minor price to pay to remain healthy. If you're tempted to drink found water, do so only if you understand the risks involved. Better yet, hydrate before your hike, carry (and drink) six ounces of water for every mile you plan to hike, and hydrate after the hike.

CLOTHING

You want to be comfortable on the trail, and that means keeping yourself cool in summer and warm in winter—especially in Texas, where temperatures can be extreme. In warm weather, a cotton T-shirt and shorts are great for urban hikes; cargo shorts are popular for their loose, comfortable fit. If you'll be in the grasslands or woodlands, a pair of hiking pants will protect your legs from ticks and snakes commonly found in these areas. You can find lightweight, quick-drying, UV-protective pants at many outdoors shops; these will keep you suitably cool. Consider a pair that converts into shorts so you can unzip them when you're done with the trail.

Hiking in cooler weather brings its own set of problems. Even though it might be cold out, you'll find yourself sweating after a little exertion. Layering is a good solution and an important part of keeping you comfortable. Wear a T-shirt or, better yet, a moisture-wicking shirt under your clothes, and top it with a lightweight fleece or sweater. In winter, wear an outer jacket. You'll more than likely find yourself taking off and putting on layers throughout the hike.

Year-round you need a good pair of hiking shoes. Day hikers are a great choice for most North Texas trails: they come in both low-top and high-top versions, are lightweight, and have good tread and support. Running/exercise shoes are suitable for paved trails but aren't ideal for dirt paths. Essential at any time of year, a hat not only keeps the hot Texas sun from burning your face but also doubles as protection against insects and low-hanging limbs. Another useful item is a rain jacket that can be compressed small enough to be stuffed in your pack; if you're caught out in the rain, you'll be thankful for it.

THE TEN ESSENTIALS

One of the first rules of hiking is to be prepared for anything. The simplest way to be prepared is to carry the "Ten Essentials." In addition to carrying the items listed below, you need to know how to use them, especially navigation items. Always consider worst-case scenarios like getting lost, hiking back in the dark, broken gear (for example, a broken hip strap on your pack or a water filter getting plugged), twisting an ankle, or a brutal thunderstorm. The items listed below don't cost a lot of money, don't take up much room in a pack, and don't weigh much—but they just might save your life.

1. **Water: durable bottles, and water treatment like iodine or a filter**

2. **Map: preferably a topo map and a trail map with a route description**

3. **Compass: a high-quality model**

4. **First-aid kit: a high-quality kit including first-aid instructions**
5. **Knife: a multitool device with pliers is best**
6. **Light: flashlight or headlamp with extra bulbs and batteries**
7. **Fire: windproof matches or lighter and fire starter**
8. **Extra food: you should always have this in your pack when you've finished hiking**
9. **Extra clothes: rain protection, warm layers, gloves, warm hat**
10. **Sun protection: sunglasses, lip balm, sunblock, sun hat**

FIRST-AID KIT

A typical first-aid kit may contain more items than you might think necessary. These are just the basics. Prepackaged kits in waterproof bags (Atwater Carey and Adventure Medical make a variety of kits) are available. Even though there are quite a few items listed here, they pack into a small space.

Ace bandages or Spenco joint wraps	**Gauze (one roll)**
Antibiotic ointment (Neosporin or the generic equivalent)	**Gauze compress pads (a half dozen 4 x 4–inch pads)**
Aspirin or acetaminophen	**Hydrogen peroxide or iodine**
Band-Aids	**Insect repellent**
Benadryl or the generic equivalent, diphenhydramine (in case of allergic reactions)	**Matches or pocket lighter**
	Moleskin/Spenco "Second Skin"
Butterfly-closure bandages	**Sunscreen**
Epinephrine in a prefilled syringe (for people known to have severe allergic reactions to such things as bee stings)	**Whistle (it's more effective in signaling rescuers than your voice is)**

HIKING WITH CHILDREN

No one is too young for a hike in the outdoors. Be mindful, though. Flat, short, and shaded trails are best for infants. Toddlers who haven't quite mastered walking can still tag along, riding on an adult's back in a child carrier. Use common sense to judge a child's capacity to hike a particular trail and always expect that the child will tire quickly and need to be carried. A list of hikes suitable for kids is provided on pages xiv–xv.

When packing for the hike, remember children's needs in addition to your own. Make sure they are adequately clothed for the weather, have proper shoes, and are protected from the sun with sunscreen. Kids dehydrate quickly, so make sure you have plenty of fluid for everyone.

GENERAL SAFETY

While many folks hit the trails full of enthusiasm and energy, eager to begin their adventures, others may find themselves more reserved about potential outdoor hazards. Although potentially dangerous situations can occur anywhere, as long as you use sound judgment and prepare yourself before hitting the trail, your hike will be as safe and enjoyable as you hoped. Here are a few tips to make your trip safer and easier.

- **Hike with a buddy.** Not only is there safety in numbers, but a buddy can help you if you twist an ankle on the trail, help if you get lost, assist in carrying lunch and water, and be there to share in your discoveries. If you'll be hiking alone, leave your hiking itinerary with a friend or relative. It's best to bring a buddy not only to infrequently traveled or remote areas but also to urban areas.

- **Stay hydrated.** North Texas heat can be brutal, and a little exertion can quickly have you sweating. Don't wait until you feel thirsty, instead drink plenty of water throughout the hike, and at regular intervals.

- **Always carry food and water,** whether you are planning to go overnight or not. Food will give you energy, help keep you warm, and sustain you in an emergency until help arrives. You never know if you'll have a stream nearby when you become thirsty. Bring potable water or treat water before drinking it from a stream. Boil or filter all found water before drinking it.

- **Stay on designated trails.** Most hikers get lost when they leave the path. Even on the most clearly marked trails, there's usually a point at which you have to stop and consider in which direction to head. If you become disoriented, don't panic. As soon as you think you may be off-track, stop, assess your current direction, and then retrace your steps to the point where you went astray. Using a map, compass, and this book—and keeping in mind what you've passed thus far—reorient yourself, and trust your judgment on which way to continue. If you become absolutely unsure of how to continue, return to your vehicle the way you came in. Should you become completely lost and have no idea of how to return to the trailhead, staying where you are and waiting for help is most often the best option for adults, and always the best option for children.

- **Be especially careful when crossing streams.** Whether you are fording the stream or crossing on a log, make every step count. If you have any doubt about maintaining your balance on a foot log, go ahead and ford the stream instead. When fording a stream, use a trekking pole or stout stick for balance, and face upstream as you cross. If a stream seems too deep to ford, turn back. Whatever is on the other side isn't worth risking your life for.

- **Be careful at overlooks.** While these areas may provide spectacular views, they are potentially hazardous. Stay back from the edge of outcrops, and be absolutely sure of your footing; a misstep can mean a nasty and possibly fatal fall.

- Standing dead trees and storm-damaged living trees pose a real hazard to hikers and tent campers. These trees may have loose or broken limbs that could fall at any time. When choosing a spot to rest or spend the night, look up.

- Know the symptoms of heat exhaustion. Excessive sweating, faintness or dizziness, clammy skin, vomiting, and paleness are all common symptoms. If symptoms arise, cool the person off by removing extra clothing, moving him or her to the shade, and give him or her water.

- Know the symptoms of hypothermia. Shivering and forgetfulness are the two most common indicators of this insidious killer. Hypothermia can occur at any elevation—even in the summer—especially when the hiker is wearing lightweight cotton clothing. If symptoms arise, get the victim shelter, administer hot liquids, and dress him or her in dry clothes or a dry sleeping bag.

- Take along your brain. A cool, calculating mind is the single most important piece of equipment you'll ever need on the trail. Think before you act. Watch your step. Plan ahead. Avoiding accidents before they happen is the best strategy for a rewarding and relaxing hike.

- Ask questions. Visitor-center and park employees are there to help. It's a lot easier to get advice beforehand than to have a mishap away from civilization when it's too late to amend an error. Use your head on the trail and treat each area as if it were your own backyard.

ANIMAL AND PLANT HAZARDS

TICKS

Ticks like to hang out in the brush that grows along trails. Hot summer months seem to explode their numbers, but you should be tick-aware all months of the year. Ticks need a host to feast on in order to reproduce. The ticks that alight onto you while you hike will be very small, sometimes so tiny that you won't be able to spot them. Primarily of two varieties, deer and dog ticks, these arthropods (not insects) need a few hours of attachment before they can transmit any disease they may harbor. Ticks may settle in shoes, socks, or hats and may take several hours to latch on. Inspect yourself every half-hour or so while hiking, do a thorough check before you get in your car, and then, when you take a posthike shower, do an even more thorough check of your entire body. Ticks that haven't attached are easily removed but not easily killed. If you pick off a tick in the woods, just toss it aside. If you find one on your body at home, kill it and then send it down the toilet. For ticks that have embedded, removal with tweezers is best.

SNAKES

Most of the snakes you might encounter on your hikes are nonvenomous and pose no threat to humans. Many folks even consider the most common snake in the area—the Texas rat snake—a welcome visitor. This snake, as its name implies, feasts on rodents, and though it may rear and act defensive if you antagonize it, its bite is harmless. Of the more than three dozen types of snakes in the area, only a handful are venomous, the most common being the cottonmouth and the copperhead. On many trails, you'll spot signs warning that you're in a snake habitat. As long as you stay on the trail and out of tall grasses, however, you're unlikely to have a problem. In fact, in all my times hiking the trails in this book, I've met only the occasional snake, and those encounters were uneventful and brief.

POISON IVY, OAK, AND SUMAC

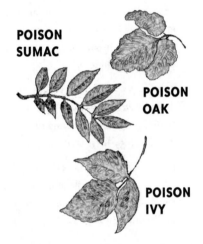

**POISON
SUMAC**

**POISON
OAK**

**POISON
IVY**

Recognizing poison ivy, oak, and sumac and avoiding contact with them are the most effective ways to prevent the painful, itchy rashes associated with these plants. In the South, poison ivy ranges from a thick, tree-hugging vine to a shaded groundcover, three leaflets to a leaf; poison oak occurs as either a vine or shrub, with three leaflets as well; and poison sumac flourishes in swampland, each leaf containing 7–13 leaflets. Urushiol, the oil in the sap of these plants, is responsible for the rash. Usually within 12–14 hours of exposure (but sometimes much later), raised lines and/or blisters will appear, accompanied by a terrible itch. Do your best to refrain from scratching, because bacteria under your fingernails can cause infection, and you'll spread the rash to other parts of your body. Wash and dry the affected skin thoroughly, applying calamine lotion or another product to help dry the rash. If the itching or blistering is severe, see a doctor. To avoid spreading the rash to others, wash not only any exposed parts of your body but also oil-contaminated clothes, gear, and pets.

MOSQUITOES

Although it's not a common occurrence, individuals can become infected with the West Nile virus if they're bitten by an infected mosquito. Culex mosquitoes, the primary varieties that can transmit West Nile virus to humans, thrive in urban rather than natural areas. They lay their eggs in stagnant water and can breed in standing water that remains for more than five days. Most people infected with West Nile virus have no symptoms of illness, but some may become ill, usually 3–15 days after being bitten.

In the Dallas–Fort Worth Metroplex, the summer months—especially August and September—bring mosquitoes, and with them the highest risk for West Nile. Mosquitoes are especially prolific on trails with tall grasses, in marshy/swampy areas, and around dusk and dawn. Anytime you expect mosquitoes to be buzzing around, wear protective clothing, such as long sleeves, long pants, and socks. Loose-fitting, light-colored clothing is best. Spray clothing with insect repellent. The U.S. Centers for Disease Control and Prevention notes that repellents containing the active ingredients DEET or Picaridin supply the best protection; the agency also suggests oil of lemon eucalyptus (a citrus-scented variety of the eucalyptus tree) as an effective plant-based repellent. Follow the instructions on the repellent, and take extra care with children. Insect-repellent clothing, available at outdoor retailers, is another source of protection against mosquitoes and other bothersome bugs.

TIPS FOR ENJOYING DALLAS AND FORT WORTH

If you plan on hiking in one of the state parks, Army Corps of Engineers sites, or national grasslands, visit a corresponding website for information to help you get oriented to the roads, features, and attractions of where you're going. General and detailed maps of the specific wilderness areas are often available online or, if you're visiting a state park, at the park office. In addition, the following tips will make your visit enjoyable and more rewarding.

- **Get out of your car and onto a trail. Auto touring allows a cursory overview of the area, but only visually. On the trail you can use your ears and nose as well. Even if you don't use the trails recommended in this guide, any trail is better than no trail at all.**

- **North Texas summers can be unbearably hot, making a day hike in late July or August seemingly impossible. If it's a nice day and you don't want to miss out on hiking because of the heat, go early in the morning. If you're on the trail at dawn, you can find temperatures 10–20 degrees lower than they'll be later in the day, and there's no better way to start your day than listening to the cheerful singing of birds along the trail.**

- **Take your time along the trails. Pace yourself. North Texas is filled with wonders both big and small. Don't rush past a tiny lizard to get to that overlook. Stop and smell the wildflowers. Peer into a clear creek for minnows. Don't miss the trees for the forest. Shorter hikes allow you to stop and linger more than long hikes do. Something about staring at the front end of a 10-mile trek naturally pushes you to speed up. That said, take close notice of the elevation maps that accompany each hike. If you see many ups and downs over large altitude changes, you'll obviously need more time. Inevitably, you'll finish some of the hikes more or less quickly than the estimated time. Nevertheless, leave yourself plenty of time for those moments when you simply feel like stopping and taking it all in.**

- **Try to hike during the week and avoid the traditional holidays, if possible.** Trails that are packed in the spring and fall are often clear during the hotter or colder months. If you're hiking on a busy day, go early in the morning; it'll enhance your chances of seeing wildlife. The trails really clear out during rainy times; however, don't hike during a thunderstorm.

- **Investigate different areas around the Metroplex.** The scenery you'll find hiking through meadows and grasslands is pleasantly different from the riparian forest alongside a fork of the Trinity River or lakeside water views. Sample a few of each to see what the area has to offer and what most appeals to you.

- **Hike during different seasons.** Trails change dramatically from spring to winter and can transform themselves into something you might not even recognize.

TOPO MAPS

The maps in this book have been produced with great care and, used with the hiking directions, will direct you to the trails and help you stay on course. However, you will find superior detail and valuable information in the USGS's 7.5-minute series topographic maps. One well-known free topo service on the Web is **Microsoft Research Maps (msrmaps.com)**. Online services such as **Trails.com** charge annual fees for additional features such as shaded relief, which makes the topography stand out more. If you expect to print out many topo maps each year, it might be worth paying for such extras. The downside to USGS topos is that most are outdated, having been created 20–30 years ago. But they still provide excellent topographic detail.

Digital topographic-map programs, such as DeLorme's TopoUSA, enable you to review topo maps of the entire United States on your computer. You can download data gathered while hiking with a GPS unit onto the software and plot your own hikes.

If you're new to hiking, you might be wondering, "What's a topographic map?" In short, a topo indicates not only linear distance but elevation as well, using contour lines. Contour lines spread across the map like dozens of intricate spiderwebs. Each line represents a particular elevation, and at the base of each topo, a contour's interval designation is given. If the contour interval is 20 feet, then the distance between each contour line is 20 feet. Follow five contour lines up on the same map, and the elevation has increased by 100 feet.

Let's assume that the 7.5-minute series topo reads "Contour Interval 40 feet" and that the short trail we'll be hiking is 2 inches long on the map and crosses five contour lines from beginning to end. What do we know? Well, because the linear scale of this series is 2,000 feet to the inch (roughly 2.75 inches representing 1 mile), we know our trail is approximately .8 miles long (2 inches equals 2,000 feet). But we also know we'll be climbing or descending 200 vertical feet because there are five contour lines and each is 40 feet. And the elevation designations written on occasional contour lines will tell us if we're heading up or down.

In addition to the outdoor shops listed in the Appendixes, you'll find topos at major universities and in some public libraries; you might try photocopying the ones you need to avoid the cost of buying them. But if you want your own and can't find them locally, visit the USGS website, **topomaps.usgs.gov.**

BACKCOUNTRY/PRIMITIVE CAMPING ADVICE

Backcountry/primitive camping is available in the LBJ National Grasslands and in many state parks and wildlife-management areas. Practice low-impact camping and adhere to the adages "Pack it in, pack it out," and "Take only pictures, leave only footprints." Practice "leave no trace" camping ethics while in the backcountry. Some backcountry areas are also public hunting areas, so research your destination before your visit.

Solid human waste should be buried in a hole at least 3 inches deep and at least 200 feet away from trails and water sources; a trowel is basic backpacking equipment.

Rules on open fires vary depending on where you go, so check before your visit; when collecting firewood, many places ask you to collect downed wood instead of chopping branches. In addition, Texas State Parks allow fires only in fire rings, fireplaces, and campsite grills. Burn bans, especially during drought periods, can restrict fires—including those at campsite grills. Double-check before your trip, because state parks may or may not be affected by a countywide burn ban.

A fishing license is required if you plan to fish. You can get one from many outdoor retailers, sports stores, and bait and tackle shops, online, or over the phone. Visit **tpwd.state.tx.us** for information on regulations, fees, permits, and how to purchase.

Following the previous guidelines will increase your chances of having a pleasant, safe, and low-impact interaction with nature. The suggestions are intended to enhance your experience. Regulations can change over time; contact the appropriate park office to confirm the status of any regulations before you enter the backcountry.

TRAIL ETIQUETTE

Whether you're on a city, county, state, or national park trail, always remember that great care and resources (from both nature and your tax dollars) have gone into creating these trails. Treat the trail, wildlife, and fellow hikers with respect.

- **Hike on open trails only. Respect trail and road closures (ask if not sure), avoid possible trespassing on private land, and obtain all permits and authorization as required. Also, leave gates as you found them or as marked.**

- **Leave only footprints. Be sensitive to the ground beneath you. This also means staying on the existing trail and not blazing any new trails. Be sure** to pack out what you pack in. No one likes to see the trash someone else has left behind.

- Never spook animals. An unannounced approach, a sudden movement, or a loud noise startles most animals. A surprised animal can be dangerous to you, to others, and to itself. Give it plenty of space.

- Plan ahead. Know your equipment, your ability, and the area in which you are hiking—and prepare accordingly. Be self-sufficient at all times; carry necessary supplies for changes in weather or other conditions. A well-executed trip is a satisfaction to you and to others.

- Be courteous to other hikers, bikers, equestrians, and others you encounter on the trails.

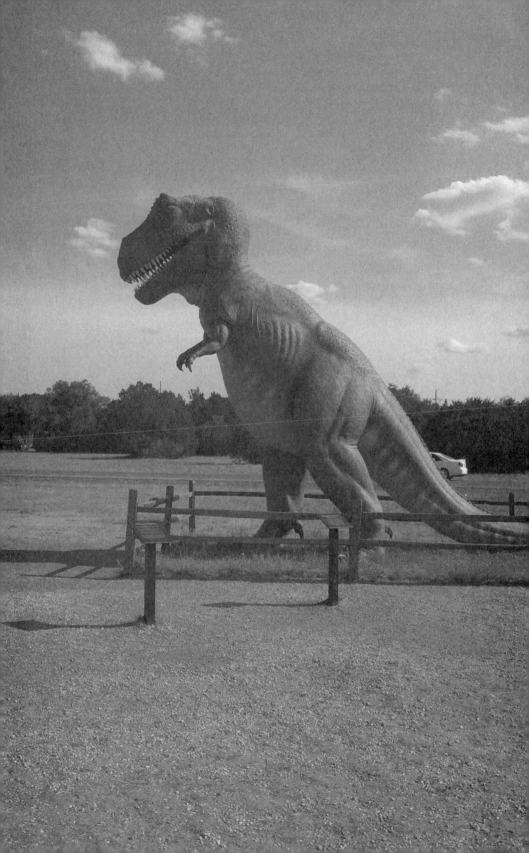

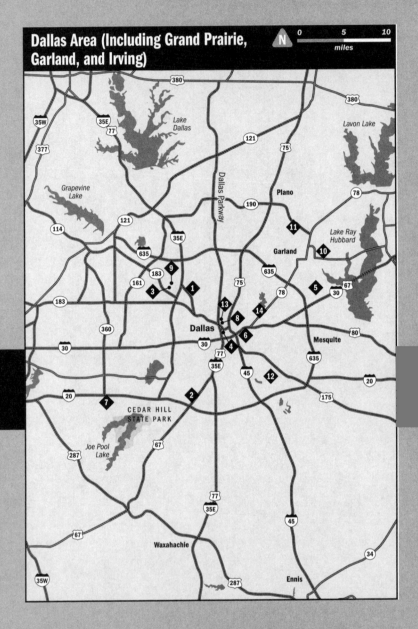

Dallas Area (Including Grand Prairie, Garland, and Irving)

N

0   5   10
miles

Lake Dallas

Lavon Lake

Grapevine Lake

Dallas Parkway

Plano

Lake Ray Hubbard

Garland

Dallas

Mesquite

CEDAR HILL STATE PARK

Joe Pool Lake

Waxahachie

Ennis

1	Bachman Lake Trail	18	
2	Boulder Park Trail	22	
3	Campion Trail	26	
4	Downtown Dallas Urban Trail	30	
5	Duck Creek Greenbelt	35	
6	Fair Park Loop	39	
7	Fish Creek Linear Trail	43	
8	Katy Trail	47	
9	L. B. Houston Nature Trail	52	
10	Rowlett Creek Nature Trail	56	
11	Spring Creek Park Nature Trail	60	
12	Trinity River Audubon Trail	64	
13	Turtle Creek Leisure Trail	69	
14	White Rock Lake Trail	73	

DALLAS AREA
(INCLUDING GRAND PRAIRIE, GARLAND, AND IRVING)

1 BACHMAN LAKE TRAIL

KEY AT-A-GLANCE INFORMATION

LENGTH: 3.23 miles

CONFIGURATION: Loop

DIFFICULTY: Easy

SCENERY: Lake

EXPOSURE: Sunny

TRAIL TRAFFIC: Heavy

TRAIL SURFACE: Paved

HIKING TIME: 1 hour 20 minutes

ACCESS: Free; open daily

FACILITIES: Restrooms, picnic tables, playground, water fountains

WHEELCHAIR TRAVERSABLE: Yes

SPECIAL COMMENTS: An airport runway nearby is slightly distracting; bring headphones.

DRIVING DISTANCE FROM MAJOR INTERSECTION: 2.5 miles from I-35E and West Northwest Highway

GPS TRAILHEAD COORDINATES

Latitude: N 32° 51' 11"

Longitude: W 96° 52' 14"

IN BRIEF

This hike winds around the perimeter of a small lake in the heart of Dallas that is popular with joggers and others. The setting is open—mowed grass is interspersed with trees, making this a very sunny trail. Without doubt you'll spot at least a few ducks and possibly egrets or herons wading to the lake edge.

DESCRIPTION

Just a stone's throw from Dallas's Love Field airport, the 205-acre Bachman Lake sits in an area that in the 1840s used to be farmland owned by the Bachman brothers. The lake was created in 1903 by damming a portion of Bachman's Creek to form a reservoir for Dallas. The larger White Rock Lake (about four times Bachman's size), however, took over this duty, leaving Bachman for recreation.

Today, the lake sits in a commercial area along Northwest Highway. Although it's not the most scenic spot, the trail encircling the lake is well maintained and provides a nice day hike for city dwellers. Because of its rather plain shoreline and shorter length, it's not as popular as nearby White Rock Lake, which also has a trail. It is, however, frequented by nearby residents, especially families, kids, and couples who find the short loop around the lake an easy and fun one to

----

Directions

Bachman Lake is just east of the former site of Texas Stadium. From I-35E toward Denton, exit Harry Hines Boulevard. Immediately bear right on Webb Chapel Extension, and after 0.5 mile turn right onto Northwest Highway. Turn right onto Bachman Drive and park in the lot next to the playground.

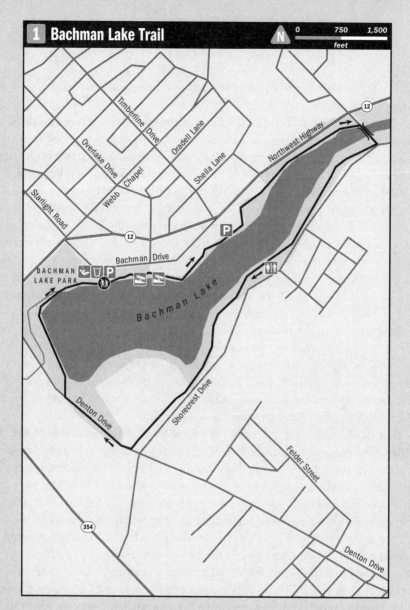

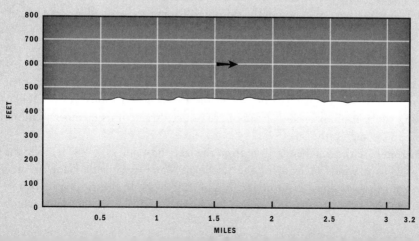

tackle on a weekend outing. Exercise stations on the southeastern shoreline also attract a few people.

The trailhead is adjacent to the busy fenced-in playground next to the recreation center and parking lot. Just ahead of you, the sun glints off the lake's dark waters. From this vantage point, the lake looks very small, the grassy slopes of the opposite side within clear view. As you turn left onto the trail and head northeast rounding the first curve, however, you'll notice that it's actually slightly bigger than you first thought—continuing northeast in a narrow band as far as you can see.

As you head down the trail, keep an eye out for ducks congregating in the shade around a grove of bald cypress trees growing along the shoreline. Ducks like to nestle into the roots of the trees, which grow up out of the water to form knobs, or "knees." On the left, you'll see a park with picnic tables and barbecue pits, which is often busy. A little farther down, some shaded benches complete the park setting.

Continue past the Bachman Lake Park picnic area at 0.75 mile. You're likely to hear loud music coming from open-air restaurants across the street to the left. The noise is slightly distracting but actually fits right into the urban vibe of the hike. Even the seagulls, of which there are dozens on the grassy banks off to your right, seem unfazed by the ever-present rumbling of the nearby cars and music. The noise fades into the background as you continue.

At 1 mile, bear right and cross the bridge to reach the other side of the lake, where, farther from Northwest Highway, you'll find it much quieter. Across the bridge, turn right, following the trail southwest. To your left is a secondary road that leads to parking places. Just across the road, behind an embankment, is Love Field; you'll undoubtedly already have seen the planes rising low over the lake after takeoff. Keep an eye out for herons and egrets standing quietly in the shallow waters on the shoreline. Signs placed along the banks discourage feeding the abundant birdlife—birds can pose a risk to landing aircraft.

As you continue, pass a few exercise stations placed at regular intervals along both sides of the trail. The stations are put to good use, and I noticed a couple of folks jogging and biking between them. Unfortunately, none of the stations include instructions, so although the purpose of some is clearly identifiable (such as log-hops or pull-up bars), the use of others is lost to many.

The trail climbs slightly. On the skyline just beyond the lake, a good view of Texas Stadium emerges in the distance. At 2 miles, reach a shady picnic area beneath a grove of huge old trees. To your left, you'll see a hangar for Southwest Airlines. To your right, just beyond the picnic area, is the boathouse for the Dallas Rowing Club. You'll probably already have noticed some of its members sculling or sweep rowing on the lake.

From here the trail bends away from the lake for 4 miles. Follow it along the sidewalk as it winds in front of the Bachman Water Treatment Plant. It then curves northwest along Denton Drive and past a small electrical grid before rejoining the lake again at 2.7 miles. From here, you'll cross the dam, which

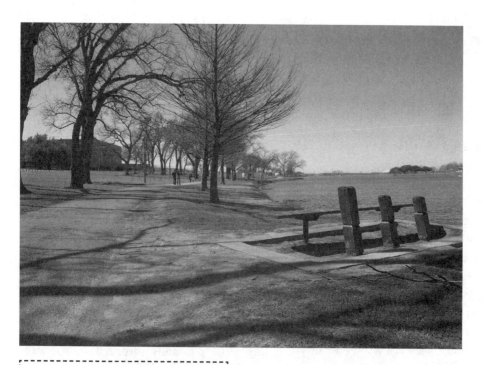

An exercise station abutting Bachman Lake

forms the lake's western side. At the far end, the trail bears back to the northeast. Pass a couple of recreational buildings used by the YMCA and reach the playground to complete the loop.

NEARBY ACTIVITIES

Just 8 miles away, the Dallas World Aquarium encompasses more than 85,000 gallons of saltwater displays, a walk-through tunnel, and exhibits on the Mayan world, South Africa, and the rainforest. For hours and fees, visit **dwazoo.com**. To get there, take I-35E south 6 miles, then take Exit 429A (I-45/US 75) toward Houston. Take the Griffin Street exit. The aquarium is at 1801 N. Griffin.

2 BOULDER PARK TRAIL

KEY AT-A-GLANCE INFORMATION

LENGTH: 2.26 miles

CONFIGURATION: Loop

DIFFICULTY: Easy

SCENERY: Woodlands

EXPOSURE: Sunny

TRAIL TRAFFIC: Moderate

TRAIL SURFACE: Dirt

HIKING TIME: 50 minutes

ACCESS: Free; open daily

FACILITIES: None

WHEELCHAIR TRAVERSABLE: No

SPECIAL COMMENTS: Don't park in the church lot.

SUPPLEMENTAL MAPS:
dorba.org/trail/boulder-park

DRIVING DISTANCE FROM MAJOR INTERSECTION: 2 miles from US 67 and I-20

GPS TRAILHEAD COORDINATES

Latitude: N 32° 40' 8"

Longitude: W 96° 52' 27"

IN BRIEF

A fun hike that twists and turns haphazardly through dense, shaded woodland. Many junctions provide ample opportunities for exploring, and color-coded trails prevent you from getting too lost.

DESCRIPTION

I am always wary of hikes with no established parking. Because of their awkward locations, they are often overly wild and little-used, not to mention overgrown and unkempt—or sometimes even closed. So it was with some skepticism that I finally visited Boulder Park, only to be pleasantly surprised with a well-maintained and clearly labeled trail network. Even better, the trail is quite pretty—offering a few deeply wooded sections that are especially lovely in the springtime, when everything is green. The park was purchased in 1967 by the city of Dallas and is near Red Bird Airport, north of Duncanville. It's maintained by DORBA—the Dallas Off-Road Bicycle Association—which has built about 6 miles of trails through its woodlands.

As previously mentioned, there is no lot to park in, so you'll have to jockey for position on one of the side streets that fill up on Sunday with churchgoers' cars. It's easy to

----

Directions

Boulder Park is adjacent to Dallas's Executive Airport, just north of Duncanville. To get there, take US 67 and exit west onto Red Bird Lane; then turn south onto Pastor Bailey Drive. The trailhead is opposite a small side street, Hallett Avenue, and usually has a cluster of cars parked along the street near it. There is no parking lot.

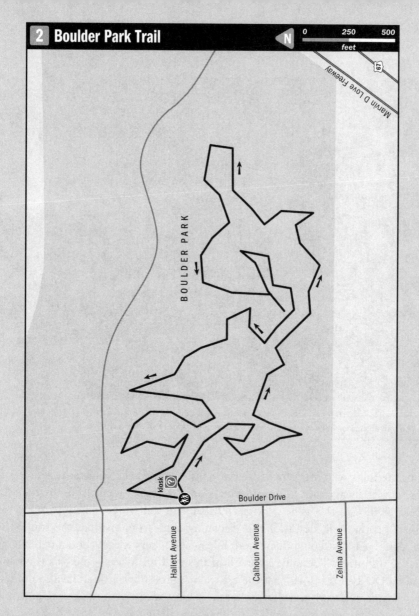

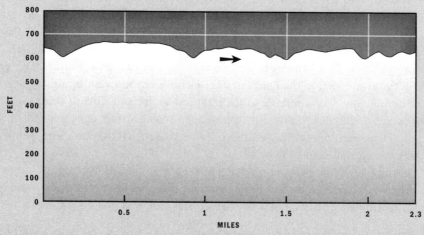

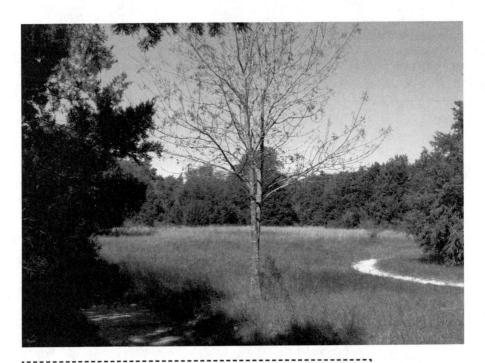

The trail alternates between open sunny sections and densely shaded portions.

spot the folks who are here visiting the trail; they tend to cluster together a few car lengths away from the parishioners and are easily identifiable by their bike racks. Although this is a favorite DORBA spot and you're likely to meet some bikers on the trail, don't let this discourage you from visiting; the trail is long enough to easily accommodate both hikers and bikers without too much inconvenience for either. The only downfall of this trail for hikers—and this is common among DORBA trails—is that the trail sometimes loops around itself pointlessly; this layout is aimed more at mountain bikers, who enjoy the twists and turns. Once you get into the woods, you may actually appreciate this, however, as it adds mileage and interest to the route.

From the trailhead, go straight past the kiosk and through the break in the trees, then turn left onto the trail. Be aware that as DORBA develops the trail, junctions outlined here can easily change and the trail can get rerouted. You're unlikely to get too lost, as the land the trail sits on is not too vast, but it's a good idea to consult any maps available at the trailhead and bring a GPS or compass to help you get oriented. On my visit, color-coded wooden trail signs marked the junctions. This trail follows the red signs. If you visit the DORBA website, you'll find an updated trail map of the park.

Heading down the path, immediately enter the woods. Above you, the trees have intertwined their limbs, welcoming you into a tunnel-like entrance. A couple of small clearings are interspersed throughout the trail, and you'll soon leave the woods and enter the first of these, where cactus dots the open ground. Be aware that DORBA has been combining and rerouting some of the older trails within the park, and you're likely to pass at least a couple of junctions that have been blocked off with branches and rocks. Stay alert and bypass any that have been closed.

As you head back into a grove of hardwood trees, the trail twists and turns a few times. The ground is relatively flat in this section, but as you continue, the terrain changes and you'll encounter a couple of small up and downs—nothing extensive, just enough to give the trail some interest.

At the next junction, go right, following the red arrow. The woods grow thickly around you, and though you're near the road—which you'll hear faintly, just beneath the birdcalls and rustling leaves, if you listen closely—you'll have no idea in which direction it is, thanks to the dense wood cover. Turn right at 0.82 mile and head slightly uphill, then back west away from the back perimeter of the park. At the next junction, continue straight; the woods part to welcome a couple of small, grassy fields dotted with yellow and white wildflowers before enveloping you once again. Go straight to get back into the woods, then go right at 1.62 miles, continuing to follow the red signs. The trail winds down a small rocky hill and enters a pocket of woods where the trees tower high above, sheltering an understory of shrubs and saplings. The ground, rich with the remains of bark and leaves, becomes soft and cushy, making for a comfortable path.

Continue straight at 1.8 miles. The trees become shorter and thinner, until they finally break and you find yourself once again in a cactus- and tree-dotted grassy clearing. No longer soft and welcoming, the ground has changed with the scenery, hardening into a chalky-white mixture that reflects the sunlight. At 2.1 miles, bear right, following the blue arrow. Wind back into the woods, and soon the sounds of the roadway will become audible. A few hundred feet farther, finally reach the western boundary fence of the park. Turn left to follow the trail just alongside the fence and back south to the trailhead.

NEARBY ACTIVITIES

Just down the street on Camp Wisdom Road, you can do some retail shopping in the Southwest Center Mall (aka Red Bird Mall) and the nearby Uptown Village at Cedar Hill. To get to Southwest Center Mall, head south on US 67, then turn right onto Camp Wisdom Road. Cedar Hill is another 7 miles south on US 67.

3 CAMPION TRAIL

 KEY AT-A-GLANCE INFORMATION

LENGTH: 3 miles

CONFIGURATION: Loop

DIFFICULTY: Easy

SCENERY: Woods, river

EXPOSURE: Partially shady–sunny

TRAIL TRAFFIC: Moderate

TRAIL SURFACE: Pavement, packed dirt

HIKING TIME: 50 minutes

ACCESS: Free; open daily, closed midnight–5 a.m.

FACILITIES: Portable toilet, benches

WHEELCHAIR TRAVERSABLE: Partially

SPECIAL COMMENTS: Bring insect repellent if hiking during warmer months.

DRIVING DISTANCE FROM MAJOR INTERSECTION: 2 miles from Loop 12 and TX 114

GPS TRAILHEAD COORDINATES

Latitude: N 32° 51' 44"

Longitude: W 96° 55' 31"

IN BRIEF

In North Irving, this pleasant trail affords easy access to river views as it follows lazily alongside the Trinity River. A packed-dirt trail and wide, paved path attract hikers, dog walkers, joggers, bikers, and skaters. Keep an eye out for a state-record elm tree on the return leg of your hike.

DESCRIPTION

When completed, Irving's Campion Trail is expected to comprise a 22-mile network of trails throughout the city. Currently about 8 miles long, the trail will eventually link to north-central Texas's much more expansive Trinity Trails System—a multicity effort to create 250 miles of accessible greenbelt along the Trinity River corridor.

Throughout the year you can choose from a variety of events along the trail: workshops, organized walks, and guided night hikes highlighting the native nocturnal critters that call the area home. On any given weekend, the trail hums with the activity of outdoors enthusiasts eager to take advantage of this little stretch of green in a city of more than 200,000 residents.

A number of parks along the trail help chronicle the pioneer settlement of the area. Kiosks along the length of the greenbelt link the past with the present. This hike starts at

----

Directions ⟶

Take TX 114 East toward Irving and exit at Riverside Drive/Rochelle Boulevard. Turn left onto Rochelle Boulevard, which becomes Riverside Drive. The trailhead is about 0.5 mile down on the right, at 5198 Riverside Dr. in Irving.

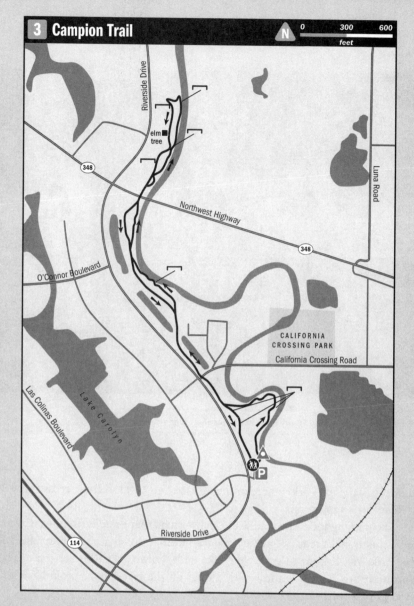

Riverside Drive

elm tree

348

Northwest Highway

348

Luna Road

O'Connor Boulevard

CALIFORNIA CROSSING PARK

California Crossing Road

Lake Carolyn

Las Colinas Boulevard

114

Riverside Drive

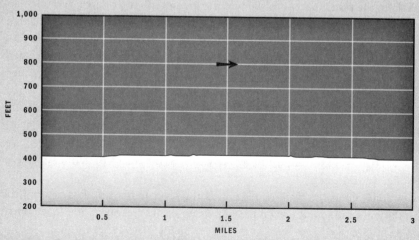

1,000
900
800
700
600
500
400
300
200

FEET

0.5   1   1.5   2   2.5   3

MILES

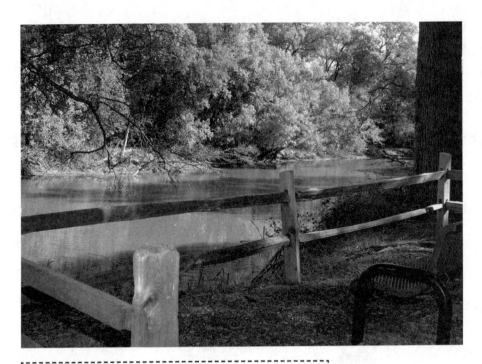

Enjoy scenic views of the Trinity River at various stops along the trail.

California Crossing Park, where in the mid- to late 1800s settlers crossed the Trinity River on wagon trains.

The parking lot at the trailhead is fairly small, but there is usually an available spot as many folks tend to pick up the trail farther down at the larger Bird's Fork Trail Park. You'll want to start your hike here, however, as this section offers the opportunity to hike a natural path alongside the river before joining with the paved portion of the greenbelt.

Pick up the trail adjacent to the parking lot and follow it north a couple hundred feet until you reach a sign advertising a river view to your right. Turn right onto this path to reach a viewpoint overlooking the sparkling waters of the Elm Fork of the Trinity River. From here, a natural trail starts just where the pavement ends on your left. Pick it up and follow it as it hugs the river and meanders through the shade.

As you hike, a smattering of small signs posted off the trail help you identify the different types of trees—green ash, American elm, and hackberry—that shelter you from the sun. To your right, the river flows quietly, disturbed only by the occasional bird flying through. You're likely to spot the tracks of native wildlife in the dirt below your feet.

Continue along the trail as it parallels the river until you emerge from the trees at 0.4 mile and join the main paved portion of the greenbelt. You'll be unprotected from the sun for a bit as the trail crosses a road at 0.55 mile, then veers back toward the woods and the river. At 0.73 mile, turn onto the nature-trail entrance and return into the woods, with the river once again accompanying you on your right. There is no shortage of benches, and at 0.93 mile you'll reach one that's ideally positioned for those who want to absorb a scenic view of the river. At 1.25 miles, cross under an overpass, then over a wooden bridge, before you bear right toward more benches and then pick up the trail alongside the river.

At 1.63 miles, reach the end of the natural trail, where you're faced with a choice. If you're not quite ready to return, you can turn right, where the Campion Trail continues for several miles, offering more greenbelt to explore. If you want to go back, the trail will take you south back down the paved trail. At 1.73 miles, come to a signpost for a state-record elm tree just off the trail. As you continue back toward the trailhead, a few intersections allow you to rejoin the natural trail by the river, if you desire. If you prefer not to retrace the path you've already taken, simply keep right at the intersections, following the paved portion of the trail, and you'll soon find yourself back at the trailhead.

NEARBY ACTIVITIES

Just down the road, in Las Colinas's Williams Square, is the largest equestrian sculpture in the world: *The Mustangs at Las Colinas,* a collection of huge, lifelike bronze mustangs racing through a fountain in the middle of a plaza. A few restaurants in the area serve lunch. To reach Williams Square, head north on Riverside Drive about 0.8 mile. Turn left onto North O'Connor Boulevard; you'll see the mustangs in about 0.3 mile.

4 DOWNTOWN DALLAS URBAN TRAIL

KEY AT-A-GLANCE INFORMATION

LENGTH: 3.08 miles

CONFIGURATION: Loop

DIFFICULTY: Easy

SCENERY: Historic landmarks, cityscape, bronze statues, fountains

EXPOSURE: Sunny

TRAIL TRAFFIC: Light

TRAIL SURFACE: Paved

HIKING TIME: 2 hours

ACCESS: Free

FACILITIES: None

WHEELCHAIR TRAVERSABLE: No

SPECIAL COMMENTS: You won't need to feed the meters on Sundays.

DRIVING DISTANCE FROM MAJOR INTERSECTION: 0.5 mile from I-35E and Commerce Street

GPS TRAILHEAD COORDINATES

Latitude: N 32° 46' 45"
Longitude: W 96° 48' 27"

IN BRIEF

This urban hike beneath the glistening skyscrapers of the Big D combines the walking routes suggested by the city's visitor center into a loop of some of the best points in the downtown jungle. Though you won't see traditional nature sights along the hike, you will be impressed as you trek past urbanized versions, including a herd of cattle stampeding over a brook, a multilevel waterfall, a sculpture garden, and an infamous grassy knoll.

DESCRIPTION

Start your hike in front of the Old Red Courthouse. One of the most recognizable buildings in downtown, the beautiful red-sandstone building, built in the late 19th century, also houses the Visitor Information Center. Stop inside and pick up brochures, pamphlets, and maps of the area. From here, head east on Main Street. At about 150 feet, pass the Kennedy Memorial Plaza, an open, grassy space in the center of which sits a huge square monument designed by the architect Philip Johnson and erected in honor of John F. Kennedy. Across the street to the left sits a treasured reminder of Dallas's history: the John Neely Bryan Cabin. The one-room log cabin is a replica of what Dallas's founder, John Neely Bryan, would have lived in around the time the city was founded.

Directions ———————————————→

Follow I-30 East toward Dallas and take Exit 44 (Industrial Boulevard). Turn left onto Industrial Boulevard and right onto Commerce Street, then continue straight onto Main Street. The Old Red Courthouse is on the right, just in front of Dealey Plaza. Park at any metered spot along the street.

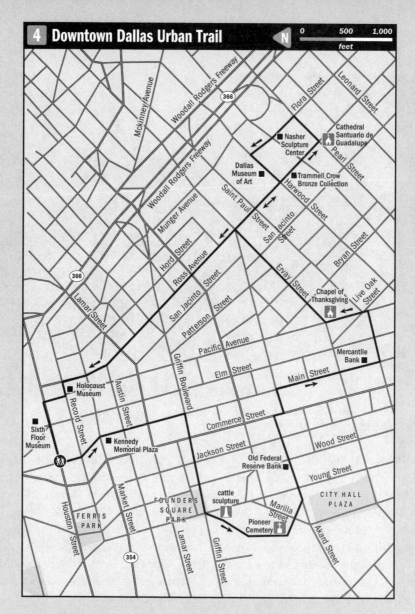

N

0   500   1,000
feet

Flora Street

Leonard Street

Mckinney Avenue

Woodall Rodgers Freeway

366

Nasher
Sculpture
Center

Cathedral
Santuario de
Guadalupe

Pearl Street

Dallas
Museum
of Art

Trammell Crow
Bronze Collection

Woodall Rodgers Freeway

Saint Paul Street

Harwood Street

Munger Avenue

San Jacinto Street

Bryan Street

366

Hord Street

Ross Avenue

San Jacinto Street

Ervay Street

Live Oak Street

Chapel of
Thanksgiving

Lamar Street

Patterson Street

Street

Pacific Avenue

Mercantile
Bank

Griffin Boulevard

Elm Street

Main Street

Holocaust
Museum

Austin Street

Record Street

Commerce Street

Wood Street

Sixth
Floor
Museum

Kennedy
Memorial Plaza

Jackson Street

Old Federal
Reserve Bank

Young Street

CITY HALL
PLAZA

cattle
sculpture

Marilla Street

Houston Street

FERRIS
PARK

Market Street

FOUNDER'S
SQUARE
PARK

Pioneer
Cemetery

Akard Street

354

Lamar Street

Griffin Street

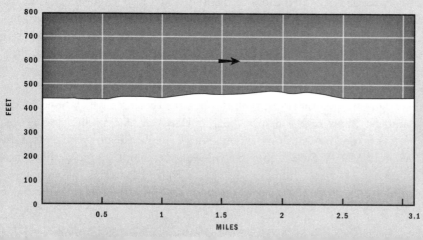

800
700
600
500
400
300
200
100
0

FEET

0.5   1   1.5   2   2.5   3.1

MILES

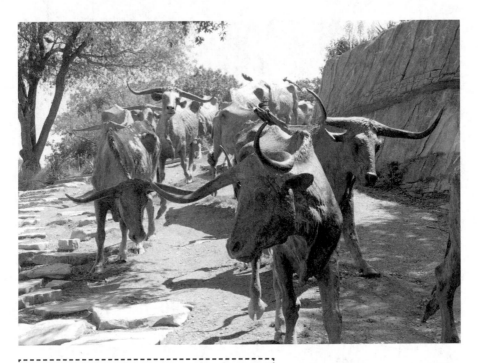

Bronze sculptures depict a cattle drive in Pioneer Plaza.

Cross Market Street, and at about 0.25 mile, just in front of the Bank of America Tower, you'll see the creation of sculptor Alexander Liberman—a huge, bright-red sculpture of circular tubes stacked atop each other. Then reach Griffin Street and turn right, following the road 0.25 mile to the Convention Center District. At 0.53 mile, come to Young Street; turn left and head toward the four-acre grassy hill where the heads of dozens of longhorn cattle are just visible.

Follow the gravel trail toward the steers, which are part of the Pioneer Plaza Cattle Drive, an amazing congregation of 70 bronze longhorn cattle driven down a hill and over a stream by three mounted cowboys. Shawnee Trail, an old route along which cowboys herded cattle in the 1800s, ran near Pioneer Plaza, which commemorates this heritage. Continue along the gravel trail, cross the stream, and turn left, heading uphill alongside the cattle. The sculptures are impressive; you can see the veins bulging in their necks and the muscles rippling beneath their bronze skin. Take a moment to examine the intricately detailed cowboys before returning to the gravel path and toward Pioneer Cemetery.

Turn left onto the short dirt path through the cemetery, which honors Dallas's founders. Many of the names, such as Harwood, Stemmons, and Flynn, have been bestowed on Dallas streets. At about 0.7 mile, the dirt path ends; turn left and cross Marilla Street. Join the sidewalk heading diagonally through a 2-acre grassy park that is home to the Dallas Police Memorial. This stainless-steel sculpture casts shadows on the ground, revealing the badge numbers of fallen officers.

At 0.75 mile, turn left onto Akard Street. To the right, you'll see the U.S., Texas, and City of Dallas flags flying in front of City Hall. To the left is an excellent view of a famous Dallas landmark, Reunion Tower—a 55-story tower topped with a dome housing a revolving restaurant and an observation deck. Cross Young Street and follow tree-lined Akard Street. Pass the historic old Federal Reserve Bank on the right. Straight ahead, if you look up you'll see a huge statue of Pegasus resting atop another famous Dallas building, the Magnolia Hotel. The building—and its logo, the winged horse—originally belonged to the Magnolia Petroleum Company and is now listed on the National Register of Historic Places. Across the street, you'll see the Adolphus Hotel, another ornate and historic building dating from 1912.

At about 0.9 mile, Akard ends. Cross the street and head through the brick plaza toward and past the Magnolia. Just beyond some patio tables where folks are enjoying the outdoors, cross Commerce Street and rejoin Akard Street on its northern section. Now turn right onto Main Street, passing Pegasus Plaza on the right, Neiman Marcus at 1.1 miles, and then a skyscraper—the Mercantile Bank building—at 1.18 miles.

Turn left onto St. Paul Street and pass the building that once housed the Titche-Goettinger department store. When you reach Elm, look to the right to see the vertical sign of the historic Majestic Theatre, here since the 1920s. Continue one block farther and head west (left) down Pacific Avenue; at 1.43 miles, make a right onto Ervay Street. Thanks-Giving Square, which celebrates the world's thanksgivings, is on the left and is a nice spot for a break. Enjoy the courtyard, the outdoor fountains, and the prominent white spiral tower, called the Chapel of Thanksgiving. Inside the chapel you can view a beautiful stained-glass design called the "Glory Window."

Continue over the trolley tracks and past the post office, until you reach Ross Avenue, at 1.7 miles. Turn right. On the left, pass the Dallas Museum of Art, fronted by a huge orange–red steel sculpture. A few hundred feet farther on the left is the Trammell Crow Bronze Collection, dozens of sculptures surrounding a tall office building. Finally, reach the Cathedral Santuario de Guadalupe, a cathedral dating to the 19th century, featuring stained-glass windows and a bell tower housing 49 bells. Turn left just in front of the cathedral onto North Pearl Street, and at 2 miles make another left onto Flora Street.

Continuing along, you'll see the Nasher Sculpture Center on your right and the Crow Collection of Asian Art on your left, which has a magnificent sculptural waterfall entrance. The road dead-ends in front of the Dallas Museum of Art; turn left onto Harwood Street. At the next intersection, at 2.18 miles, turn right to get back onto Ross Avenue.

At 2.4 miles, walk past Fountain Place on the right—a prism-shaped skyscraper at the base of which is a waterfall with ledges and pools. This is a nice place to explore, with a few acres of fountains and waterfalls. Cross Lamar Street and then see redbrick buildings, indicating you've reached the West End Historic

District, an attractive area of old warehouses that have been converted into stores and restaurants. At 2.83 miles, turn left onto Record Street and pass the Holocaust Museum, then turn right onto Pacific Avenue, following the trolley tracks.

A block down, turn left onto Houston Street. On the right is the former Texas School Book Depository, where on November 22, 1963, Lee Harvey Oswald shot and killed President John F. Kennedy from its sixth floor. Today, the building houses the Sixth Floor Museum, which harbors exhibits on JFK's life and death. A few steps farther, and you're at the entrance to Stemmons Freeway and in the middle of Dealey Plaza, a National Historic Landmark. Here lies the infamous "grassy knoll"—the controversial hill where some theorize another shooter in the Kennedy assassination was hidden. Crowds always gather in this spot, reading brochures and pamphlets about the incident. An X in the street marks where the motorcade was at the time of the shooting.

Cross the street and find a reflecting pool and a statue honoring George Bannerman Dealey, the Dallas businessman and civic planner after whom the plaza is named. From here, turn left back onto Main Street to reach the trailhead.

NEARBY ACTIVITIES

A few blocks east of downtown, visit Deep Ellum, Dallas's arts and entertainment district, where retail shops sell artsy and unusual items and an array of restaurants beckons you to grab a bite to eat. In the evenings, the area is a popular nightlife hub. To get to Deep Ellum, head east down Elm Street—it's just past the Central Expressway.

DUCK CREEK GREENBELT 5

IN BRIEF

Winding through a greenbelt alongside the murky green waters of Duck Creek, this trail is a great hike for bird-watchers.

DESCRIPTION

Part of the Garland Parks and Recreation Department, the Duck Creek Greenbelt cuts a green swath of wilderness through a populated urban area, offering locals a pleasant hike through the woods alongside the creek. I've started this hike on the southeastern end of the greenbelt, although a couple of different parking areas provide alternate access along its length. Adjacent to the parking area, a huge pavilion offering shade and tables is available for rent; contact the parks department at (972) 205-2750. While this isn't the most scenic hike you'll find in this book, it should appeal to folks who live in the area and are looking for a quick outdoor escape.

The trailhead is on the north side of the parking area, next to a box offering cleanup baggies for folks who have brought their dogs. The trail heads northwest, following alongside Duck Creek Drive, which peeks in and out of view through the trees to your right. On your left, trees grow thick alongside a deep gully formed by Duck Creek. The low rumble of cars driving by on the nearby roadway is only

KEY AT-A-GLANCE INFORMATION

LENGTH: 2.95 miles

CONFIGURATION: Balloon

DIFFICULTY: Easy

SCENERY: Woods

EXPOSURE: Partially shady

TRAIL TRAFFIC: Moderate

TRAIL SURFACE: Paved

HIKING TIME: 1 hour

ACCESS: Free; open daily

FACILITIES: Picnic tables

WHEELCHAIR TRAVERSABLE: Yes

SPECIAL COMMENTS: Dogs are permitted but should be kept leashed.

DRIVING DISTANCE FROM MAJOR INTERSECTION: 3 miles from I-635 and I-30

Directions

Take I-30 East to Exit 56B onto I-635 North. Go 1 mile and take Exit 9A, turning right onto Oates Drive. After about 1.7 miles, turn left onto Duck Creek Drive. The parking lot, on the left at 4917 Duck Creek Dr., is marked with a CAMP GATEWOOD sign.

GPS TRAILHEAD COORDINATES

Latitude: N 32° 51' 11"

Longitude: W 96° 36' 43"

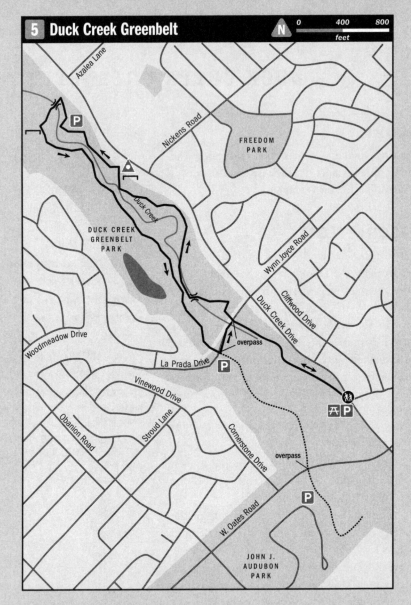

N

0   400   800
feet

Azalea Lane

P

Nickens Road

FREEDOM PARK

Duck Creek

DUCK CREEK GREENBELT PARK

Wynn Joyce Road

Cliffwood Drive

Duck Creek Drive

overpass

Woodmeadow Drive

La Prada Drive

P

Vinewood Drive

Obanion Road

Stroud Lane

Cornerstone Drive

overpass

P

W. Oates Road

JOHN J. AUDUBON PARK

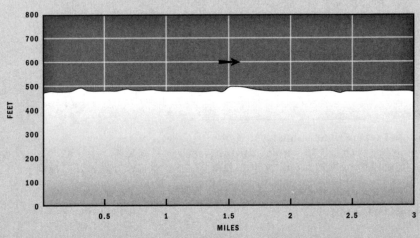

FEET

800
700
600
500
400
300
200
100
0

0.5   1   1.5   2   2.5   3

MILES

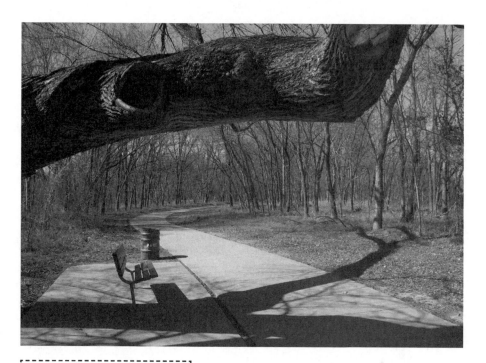

A shady rest spot on the greenbelt

slightly distracting, and as you walk farther along the path, the cheery chirping of birds in the trees will turn your attention away from the sounds of urban life.

The woods brush the trail, blessing it with partial shade for most of the hike. They also provide an ideal haven for vines, which climb the trunks and hang loosely from the branches of some of the trees. At 0.86 mile, cross a small bridge and continue northwest through the tall trees. You'll catch glimpses of the creek through the woods a couple dozen feet to the left before you reach an overlook at 1.43 miles. The setting is pretty: a deep gully through which the greenish waters of the creek laze. Trees loom overhead and cling to the creek's edge, creating the ideal haven for birds and frogs—easy to spot here.

Though charming, the gully does unfortunately collect loose trash blown in by the wind. Nevertheless, the trail is popular among local residents, who look beyond the distracting refuse to see the justifiable charm of the creek. Many come with binoculars to spot birds; others come with strollers and dogs, while still others bring their kids, who dip their feet in the water and hunt for turtles. I also spotted a number of older folks, attracted by the trail's flat, shaded, paved surface. Remind kids that swimming or wading in the creek is prohibited.

At 1.71 miles, pass the parking lot of an alternate trailhead on the right. A few hundred feet farther, a bridge spans Duck Creek, allowing you to cross. Once across the creek, bear left, following the path back the way you came but along the opposite side of the creek. On this side of the creek, the trail is much quieter, as the sound of cars completely fades from hearing. You'll find yourself winding back southwest on the southern side of the woods and creek. A variety of small and large nests in the trees provides evidence of a wide array of birdlife.

Soon, reach a sunny section and, off to your right, pass a wide field that abuts a small pond. As I hiked past, dozens of gulls and groups of ducks had taken over the banks of the small oasis, waiting for handouts from a couple of young kids. In the distance beyond the pond, you'll see the backside of local residences. Continue past the field and into the woods. At 2.83 miles, come to an overpass. Cross under the overpass, then bear right (away from the creek) and follow the path as it winds uphill to street level. If you instead continue straight, you'll pass through a section of woods cleared for Frisbee golf before reaching another access point to the greenbelt, directly across the creek from the pavilion and trailhead where you started. Proximity to the Frisbee area brings a little more traffic to this side of the creek than the opposite side.

Once you're at street level, turn around and head back northeast, crossing atop the overpass along the fenced-in sidewalk on the bridge's side. This will take you back across the creek. Once you've crossed over, turn right, picking the path up again as it heads southeast alongside the creek. This is the path you started on. From here retrace your steps back to the trailhead.

NEARBY ACTIVITIES

Just 8 miles north is the Firewheel Town Center, an open-air complex of department stores, retail shops, and restaurants—a good spot to grab a bite to eat and do some shopping. To get there, take Duck Creek Drive north, where it turns into South First Street. Turn right onto TX 78/Lavon Drive and go 3 miles. The mall is at the intersection of TX 78 North and the President George Bush Turnpike (TX 190).

FAIR PARK LOOP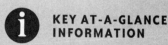

IN BRIEF

This trail loops through the fairgrounds, passing historic Art Deco buildings, the Cotton Bowl football stadium, the Texas Vietnam Memorial, various statues and museums, and a small lagoon.

DESCRIPTION

Listed as a National Historic Landmark, the Fair Park Buildings in Dallas are a group of Art Deco structures built in the 1930s for the Texas Centennial Exposition. According to the National Historic Landmark Registry, they form one of the largest such collections in the country. Today the area is the site of the State Fair of Texas. Its mascot—Big Tex, a statue more than 50 feet tall depicting a Texan complete with a cowboy hat and a Lone Star shirt—sits at the entrance while the fair is in attendance, greeting millions of visitors each year during its annual three-week run. When the fair is not on the grounds, Big Tex is taken down and the visitors dwindle. The buildings, gigantic Ferris wheel, and permanent exhibits and displays, however, remain; entrance to the area is free, and visitors are welcome to roam around. A pretty lagoon with swan boats and fountain, the Texas Vietnam Memorial, and an esplanade decorated with huge sculptures—not to mention the Cotton Bowl and various museums—make for an enjoyable hike.

- -

Directions   ⟶

Take I-30 East to Exit 47, Second Avenue/Fair Park. Continue straight to reach Fair Park. Park at the Grand Avenue entrance in front of the Dallas Museum of History.

ⓘ KEY AT-A-GLANCE INFORMATION

LENGTH: 2.95 miles

CONFIGURATION: Loop

DIFFICULTY: Easy

SCENERY: Lagoon, Art Deco buildings, fairgrounds

EXPOSURE: Sunny

TRAIL TRAFFIC: Moderate

TRAIL SURFACE: Paved

HIKING TIME: 1 hour

ACCESS: Free; open daily when fair not in town

FACILITIES: Restrooms, water fountains

WHEELCHAIR TRAVERSABLE: Yes

SPECIAL COMMENTS: There is an admission charge for the grounds when the State Fair of Texas is in town; in the off-season, there is no charge. Museums are open year-round (with admission), so plan for a whole day if you intend to visit some after the hike.

DRIVING DISTANCE FROM MAJOR INTERSECTION: 1.3 miles from I-30 and US 75

GPS TRAILHEAD COORDINATES

Latitude: N 32° 46' 42"

Longitude: W 96° 45' 51"

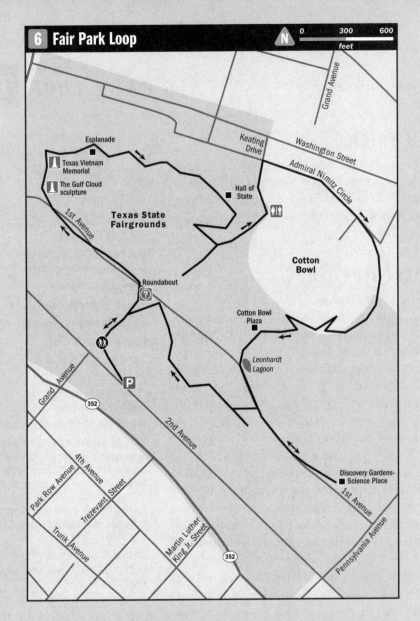

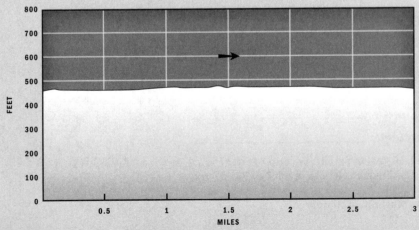

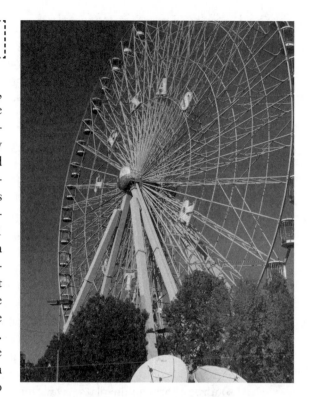

The famous Texas Star Ferris Wheel looms above the last part of the hike.

From the parking lot, head to the pedestrian gate at the Grand Avenue entrance. Start the hike by heading northeast on Grand and down a wide promenade, keeping the Dallas Museum of Natural History to your right. At 0.1 mile, reach a kiosk with a map of the grounds. Continue straight, then turn left onto First Avenue at the roundabout, keeping the Old Mill Inn on your right. Established in 1936, the building was originally a flour-mill exhibit, built to resemble an 1836 mill. Today the structure, complete with waterwheel, houses a restaurant.

Continue along the redbrick path, the Dallas skyline rising in the distance. At 0.42 mile, reach a metal sculpture called *The Gulf Cloud,* erected in 1916 in memory of the first secretary of the State Fair of Texas, Captain Sydney Smith. The sculpture depicts a woman and her daughters, each representing an aspect of Texas's geography—the prairies, the mountains, and the Gulf Coast. Beyond the sculpture is a short field of grass and, beyond that, the Texas Vietnam Memorial. To get there, turn right, heading down the half-circular driveway, and turn left onto the memorial's walkway. The walls list the names of more than 3,000 casualties of the war.

Continue by turning right to follow the walkway out. Ahead is the Women's Museum. Walk a few hundred feet, then turn right at the statue and head down the walkway. To your left is the Continental DAR House, a small, white Colonial-style house with green trim. During the fair, the DAR (Daughters of the American Revolution) House is open to the public, displaying exhibits on American history.

Continue straight, and at 0.75 mile reach the esplanade, a long corridor lined with buildings and six huge sculptures surrounding a reflecting pool. At the far end of the esplanade rises the Hall of State. As you walk through the esplanade, you'll see some magnificent murals by the artist Pierre Bourdelle on the buildings. During the winter holidays, the esplanade is lined with lights and Christmas trees.

At 1 mile, reach the Hall of State, a magnificent Art Deco building in front of which stands a gold archer. Along the frieze, the names of dozens of important Texas figures—among them Travis, Hogg, Ellis, Lamar, and Milam—adorn the building. A column of statues at the front steps representing Spain, France, Mexico, the Republic of Texas, the Confederate States, and the United States, compose the Six Flags of Texas.

From the state hall, turn right, heading south. At the end of the building, head left onto the walkway, keeping the Tower Building on your right. Ahead, seemingly out of place, looms the historic Cotton Bowl, a huge football stadium dating back to 1932. The stadium has a long and rich history, not only having hosted such popular football teams as the Dallas Cowboys and SMU Mustangs but also having been the site of events such as the 1994 Fifa World Cup and concerts by performers such as Elvis Presley and Aerosmith. At 1.4 miles, turn left onto the drive encircling the Cotton Bowl. After a couple hundred feet, take a left onto Keeting Drive and then the first right onto Nimitz Drive.

Follow Nimitz past some exhibition halls and the Creative Arts Show Place Theatre to head toward the Children's Petting Zoo, which is open during the fair. On your right, you'll see the backside of the Cotton Bowl. Continue walking down the road toward the Ferris wheel. You'll soon see a MIDWAY sign atop a closed-off entrance to a section holding the fair's amusement rides and games. The road curves to the right and comes out onto a plaza in front of the Cotton Bowl.

Head southwest through the plaza, away from the Cotton Bowl and toward the Leonhardt Lagoon. Take a left at the benches in front of the water. Along the water's edge, you'll see oddly shaped red walkways, which actually make up a sculpture designed to resemble a fern. Kids can often be seen leaning from its edges looking into the waters for the many turtles that inhabit the lagoon. Among the fish are yellow bluehead and longear sunfish; the plants include lizard tail, water hyacinth, and cattails. Swan boats regularly circle the lagoon, completing the tranquil scene.

Continue following the walkway southeast alongside and past the lagoon. As you walk, you'll get closer to the gigantic Texas Star Ferris Wheel to the left, allowing you to appreciate its beauty and size. The pathway continues past the Science Place and the Discovery Gardens before ending at a parking lot. From here, turn back, retracing your steps to the lagoon, this time turning left to follow the walkway along the opposite side of the lagoon, past the IMAX, and back toward the trailhead.

NEARBY ACTIVITIES

You could spend the entire day here after the hike enjoying the sights, including the Dallas Aquarium at Fair Park, the Women's Museum, the African American Museum, and the Texas Discovery Gardens. If you intend to visit multiple museums, ask about purchasing a ticket that allows entrance to all of them. For a bite to eat, stop by the Old Mill Inn, open year-round from 11 a.m. until 2:30 p.m.

FISH CREEK LINEAR TRAIL 7

IN BRIEF

A sunny hike through a cheery wooded greenbelt frequented by birds and enjoyed by local residents. A plaque in the middle of the new trail marks the Arlington–Grand Prairie city line.

DESCRIPTION

The neighboring cities of Grand Prairie and Arlington have worked together to connect with a linear park and trail alongside Fish Creek. In Arlington, the Fish Creek Linear Park extends from TX 360 west to Cravens Park. The park and trail continue into Grand Prairie, on a previously established section certified as the Nancy Dillon National Recreation Trail. Here, the trail follows Fish Creek about 2.5 miles, heading west past Great Southwest Parkway. Parking spots are plentiful along the entire length of Grand Prairie's trail, allowing access from just about anyplace you'd like to start. I began this hike on the western end of the trail, which is very near the gateway into Arlington.

Folks on this trail are exceedingly friendly—they go out of their way to smile and say hi, ask how you're doing, and give advice. Much of this probably owes to the fact that the trail abuts the backyards of people's homes, and residents have taken a personal responsibility for the trail's upkeep. Even at the trailhead, you'll notice that you're just behind a

KEY AT-A-GLANCE INFORMATION

LENGTH: 3.08 miles

CONFIGURATION: Out-and-back

DIFFICULTY: Easy

SCENERY: Trees, birds

EXPOSURE: Sunny

TRAIL TRAFFIC: Moderate

TRAIL SURFACE: Paved

HIKING TIME: 1 hour

ACCESS: Free; open daily, 5 a.m.–midnight

FACILITIES: Playground, benches

WHEELCHAIR TRAVERSABLE: Yes

SPECIAL COMMENTS: Bring a hat and sunscreen.

DRIVING DISTANCE FROM MAJOR INTERSECTION: 2.1 miles from I-20 and TX 360

Directions

Take I-20 toward Grand Prairie and exit onto South Great Southwest Parkway, heading south. Turn right onto Claremont Drive, then left onto Largo Drive. The parking lot is at the end of Largo, adjacent to the trail.

GPS TRAILHEAD COORDINATES

Latitude: N 32° 39' 57"

Longitude: W 97° 3' 35"

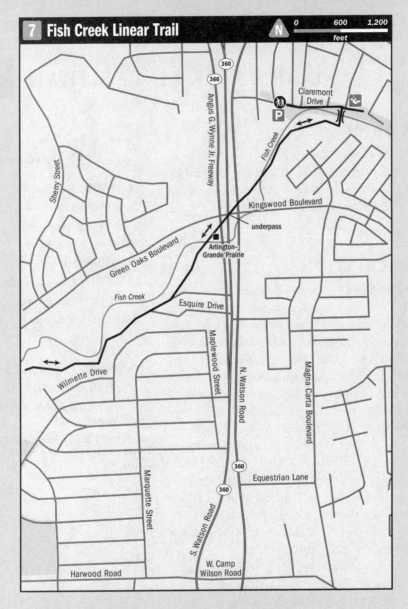

360

360

Claremont
Drive

Fish Creek

Kingswood Boulevard

underpass

Arlington–
Grande Prairie

Angus G. Wynne Jr. Freeway

Sherry Street

Green Oaks Boulevard

Fish Creek

Esquire Drive

Wilmette Drive

Maplewood Street

N. Watson Road

Magna Carta Boulevard

Marquette Street

S. Watson Road

360

360

Equestrian Lane

Harwood Road

W. Camp
Wilson Road

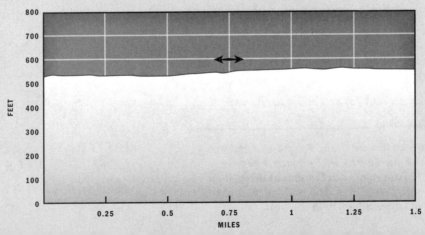

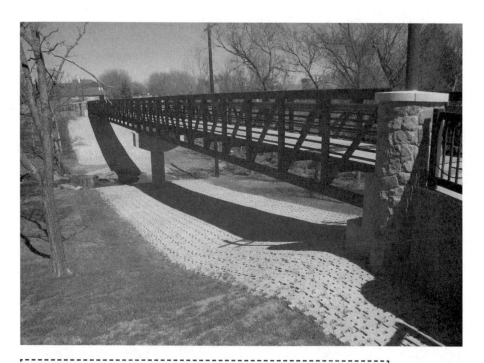

A sun-drenched bridge leads towards the Grand Prairie–Arlington city boundary.

quiet neighborhood where the locals simply step out their front doors and onto the trail. This pleasant sense of community sets this trail apart from other greenbelts of its kind.

From the trailhead, turn left onto the trail and head east. To your right, a couple dozen feet off the trail and hidden behind tall trees, is the creek—a sparkling green ribbon of water running parallel to the trail. Peeking down its banks, you're likely to see toads and frogs hopping into the water and out of sight. A large playground to the left gives kids a chance to burn some energy; if it's a sunny day, be sure to coat them with plenty of sunscreen, because the play area has no shade.

At 0.23 mile, reach a junction; if you go straight, you'll continue through Grand Prairie. A jogger I met here commented that there was a Mexican bakery with tasty treats at the end, a fact that kept her motivated to finish her run. Although the bakery might sound tempting, you'll want to bear right to get to Arlington. Cross over the beautiful, huge, rust-colored bridge spanning the narrow creek. On the other side of the bridge, bear right and follow the trail as it winds onto a sunny peninsula sandwiched between the backyards of homes to your left and the narrow creek to your right. Ahead and above you is a network of crisscrossing overpasses. Here, in the shadow of TX 360, adjacent to the creek, a huge round plaque in the ground marks the Arlington–Grand Prairie city boundary. Around you, the trail is new and well maintained; litter and graffiti you might find beneath other bridges is notably absent. Teenagers jog and skate by, contributing to the trail's friendly vibe.

The trail continues southwest, deeper into Arlington. The smooth, paved path is clearly marked with a yellow stripe down its center. To your right, the creek winds through a deep gully. Just across the gully, glimpse a shopping complex before you head slightly uphill and the woods screen the buildings from view. To your left, the backyards of houses in a small residential subdivision are quickly overtaken by woodland.

On my hike, the unmistakable sounds of woodpeckers tapping the upper trunks of the trees filled the air, outdone only by the chirping of other birds flitting from branch to branch. It's a peaceful, upbeat setting, in which you'll find friendly older folks out enjoying a walk in the fresh air and younger ones biking happily along. One cyclist who had stopped for a sip from her water bottle greeted me as I walked by and enthusiastically described how amazed she was that she could bike from Tarrant County in Arlington, where she lived, straight into Dallas County. This was her first foray down the trail, and she was surprised and impressed with its beauty and charm, especially since it runs through such a busy city.

Continue southwest through much of the same woodland scenery. At 1.54 miles, reach the back fence of an elementary school set a few hundred feet off the trail to the left. This is a nice spot for taking a quick breather before you turn around and retrace your steps to the trailhead. Alternatively, you can continue straight down the trail through more woodlands. You'll eventually reach Cravens Park at the far western end.

NEARBY ACTIVITIES

Just 7 miles away, the planetarium at the University of Texas at Arlington offers simulated views of the current night sky and constellations in a 1-hour star or music show. The schedule includes afternoon showings on weekends; check the discounts for students and seniors. Visit **uta.edu/planetarium** for more information and showtimes. To get there, take TX 360 North, exit at Park Row Drive, and go west 3 miles. Turn right onto Cooper Street, then right again onto Mitchell Street. Turn left onto West Street. Two blocks along, you'll find the parking garage. Walk out the opposite side of the garage onto Planetarium Place.

KATY TRAIL 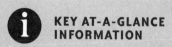 8

IN BRIEF

Popular with a young, urban crowd, this linear trail creates a pedestrian-friendly corridor between downtown Dallas and the Mockingbird DART station and has become a place to see and be seen. Always lively, this trail will appeal to those who don't mind a constant bustle of activity.

DESCRIPTION

No trail is more well known in Dallas than the Katy Trail. Without question, it is one of the most popular trails in the Metroplex. Crowds of people overtake it on weekends and holidays, offering the adventurous visitor an always-lively experience. And if you think you can

---

Directions ⟶

The trail is behind the American Airlines Center, at Victory Park in Dallas. When there are no events at the center, you can park free in its north parking lot; at other times, you can park in a metered space in the nearby West End. If you're traveling south from I-35E toward downtown Dallas, you can get directly to the center by taking the Oaklawn/Victory Avenue/Hi Line Drive exit. Stay on the service road, then turn left onto Victory Avenue.

To get to the parking in the West End from I-35E South, take the Continental Avenue exit and turn left onto Continental, which turns into Lamar Street. At the intersection of Lamar and McKinney Avenue, the West End will be on the right. Continue one more block to Munger Avenue and turn right. Park in any lot or metered space, and walk north down North Houston Street (which runs parallel to Lamar on its west) toward the American Airlines Center. The trailhead is across the street from the parking lot of the American Airlines Center on North Houston.

KEY AT-A-GLANCE INFORMATION

LENGTH: 5.64 miles

CONFIGURATION: Out-and-back

DIFFICULTY: Easy

SCENERY: Trees, city views

EXPOSURE: Mostly sunny, some shade

TRAIL TRAFFIC: Heavy

TRAIL SURFACE: Concrete path

HIKING TIME: 1.75 hours

ACCESS: Free; open daily, 5 a.m.–midnight

WHEELCHAIR TRAVERSABLE: Yes

SPECIAL COMMENTS: If you can't find a spot near the trailhead, try parking at one of the parks adjacent to the trail.

SUPPLEMENTAL MAPS: katytraildallas.org (click "Download a Map" on the home page)

DRIVING DISTANCE FROM MAJOR INTERSECTION: 1.4 miles from Woodall Rodgers Freeway and I-35E

GPS TRAILHEAD COORDINATES

Latitude: N 32° 47' 33"

Longitude: W 96° 48' 39"

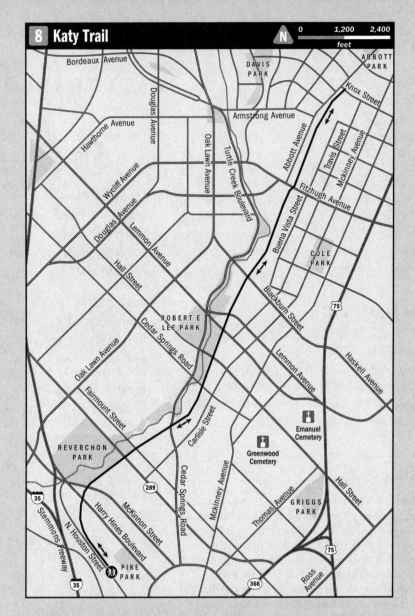

N

0   1,200   2,400
feet

Bordeaux Avenue

DAVIS
PARK

ABBOTT
PARK

Knox Street

Douglas Avenue

Hawthorne Avenue

Armstrong Avenue

Abbott Avenue

Travis Street

McKinney Avenue

Oak Lawn Avenue

Turtle Creek Boulevard

Wycliff Avenue

Fitzhugh Avenue

Buena Vista Street

Douglas Avenue

Lemmon Avenue

COLE
PARK

Hall Street

75

Blackburn Street

ROBERT E
LEE PARK

Cedar Springs Road

Lemmon Avenue

Haskell Avenue

Oak Lawn Avenue

Fairmount Street

Carlisle Street

Emanuel
Cemetery

REVERCHON
PARK

Cedar Springs Road

McKinney Avenue

Greenwood
Cemetery

Hall Street

289

McKinnon Street

Harry Hines Boulevard

McKinney Avenue

Thomas Avenue

GRIGGS
PARK

35

75

Stemmons Freeway

N. Houston Street

PIKE
PARK

366

Ross
Avenue

35

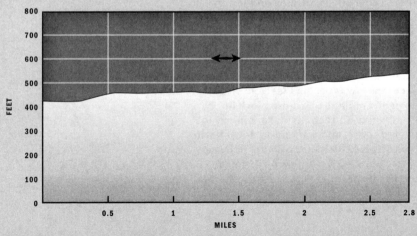

800

700

600

500

400

300

200

FEET

100

0

0.5   1   1.5   2   2.5   2.8

MILES

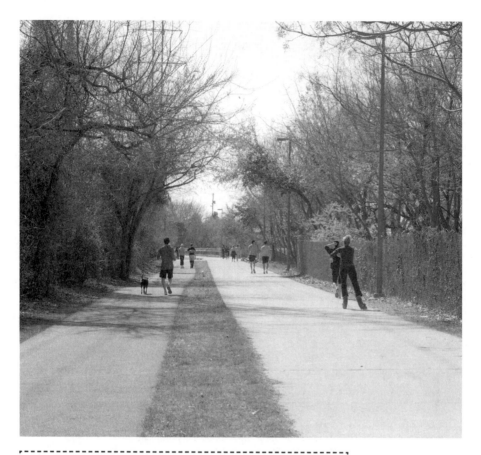

Don't plan to be alone on the Katy Trail—it's always bustling with activity.

avoid the crowds by visiting during the scorching summer months—well, think again. This trail is always hopping, thanks in part to its easy accessibility in highly populated areas of the city. In fact, according to the Friends of the Katy Trail, a nonprofit organization dedicated to the trail's expansion and development, more than 300,000 people live within 1 mile of the trail.

To accommodate the many folks who live in the area, the trail has a number of access points along its length. In addition, it passes several city parks and intersects a couple of major streets, affording further access. Because of its popularity, you'll encounter a wide assortment of outdoor types along its length: expect to share the trail with other hikers, walkers, joggers, bikers, dog walkers, skateboarders, and inline skaters. The trail is about 5.6 miles out-and-back, stretching from the American Airlines Center to Airline Road, near the Southern Methodist University campus.

In recent years, a massive publicity campaign to promote safety along the trail has been implemented with the help of names such as former Dallas Cowboys quarterback Troy Aikman (a high-profile user of the trail). In particular, the

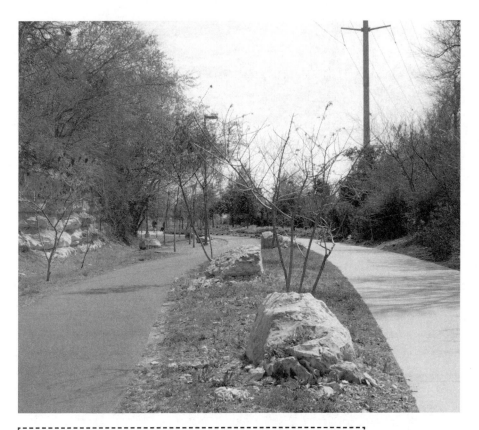

The trail is divided to accommodate both bicycle and pedestrian traffic safely.

campaign focuses on trail etiquette and safety awareness so that visitors know how to share the trail when there is both biker and pedestrian traffic.

The trail's history dates back to the late 1800s, when the Missouri–Kansas–Texas (MKT) Railroad began operating a passenger and freight line into Texas, connecting it with states to the north. The MKT, nicknamed the "Katy," eventually connected St. Louis with Dallas and Fort Worth and extended as far south as Galveston. In the late 1980s, to avoid financial losses, the MKT merged with the Missouri Pacific Railroad Company, part of the Union Pacific Railway. Dallas's Katy Trail owes its existence in part to Union Pacific, which donated the abandoned tracks to the city. In Missouri, another old abandoned section of the Katy Trail has been similarly donated and forms a 225-mile trail known as Katy Trail State Park.

The trailhead for this hike is in Victory Park behind the American Airlines Center, across the street from the facility's parking lot. A plaque identifying this entrance point as Victory Promenade marks the trailhead. If you prefer not to drive into downtown Dallas and the West End, other entrance points for the trail include Reverchon Park (see Hike 13, page 69), David's Way Plaza, and the Dallas Theater Center.

From the Victory Park trailhead, the path ascends a small incline to reach the elevated trail bed, from the top of which you have a decent, though slightly obstructed view of the Dallas skyline if you turn around. Because of its old railway status, the trail from here to the end is relatively level, having only a few gentle turns. The scenery is mostly a thick curtain of trees obscuring the highways, streets, and autos only a short distance below. If you're interested in orienting yourself, the trail runs roughly between Oaklawn Avenue and Stemmons Freeway to the left, and the busy Central Expressway to the right. Surprisingly, the sounds of urban life do not overwhelm, and at many points you'll even be unaware that you're hiking through the busiest part of Dallas.

The trail is about 12 feet wide and divided into two lanes—one for bikers, the other for pedestrians. You'll find the division of lanes a welcome feature, as the trail is always heavily trafficked. The path is very nicely maintained; you'd be hard-pressed to find any litter, or even a spot where the grass comes close to encroaching on the path. The trail developers have also done an excellent job marking the trail: when you cross a highway or pass a park, you'll see signs telling you exactly where you are.

You won't find much wildlife along the path, though you may spot a few squirrels scurrying in front of you or a stray cat walking along the path's edge. The backyards of condos and homes abut the trail at various spots along the way, serving as a reminder of the trail's urban location.

At 0.6 mile, just after you pass over Harry Hines Boulevard and McKinnon Street, look for Reverchon Park (conceived as Dallas's version of Central Park) to the left. The park is named in honor of James Reverchon, a renowned botanist from the late 19th century who lived nearby.

From here, the trail passes over Maple and Cedar Springs roads. At about 1.6 miles, just after you cross Lemmon Avenue, pass Turtle Creek Park on the left. As you continue northeast, you'll reach the Highland Park area. The intersection of David's Way and Travis Street, at 2.8 miles, is a good turnaround spot. If you need to cool off or grab a drink before the hike back, a couple of restaurants and a convenience store are just within reach. To extend the hike, you can continue straight another mile, where the trail ends at some bike lockers not far from SMU and Mockingbird Station.

NEARBY ACTIVITIES

The West End is a pedestrian-friendly walking district with several restaurants. Once the hub of Dallas's commercial activities, today the renovated warehouses make up one of the city's main entertainment areas. Listed on the National Register of Historic Places, the West End is also the home of Dealey Plaza, where John F. Kennedy was shot in 1963.

9 L. B. HOUSTON NATURE TRAIL

KEY AT-A-GLANCE INFORMATION

LENGTH: 1.61 miles

CONFIGURATION: Loop

DIFFICULTY: Easy

SCENERY: Cedar, elm, oak woodlands, river views

EXPOSURE: Shady

TRAIL TRAFFIC: Heavy on weekends

TRAIL SURFACE: Packed dirt

HIKING TIME: 40 minutes

ACCESS: Free; open daily

FACILITIES: None

WHEELCHAIR TRAVERSABLE: No

SPECIAL COMMENTS: Rains cause the trail to become muddy and impassable. If it rained the day before you plan to hike, choose a different trail.

DRIVING DISTANCE FROM MAJOR INTERSECTION: 2.7 miles from TX 114 and TX Loop 12

GPS TRAILHEAD COORDINATES

Latitude: N 32° 51' 59"

Longitude: W 96° 55' 22"

IN BRIEF

This flat trail through the woods offers glimpses of the Elm Fork of the Trinity River and is a cool, shady hike for a hot summer's day.

DESCRIPTION

Tucked away in a corner of North Irving, this fun little trail offers locals easy access to a little bit of wilderness close to home. To me, this trail is a perfect example of how city dwellers craving the outdoors can turn an otherwise unremarkable location into a happening weekend spot. If it's nice out, you're likely to find the trailhead hopping with all kinds of activities: kayakers prepping their gear for an outing along the nearby river, fishermen meandering down to the water with poles and tackle box in hand, joggers stretching in preparation for a run, or bikers readying their bikes for a spin along the trail.

Maintained by DORBA, the Dallas Off-Road Bicycle Association, the several miles of trails here are open to both bikers and hikers. An impressive amount of energy has been put into the trail's maintenance, and though in years past the vicinity had a reputation for attracting vagrants and partiers, the care and maintenance of volunteers have

----

Directions

From TX 183, take the TX 114 exit toward Grapevine and then the Tom Braniff Drive/Loop 12 exit. Turn north onto Tom Braniff Drive, which becomes Wildwood Drive. The trailhead is about 1 mile ahead on the right, at the intersection of Wildwood Drive and California Crossing Road, across the street from the National Guard Armory.

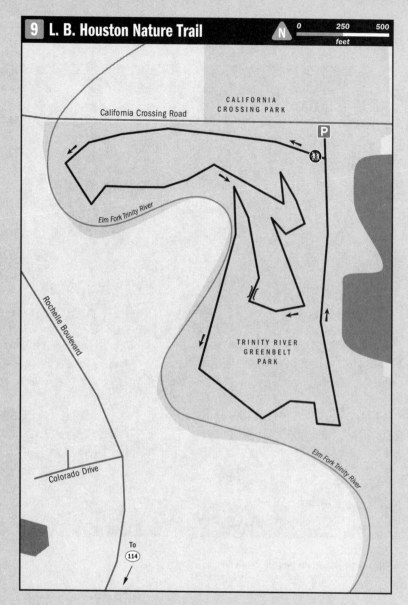

CALIFORNIA
CROSSING PARK

California Crossing Road

Elm Fork Trinity River

Rochelle Boulevard

TRINITY RIVER
GREENBELT
PARK

Elm Fork Trinity River

Colorado Drive

To
114

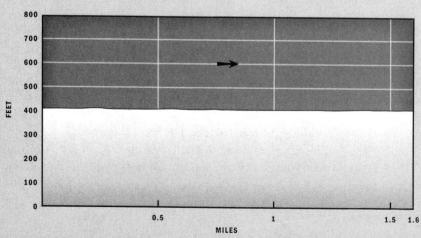

FEET

800
700
600
500
400
300
200
100
0

0.5   1   1.5 1.6

MILES

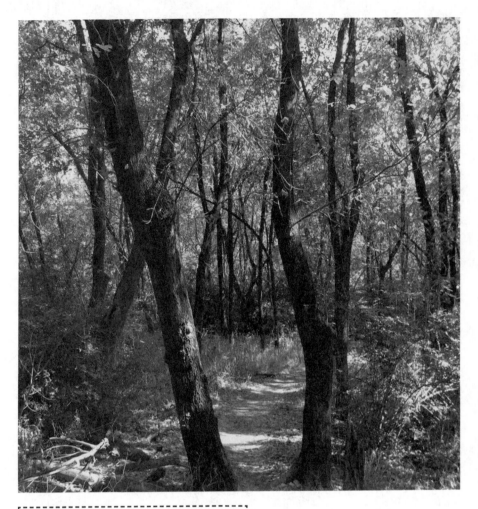

The narrow dirt path winds through dense foliage.

completely turned the area around. You'll find the trail clean, well maintained, and well frequented.

As you approach from the parking lot, to your left you'll see a pond whose still waters attract birds, such as herons and egrets, searching for a meal. When the water is low, a sandbar attracts local kids looking to hone their fishing skills. Straight ahead, you'll see a tree-lined wide grassy lane down which trickles a steady stream of folks exiting the trail from both sides of the wood.

To the right, you'll see the trailhead. A small kiosk in front of it bears a trail map. The trail is intended to be one long loop, encouraging traffic to flow in one direction. The first part, however—which is ideal for hikers because of its smooth, level terrain—comes back out onto the grassy median before continuing. This allows for a pleasant walk while avoiding the more technical sections of the latter half of the trail. If you were to venture on, the trail crosses the central grass strip into the southeast section. The dips in these sections appeal to mountain bikers.

Begin the hike by entering the trail as it heads right and disappears into the woods. Keep right to follow the main trail. The trail immediately starts to twist and turn gently as it haphazardly makes its way through the trees. Off to the right, catch glimpses of California Crossing Road. At first you'll hear the background hum of the occasional car, but that quickly gives way to the chirping of birds and the rustling of trees. The trees are closely packed all along the trail, bathing most of the path in shade. At some points the branches converge tightly just overhead, enveloping the walkway in lovely tunnels of foliage. In other parts, the trees are a little more spaced apart, allowing wild grass to grow tall and thick at their bases.

The trail itself is narrow, allowing for only single-file walking. It approaches trees only to curve away at the last minute, keeping the hike interesting as your attention is naturally drawn outward to the cedar, elm, oak, and other trees and plants you pass. Stay to the right, following the outer trail as it makes a rough loop along the banks of Elm Fork of the Trinity River. At a couple of spots, you can glimpse the river through the trees to the right. Birds are often seen flying over the water before disappearing into the trees on the far side of the river.

The day of our hike, DORBA volunteers were on the trail cutting back limbs, clipping bushes, and cleaning debris. Judging from the excellent condition of parts of the trail they had not yet reached, this is not a one-time undertaking, but rather a continual effort.

At about 0.95 mile, reach a nice vantage point for viewing the wide expanse of river, whose waters are a muddy greenish-gray. In the spring and summer, colorful butterflies flutter through the foliage at the river's edge.

The trail crosses a short wooden footbridge, heads slightly uphill, and, at 1.3 miles, leaves the woods, whereupon you'll find yourself again on the wide, grassy lane just south of the trailhead. Turn left and follow the trail 0.25 mile back to the trailhead. Pass the pond on the right before arriving back at the parking lot.

NEARBY ACTIVITIES

In nearby Williams Square in Las Colinas, a section of North Irving, is the largest equestrian sculpture in the world: *The Mustangs at Las Colinas,* a collection of huge, lifelike bronze mustangs racing through a fountain in the middle of a plaza. A few restaurants in the area serve lunch. To get to Williams Square, head west on California Crossing and turn right onto Riverside Drive. Turn left onto North O'Connor Boulevard; you'll see the horses about 0.5 mile ahead on the right.

10   ROWLETT CREEK NATURE TRAIL

KEY AT-A-GLANCE INFORMATION

LENGTH: 4 miles

CONFIGURATION: Double loop

DIFFICULTY: Moderate

SCENERY: Woodland, creek

EXPOSURE: Shady with a section of sun

TRAIL TRAFFIC: Heavy

TRAIL SURFACE: Packed dirt

HIKING TIME: 1.5 hours

ACCESS: Free; open daily

FACILITIES: Portable toilets, water fountain, picnic tables

WHEELCHAIR TRAVERSABLE: No

SPECIAL COMMENTS: Watch for snakes sunning on the trail.

DRIVING DISTANCE FROM MAJOR INTERSECTION: 8.3 miles from I-30 and I-635

GPS TRAILHEAD COORDINATES

Latitude: N 32° 55' 12"

Longitude: W 96° 35' 44"

IN BRIEF

This heavily traveled trail is an excellent choice for a hot, sunny day because most of it is shaded by woods. Because of the dense woodland along the entire length of the trail, this hike will appeal more to those looking for exercise than to those looking for scenic views.

DESCRIPTION

You'll be lucky if you can find a parking space in the Rowlett Creek Preserve in Garland. If you look closely, however, you're likely to see bike racks, helmets, and aerodynamic clothing—indicators of the activity that's most popular on this trail: mountain biking. The trails are, however, open to hikers, and because there are more than 10 miles of trails, it does not feel overwhelmingly crowded (though you certainly won't feel lonely). The trails are arranged in numbered loops; the higher the number, the more difficult the trail for a biker. What makes this trail particularly appealing is that almost all of it is shaded, making for an ideal summer hike.

This hike starts with the Loop 1 Trail. Find the trailhead on the north side of the parking lot, to the left of a gazebo and just behind a kiosk displaying a map of the preserve. The narrow dirt path disappears north

----

Directions ⟶

Take the President George Bush Turnpike (TX 190) to its end, at TX 78 North. Turn right onto 78 North (Lavon Drive), heading toward Garland. Go about 2 miles and turn left onto Castle Drive to Rowlett Creek Preserve. The parking lot is about 1.7 miles ahead, at the intersection of Castle Drive and East Centerville Road.

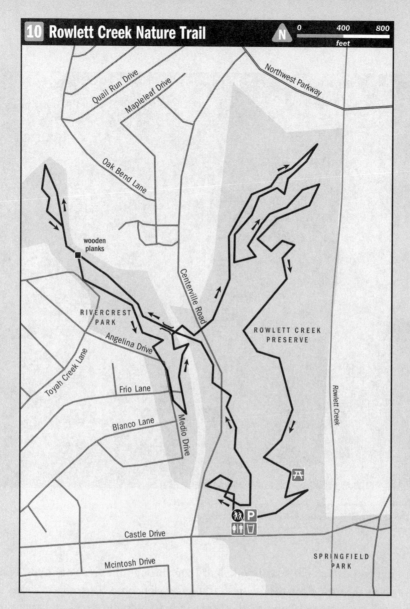

N

| 0 | 400 | 800 |

feet

Quail Run Drive

Mapleleaf Drive

Northwest Parkway

Oak Bend Lane

wooden planks

Centerville Road

RIVERCREST PARK

ROWLETT CREEK PRESERVE

Angelina Drive

Toyah Creek Lane

Frio Lane

Blanco Lane

Medio Drive

Rowlett Creek

P

Castle Drive

SPRINGFIELD PARK

Mcintosh Drive

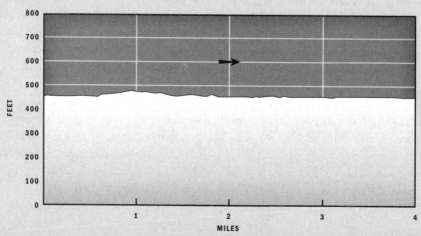

FEET			
800			
700			
600			
500			
400			
300			
200			
100			
0	1	2	3	4

MILES

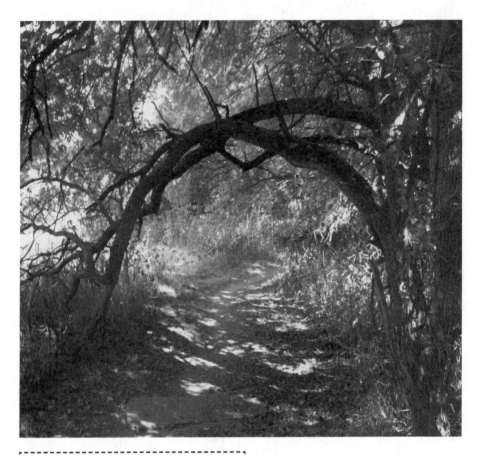

The shady trail passes through dense woodlands.

into the woods and curls lazily in a half-loop through the trees until you reach a turnoff at 0.57 mile for the Loop 7 Trail. Turn left onto the trail; at about 0.63 mile, the path crosses beneath the bridge for Centerville Road and then heads into more woods. The trail then follows a narrow creek north toward the northern edge of the preserve. Dense woods in this section cast a deep shade over the trail, providing welcome relief during a sunny day. To the right, the woods end at the backyards of private homes that abut the opposite side of the creek.

Continue on the trail, reaching a fence and a small sign at the edge of the preserve; the trail winds along this fence before coming to a junction at 1 mile. Take the trail to the left, heading downhill. The trails that cut through this section are close enough together that you're likely to glimpse bikers or hikers winding through the woods on trails completely obscured by the dense trees. This gives the confusing illusion that people might be heading toward you or coming up from behind you, when in fact they are on a completely different part of the trail. Keep alert, because when a rider is on the same trail, the path's twists and turns prevent you from knowing it until he or she is right in front of you, leaving you little time to step aside.

Reach the next junction at 1.1 miles, where trails head to the left and right while one continues straight ahead; choose this middle path to avoid the steep hills intended for mountain bikers. At 1.23 miles, go right and follow a long wooden boardwalk overlaying the trail. You'll dodge a couple of low-hanging limbs, then reach the end of the boardwalk's wooden planks. At 1.4 miles there is yet another junction—head right. At this point, the trail climbs out of the woods and onto a small, sun-drenched ridge, where Centerville Road stretches in front of you. Bear right, heading downhill; the path curls in a short loop through another section of woods, then, at 1.8 miles, comes back up onto the sunny, tree-less ridge. Follow the trail back into the woods; the trees lean together, forming a cavelike entry into the inviting relief of deep shade.

A couple hundred feet farther and you'll be back at the bridge. Just after the overhang, stay to the right to pick up a trail that brings you back to the Loop 7 turnoff. At about 1.9 miles, approach the split and bear left. At about 2 miles, bear left again, following the sign for Loop 1a. Cross a small brook; follow it for 2.25 miles and then bear right, continuing on Loop 1a. The trail is level for the rest of the hike, making for easy walking. Keep your eyes peeled for snakes—it isn't unusual to spot them curled in the middle of the trail, and I once spied a 3-foot one just barely slithering out of the way as bikers whizzed past.

At 2.9 miles, join Loop 1. The trail passes straight through a wide field, the only sunny portion of the trail. At 3.88 miles, come to a picnic table set conveniently in the shade of a huge lone tree—a nice spot at which to stop and eat lunch before heading home. From the picnic table, the trail merges onto a paved pathway that ends at the parking lot.

NEARBY ACTIVITIES

Just a few miles away, the Firewheel Town Center—an open-air complex of department stores, retail shops, and restaurants—is a good place to grab a bite to eat and do some shopping. It's about 2 miles northwest, at the intersection of TX 78 North and the President George Bush Turnpike (TX 190).

11 SPRING CREEK PARK NATURE TRAIL

KEY AT-A-GLANCE INFORMATION

LENGTH: 1.02 miles

CONFIGURATION: Loop

DIFFICULTY: Easy

SCENERY: Woodland forest, birds, creek

EXPOSURE: Shady–sunny

TRAIL TRAFFIC: Light

TRAIL SURFACE: Packed dirt

HIKING TIME: 30 minutes

ACCESS: Free; open daily

FACILITIES: None—bring water.

WHEELCHAIR TRAVERSABLE: No

SPECIAL COMMENTS: For additional information, go to springcreek forest.org.

DRIVING DISTANCE FROM MAJOR INTERSECTION: 5.2 miles from TX 190 and US 75

GPS TRAILHEAD COORDINATES

Latitude: N 32° 57' 52"

Longitude: W 96° 39' 25"

IN BRIEF

This flat, well-maintained forest trail follows a creek toward a bench nestled in the shade beneath the trees. With a keen eye, you can catch sight of the variety of resident and migrant birds that make this a popular spot with birders. Note that neither Spring Creek Forest nor Spring Creek Park has restrooms or drinking water, so come prepared.

DESCRIPTION

The Spring Creek Forest Preserve and the Spring Creek Park Preserve, which straddle Holford Road in North Garland within about 500 feet of each other, offer hikers quiet patches of remarkably preserved forest wilderness less than a mile from the George Bush Highway. The Spring Creek Forest Preserve, which is popular with naturalists and plant enthusiasts, boasts a unique occurrence of bur, chinquapin, Shumard, and Texas red oaks growing in community with various types of elm, ash, and hackberry. More than 150 different species of birds have been identified here. A short, paved path to a bench overlooking the creek makes for a pleasant stroll. Across the street, the Spring Creek

---

Directions ————————→

From Dallas, take TX 75 North to Garland, and take Exit 24 toward Belt Line Road. Turn right on Belt Line and go 1 mile, then make a left onto North Grove Road, then a right onto Arapaho Road. Go about 3 miles and turn left onto Holford Road. The Spring Creek Park Preserve is about 0.5 mile ahead on the left; Spring Creek Forest Preserve is 0.1 mile farther on the right. Park at Spring Creek Park Preserve.

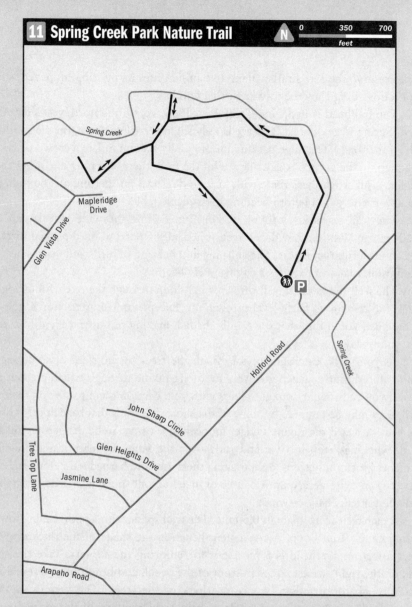

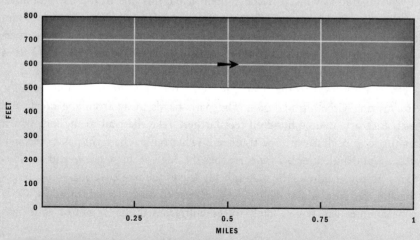

Park Preserve shelters similar plant and animal life. Its inviting, unpaved, shady trail loops along the creek through the woods.

The trailhead is in Spring Creek Park Preserve, on the northwest side of the road (Spring Creek Forest Preserve is only slightly farther down, on the southeast side of the road.) The huge parking lot can easily accommodate a crowd of hikers, although on the gorgeous day that we hit the trail, there was only one other car in the lot. A hiker who was there with his two dogs was just getting off the trail, giving us a friendly nod before heading for a picnic table.

The trail starts just off the parking lot. Follow the wide gravel path that heads north. Within a few dozen feet, it becomes a narrow, hard-packed dirt trail and enters a riparian forest. The chirping and buzzing of birds and insects perfects the illusion that you're miles away from civilization.

The well-maintained trail curls in a half-loop through the trees, following the creek and remaining fairly level throughout. Except for a short section at the end of the hike, you'll find that the trail is shaded, making this an excellent hike for a hot, sunny day.

As you walk, catch glimpses through the trees to the right of some ragged sand-colored bluffs, which give way to a long ravine through which a creek gurgles. If you've brought younger hikers with you, caution them to stay on the main trail; they may be tempted by some of the short side trails that branch off through the brush toward the ravine's edge. Innocent curiosity can be dangerous for children, who may step too far and slide over the edge. In many cases, logs and branches block these trails, discouraging their use, and barbed wire along the edge serves as an extra deterrent. A couple of nice lookout spots farther down the trail provide for safe, easy viewing.

Reach a clearing at about 0.5 mile. The trail splits, with a path leading toward Spring Creek Trail Loop. A convenient bench in the shade of the thick grove of trees towering overhead is a nice spot for enjoying the scenery. Take the short trail on the right, which passes in front of the bench and heads north a few dozen feet through the woods to a nice overlook of the creek. The various summer, winter, and migrating winged residents help make this one of the more popular birding spots in the Metroplex. Keep an eye out for these short- and long-term residents, which include bluebirds, woodpeckers, finches, warblers, owls, sparrows, and kinglets. The most common wildlife you're likely to see, aside from birds, is a few squirrels scurrying beneath the trees.

Retrace your steps to the bench and take the opposite trail, following the signs for Spring Creek Trail Loop. The path heads away from the creek and reaches a fork at a couple hundred feet farther. Take the trail to the left, which finishes the loop back toward the trailhead. (The trail to the right passes through a small grassland and, after 0.2 mile, reaches the edge of the preserve and an alternate exit.) As you continue, the path quickly leaves the tree covering and emerges into the sun, heading in a straight line southeast through a small meadow. On a spring or summer day, you're likely to see butterflies fluttering out of your path

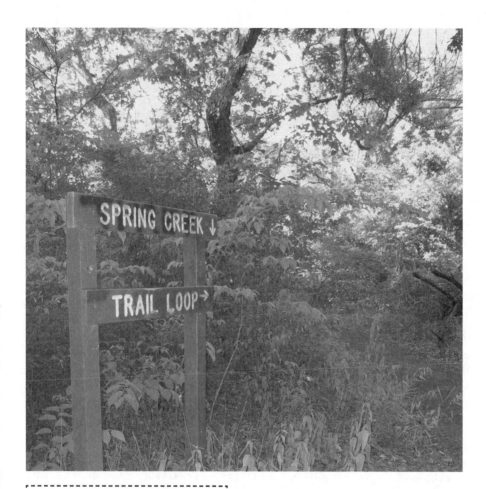

The well-maintained trail is clearly marked.

as you make your way down the narrow trail. After 0.3 mile, you'll see the picnic table and the parking lot from which you started.

The Preservation Society for Spring Creek Forest (**springcreekforest.org**) has a wealth of information on the plant and animal habitats of the area (including logs of the various bird species sighted), along with information on nature walks and talks.

NEARBY ACTIVITIES

Just a few miles to the southeast, the Firewheel Town Center—an open-air complex of department stores, retail shops, and restaurants—is a good place to grab a bite to eat and do some shopping. To get there, head northeast on Holford Road, and turn south onto President George Bush Turnpike, traveling about 1.3 miles. Take the TX 78 North exit toward Sachse/Wylie, and turn right onto Lavon Drive.

12 TRINITY RIVER AUDUBON TRAIL

KEY AT-A-GLANCE INFORMATION

LENGTH: 2.5 miles

CONFIGURATION: Loop

DIFFICULTY: Easy

SCENERY: Forest, wetlands, river

EXPOSURE: Sunny

TRAIL TRAFFIC: Moderate

TRAIL SURFACE: Packed dirt

HIKING TIME: 45 minutes

ACCESS: Tuesday–Saturday, 9 a.m.–4 p.m., Sunday, 10 a.m.– 5 p.m.; $6 adults, $3 children, $4 seniors (60+)

FACILITIES: Restrooms, water fountain, picnic tables, benches

WHEELCHAIR TRAVERSABLE: No

SPECIAL COMMENTS: Admission is free on the third Thursday of the month.

DRIVING DISTANCE FROM MAJOR INTERSECTION: 3 miles from I-45 South and Loop 12

GPS TRAILHEAD COORDINATES

Latitude: N 32° 42' 13"

Longitude: W 96° 42' 18"

IN BRIEF

The Audubon Center will do its best to keep you entertained with hands-on indoor exhibits and displays. When you finally venture outside, you'll find well-maintained trails that explore the diversity of the Great Trinity Forest. Bird-watching areas, picnic tables, and signage combine for a fun, family-friendly afternoon on the trail.

DESCRIPTION

Opened in October 2008, the Trinity River Audubon Center is an exciting collaboration between the City of Dallas and the National Audubon Society to make the surrounding area—the Great Trinity Forest—accessible to hikers, birders, and other outdoors enthusiasts. The forest is one of Dallas's special natural features: a forested urban park, one of the largest such parks in the country. Situated primarily south of Dallas, the preserve consists of 6,000 acres of bottomland forest and is part of the Trinity River Project, an effort to develop transportation and flood protection, foster nature preservation, and provide recreation for area residents.

The Trinity River Audubon Center was constructed to showcase the Great Trinity Forest and its resources, and it does so spectacularly. Designed with the nature lover in mind, the center contains displays and interactive

---

Directions ————————————————————➤

The trail is at the Trinity River Audubon Center, 6500 Great Trinity Forest Way, in Dallas. To get there from downtown Dallas, take I-45 South and exit at Loop 12 East/ East Ledbetter Drive. Go about 2 miles to reach the entrance, on the right.

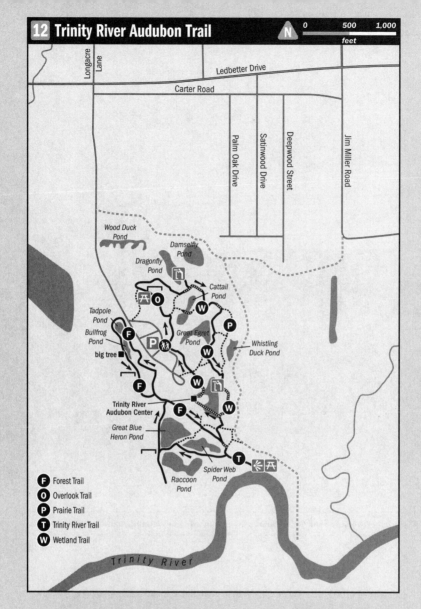

N

| 0 | 500 | 1,000 |

feet

Longacre Lane

Ledbetter Drive

Carter Road

Palm Oak Drive

Satinwood Drive

Deepwood Street

Jim Miller Road

Wood Duck Pond

Damselfly Pond

Dragonfly Pond

Cattail Pond

O

W

P

Tadpole Pond

F

Bullfrog Pond

big tree ■

P

Great Egret Pond

W

Whistling Duck Pond

F

W

W

Trinity River Audubon Center

F

Great Blue Heron Pond

T

Spider Web Pond

Raccoon Pond

F Forest Trail
O Overlook Trail
P Prairie Trail
T Trinity River Trail
W Wetland Trail

Trinity River

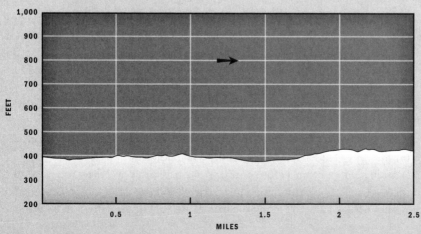

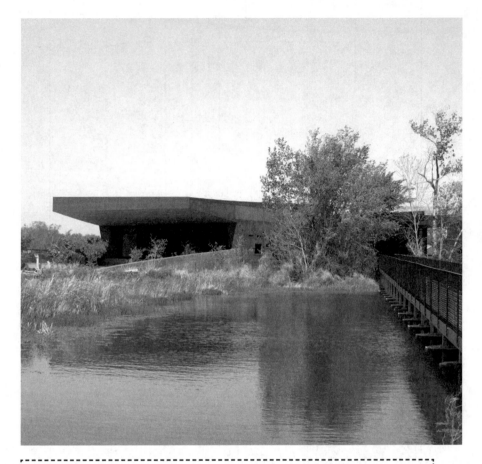

The Trinity River Audubon Center guards the entrance to the Wetland, Prairie, and Forest trails.

exhibits, as well as a network of well-laid-out trails that entice you to explore the forest beyond.

As you walk into the center's beautifully designed building, you'll be hard-pressed to imagine that not so long ago the area was uninviting. Today, the landscape of rolling hills and dense green forest betrays no hint of its rocky past, but rather welcomes you to hike through native Texan wetlands, grasslands, and bottomland hardwoods.

The starting point for the trails is the center itself: a beautiful LEED-certified facility uniquely designed to resemble a bird in flight. A small admission fee entitles you to explore the center and access the trails. If you're with a group, consider going on the third Thursday of the month, when admission is free.

Set aside plenty of time before or after your hike to peruse the various exhibits and displays. The largest exhibit is an interactive flood simulator, demonstrating the flooding that occurs naturally along the Trinity River. With the press of a button, a narrator starts talking as water seeps onto the large display, showing what happens during a 100-year flood, a 500-year flood, and a catastrophic flood. Nearby, an equally compelling exhibit targeted to kids shows how to shape and route a river.

Plenty of other diversions will catch your interest—informational plaques on the birds and animals of the forest, wetlands, tall-grass and blackland prairies, and floodplains abound. Kids and parents alike will be enthralled by displays of specimens such as skulls, spiders, and snakeskins. Small aquariums built into the walls housing catfish and turtles will keep you mesmerized; exhibits emitting the sounds of river animals such as frogs, crickets, and birds will keep you entertained.

When you paid your admission fee, the attendant provided you with a small orientation map, which directs you to pick up the trails behind the main building. For this hike, I've combined several trails into one trek that takes you through different landscapes.

From the back of the center, head down the raised walkway to the first junction. Signs point out the Wetland Trail to your left and the Forest Trail to your right. Turn right, following the Forest Trail until you reach the intersection marked TRINITY RIVER VISTA. Turn left, winding past wildflowers, over a small bridge, into the shelter of the forest, and out toward picnic tables and a view of the Trinity River as it bends around a curve. I've yet to see a prettier river vista in the Metroplex.

When you're done admiring the view, retrace your steps to the Trinity River Vista junction and bear left back onto the Forest Trail. Pass two small junctions; continue straight on the main trail until you reach an intersection at 0.85 mile into the hike. From here, make a right up the steps built into the trail and enter the cool shade of the woods. Tall trees surround you, and a pleasant feeling of solitude envelops you as you hike through the quiet forest. The trail makes a short loop before reaching a huge tree surrounded by benches where programs and presentations are held. Continue past the tree and bear right when you rejoin the main trail.

Quickly loop out of the shade and back into the sun, bearing right at the next junction to head down around a pond and over to a well-positioned bench at about 1.4 miles. When you're ready to continue, turn right onto the trail heading between the ponds. Butterflies will flutter out of your way and birds will chirp from above as this trail merges onto the Trinity River Trail. The path here should look familiar—just follow it until you've returned to the Wetland–Forest Trail junction, where your hike began.

From here, explore the northern trails by following the WETLAND TRAIL sign. This section of trail is a boardwalk constructed above the swampy wetlands. A few hundred feet from the junction, arrive at a lookout platform where you can survey the wetland habitat of creatures you may have seen in the visitor center, such as frogs, turtles, and fish. From the lookout, continue following the Wetland Trail past a pond and to a junction about 1.9 miles into the hike. Bear left, following signs pointing the way to the Overlook Trail.

It's hard to imagine now, but the land you're trekking on was formerly known as the Deepwood Landfill—an illegal dumping ground for more than 1.5 million tons of construction debris. The land was reclaimed and the debris molded and shaped to provide an area upon which native flora fauna could grow and thrive.

About 500 feet farther, come to another junction; turn right, following the WETLAND TRAIL sign. A couple hundred feet ahead, reach a well-designed bird blind where you can survey the native birds that populate the surrounding ponds.

From the bird blind, continue to the next trail junction and turn right, following the OVERLOOK TRAIL signs. The trail climbs slightly, looping around until you reach the top of a small hill where, in addition to a cool breeze and commanding view, you'll find picnic tables, benches, and a kiosk. This is an excellent spot to break for lunch.

Return to the trailhead by bearing right at the junction, past the kiosk, and retracing you steps until you reach the center.

NEARBY ACTIVITIES

Fair Park is only 8 miles away. When you're done with your hike, visit one of its museums or gardens, including the African American Museum, the Museum of the American Railroad, the Texas Discovery Gardens, and the Women's Museum. For more information, call (214) 426-3400 or visit **fairpark.org**. To get to Fair Park from the Trinity River Audubon Center, head northeast on Loop 12 East/East Ledbetter Drive. Take I-45 North to Dallas/Sherman. Take Exit 284A to merge onto I-30 East, then take Exit 47 (Second Avenue/Fair Park) and follow the signs.

TURTLE CREEK LEISURE TRAIL 13

IN BRIEF

This scenic trail winds alongside Turtle Creek and Turtle Creek Boulevard, heading northeast through a greenbelt that passes through a couple of parks. In several sections, the trail runs atop wooden bridges. Hike this trail in the fall for brilliant displays of fall foliage.

DESCRIPTION

Named after the renowned French botanist Julien Reverchon, Reverchon Park in Dallas serves as the trailhead for this hike. The park was modeled after Central Park in New York City. In its 46 acres of open space, you'll find tennis and basketball courts, a recreation facility, and picturesque narrow staircases that wind up small landscaped hills to stone-bench seating areas. You'll also find access to the nearby Katy Trail (see page 47). On the trail, traffic is light; most of the people there are joggers who live in the nearby condos and couples strolling along the creek. The path—which in some sections is built onto wooden trestle bridges suspended above the water—is slightly below street level and hidden from view in a few sections. As you would in any large city park, hike this trail with a pal.

The trailhead is to the south of the recreation center, adjacent to a smaller parking lot. Cross the short bridge and turn left. The paved path leads onto a long wooden bridge with

KEY AT-A-GLANCE INFORMATION

LENGTH: 3 miles

CONFIGURATION: Out-and-back

DIFFICULTY: Easy

SCENERY: Fall foliage, creek, turtles

EXPOSURE: Partially sunny

TRAIL TRAFFIC: Light

TRAIL SURFACE: Paved path

HIKING TIME: 1.5 hours

ACCESS: Free; daily

FACILITIES: Restrooms, water fountains

WHEELCHAIR TRAVERSABLE: No

SPECIAL COMMENTS: Avoid this trail after heavy rains—the creek can be flooded, resulting in trail closures. Some sections of trail are secluded; hike with a pal.

DRIVING DISTANCE FROM MAJOR INTERSECTION: 1 mile from Oak Lawn Avenue and Stemmons Freeway

Directions

Take I-35 to Oak Lawn Avenue and turn right. Turn right onto Maple Avenue. Reverchon Park is 0.25 mile down on the right. Park in the lot in front of the main entrance and recreation center.

GPS TRAILHEAD COORDINATES

Latitude: N 32° 48' 1"

Longitude: W 96° 48' 41"

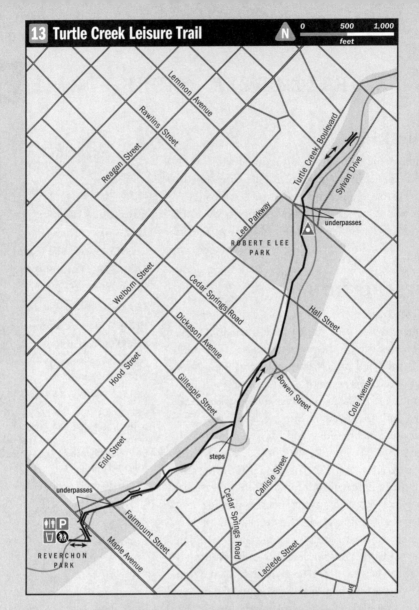

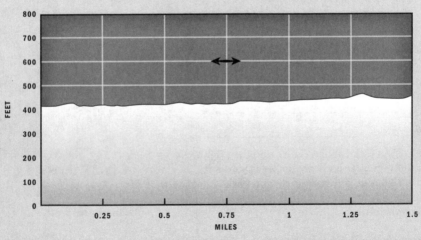

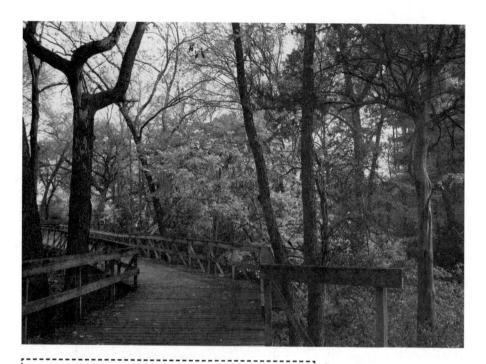

One of the many wooden walkways suspended above the creek

wooden trestles suspended a few feet above Turtle Creek, then rounds a curve and goes under an overpass. The trail continues northeast at creek level and crosses another bridge at 0.15 mile, staying on the western bank of the creek.

A few hundred feet farther, bear right to reach another underpass at 0.23 mile. The trail rises to street level, then winds atop another long trestle bridge. On your left is Turtle Creek Boulevard, lined with condos and apartments. On your right the creek, actually a tributary of the Trinity River, is still within view.

At 0.38 mile, cross Park Bridge Court and follow the sidewalk past a wide grassy field, on the far side of which is the creek. The sidewalk curls to the right, approaching the creek, then goes over another wooden bridge. The trail then splits to the right and left. To the right, the trail winds downhill to go below street level and under an overpass. The city has closed off this section, so you stay to the left and cross Cedar Springs Road at the crosswalk. Across the street, head about 400 feet to the right to find an entrance through the railing with steps leading back below street level to the creek, where you can pick the trail up again. A wooden walkway suspended above the water continues for several hundred feet alongside the creek. To your right, the far side of the creek's shores is densely covered with trees. As you walk along, it quickly becomes apparent why the creek was named after turtles: you can often spot their heads or shells popping out of the clear water as they laze about. In the afternoon, shade from the wall to your left shields you from the blazing sun on a hot day.

The trail ascends to street level at 0.88 mile and continues alongside the boulevard. Cross North Hall Street and enter a park. A plaque posted alongside the trail confirms that you're still on Turtle Creek Leisure Trail. To your right, a dam built into the creek helps pool its waters. The creek is wide enough here that it almost forms a pond—a perfect backdrop for the beautifully manicured park grounds. The surroundings are so attractive and distracting that you'll hardly notice the slow-moving cars on the boulevard to your left. A circular fountain has been placed in the creek's center, and the gentle sound of falling water drowns out the sounds of city life. Dozens of ducks are often seen circling the waters or nestled along the green bank.

On the far side of the creek, the bank slopes gently to the water's edge. Narrow stairs at intervals along the banks provide nature lovers easy access to the water. Stone benches at the water's edge complete the tranquil scene. In the fall, the leaves of the trees along both sides of the creek turn brilliant shades of yellow, red, orange, and gold. As you walk along, you'll feel as though you've entered a painting, and you may find it impossible not to let the beauty of your surroundings lift your spirits.

Before long, you'll leave the park, still continuing along the creek. Go through two underpasses, then pass through William B. Dean Park. A bridge at the far end of the park is a congregating place for ducks and a good place to stop and check the creek for turtles before turning around and retracing your steps to the trailhead.

NEARBY ACTIVITIES

Check out Uptown's West Village, known for its boutiques, restaurants, and nightlife. To get there, go 0.8 mile southeast down Maple Avenue and turn left onto McKinney Avenue.

WHITE ROCK LAKE TRAIL

IN BRIEF

Popular with joggers, bikers, walkers, and hikers, this lengthy trail runs along White Rock Lake. The hike starts just past the waterfall-like spillway and hugs the shoreline, offering constant views of the water as it winds past the Dallas Arboretum.

DESCRIPTION

White Rock Lake is one of the most well-known outdoor spots among Dallasites. Its 9-mile trail circumnavigates the lake and attracts joggers, walkers, hikers, bikers, and skaters. One of the lake's draws is that it's only 6 miles northeast of Dallas, in a populated area just 4 miles east of Highland Park.

Completed in 1911, the lake was originally intended as a primary reservoir for the city of Dallas. The city quickly outgrew the lake, though, and eventually the larger Lake Dallas was created to supply water. In its early days, the lake was also a popular local swimming hole; I even ran into an older gentleman by the trailhead who reminisced about the days he spent as a child with his father playing in the waters. Swimming there was banned in the early 1950s and hasn't been permitted since. The lake is also widely known for the annual White Rock Marathon, which started in 1971. The route runs a loop from downtown to the lake and back.

KEY AT-A-GLANCE INFORMATION

LENGTH: 4.66 miles

CONFIGURATION: Out-and-back

DIFFICULTY: Easy

SCENERY: Lake, spillway

EXPOSURE: Sunny

TRAIL TRAFFIC: Heavy

TRAIL SURFACE: Paved

HIKING TIME: 1.75 hours

ACCESS: Daily; free

FACILITIES: Water fountains, benches

WHEELCHAIR TRAVERSABLE: Yes

SPECIAL COMMENTS: Bring a windbreaker if it's windy out—the wind can really pick up over the water.

SUPPLEMENTAL MAPS: whiterock lake.org/pdf/wrlmap_.pdf

DRIVING DISTANCE FROM MAJOR INTERSECTION: 4.5 miles from I-30 and US 75

Directions ──────────→

Follow I-30 East toward I-45 South, and take Exit 488 (Barry Avenue) onto E. R. L. Thornton Freeway toward East Grand Avenue. Turn left onto East Grand and drive 2 miles. East Grand will become Garland Road. Turn left onto Winsted Drive and you'll see a sign for White Rock Park. Park in the lot on the right.

GPS TRAILHEAD COORDINATES

Latitude: N 32° 48' 51"

Longitude: W 96° 43' 38"

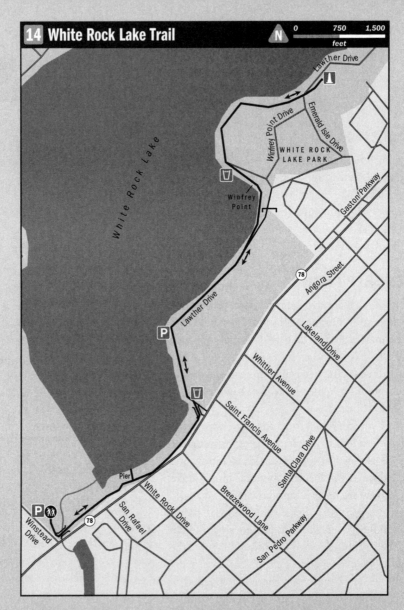

0 · 750 · 1,500
feet

N

White Rock Lake

Lawther Drive

Winfrey Point Drive

Emerald Isle Drive

WHITE ROCK
LAKE PARK

Gaston Parkway

Winfrey
Point

Lawther Drive

78

Angora Street

Lakeland Drive

Whittier Avenue

Saint Francis Avenue

Santa Clara Drive

P

Pier

White Rock Drive

Breezewood Lane

San Pedro Parkway

P

Winstead
Drive

78

San Rafael
Drive

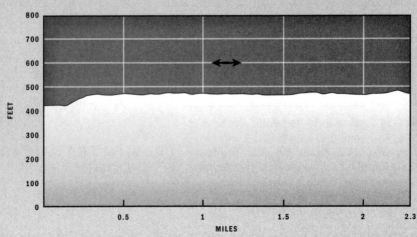

FEET

800
700
600
500
400
300
200
100
0

0.5 · 1 · 1.5 · 2 · 2.3

MILES

In years past, the lake's urban location gave it a reputation for being unsafe. Its image has been rehabilitated, however, thanks in large part to a volunteer group known as For the Love of the Lake (FTLOTL), which has worked hard to clean and renovate the lake. Because of FTLOTL's efforts, it is very well kept, feels safe, and is surprisingly scenic. Also contributing to the feeling of safety is the fact that this section of the trail is not isolated and well exposed. During the day, you'll find it very busy—there are folks with baby strollers, dogs, and kids. Remember, though, that this is an urban trail, and heed the signs by the parking lot advising you to keep your valuables in your trunk. It's also a good idea for women and kids to bring a buddy along.

The land surrounding the lake is part of White Rock Park, which has several entrances. This hike starts from the southern end of the lake, at an entrance near the spillway. The small parking lot stays fairly full on weekends, although you can almost always manage to find at least one spot to squeeze your car into. The path comes into view to the left, running just in front of the spillway. Get on the trail and turn right, heading away from the parking lot toward Garland Road. The trail immediately curves left, crosses a concrete bridge that bounces as folks jog by, and takes you directly alongside the massive, tiered spillway. Water cascades down its huge steps, which creates a thunderous noise. Ducks can often be spotted paddling on the top level, ignoring the nearby waterfall.

Just across the bridge, the trail, which once wound very close to the edge of the lake, has been rerouted along Garland Road. This is the loudest and least pleasant section of the trail, because for a few hundred feet you'll find yourself essentially on the sidewalk of a busy road. The trail soon curves downhill, away from the road and back toward and alongside the shoreline to your left. You'll have a good view of the path curving out before you, following the shoreline until it disappears around a bend in the shore. Expect the path to be busy. Bikers and joggers are constantly coming and going, and if you stop for a minute or two, expect to be overtaken by other hikers or dog walkers.

At 0.4 mile, pass a pier; walk out to the water and you might see ducks just around the shore. Thanks in part to the Adopt-a-Shoreline program, you'll find the shore well kept. Through this program, various groups agree to be caretakers of certain sections of the trail. You'll see wooden signs along the shore as you hike, identifying the group—such as Boy Scout troops and REI—whose section you're in. Trash receptacles along the trail also help keep the area clean.

As you continue, you'll catch sight of a few very nice residences bordering Garland Road on your right before the trail curves northwest away from the street and over a bridge at 0.78 mile. Take a moment to glance over your shoulder for a nice view of the Dallas skyline. A couple hundred feet farther, reach a water fountain where you can refresh yourself and read a nearby historical marker.

Continue down the trail, following the shoreline. To your right, a fence runs behind the Dallas Arboretum; to your left, you'll have a complete view of the

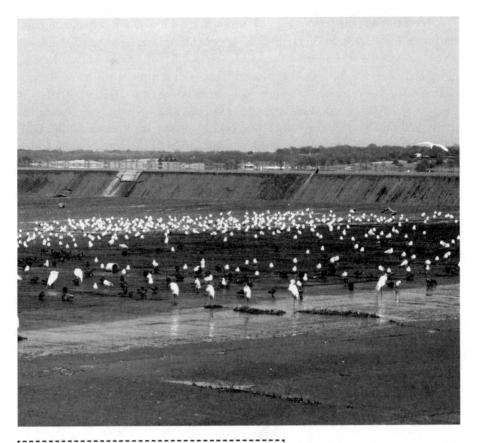

Hundreds of birds gather in the spillway alongside the trail.

lake's grassy, tree-dotted shoreline. The trail is mostly sunny and exposed, allowing great visibility wherever you are on the trail; at 1.55 miles, however, you'll reach one of the few sections with a small grouping of trees, providing some much-needed shade.

At 1.63 miles, note a parking lot to your right and kids playing on the shoreline to your left. This lake entrance is known as Winfrey Point. Joggers joining the trail here are likely to merge and pass you on their quest for fitness. The trail then turns into a wide path painted with double lanes on each side. Continuing north, you'll soon round another curve and see a densely wooded section ahead. A playground on your right marks yet another entrance. To your left, a shallow inlet attracts wading and shorebirds. A short dock extends into the waters, offering a good spot from which to view the birdlife. Here you'll also find a statue honoring the Civilian Conservation Corps, which worked at White Rock Lake from 1935 to 1942. Take a few minutes to rest before turning and retracing your steps to the trailhead. If you want to extend the hike, the trail continues another 6.5 miles, looping the rest of the way around the lake before returning you to the trailhead.

NEARBY ACTIVITIES

Head into downtown Dallas and explore the Arts District. The Dallas Museum of Art is renowned for its collection of European paintings. Visit **dallasmuseumofart .org** for lists of the current exhibitions. Other nearby museums include the Nasher Sculpture Center, which houses pieces by Matisse, de Kooning, Picasso, and Rodin, and the Crow Collection of Asian Art. From White Rock, take I-30 West about 2 miles, then exit onto I-45 South/US 75 North to reach Elm Street. Turn right on North Central Expressway, then left onto North Pearl Street. Drive about 0.5 mile. Turn left onto Flora Street, then left again onto North Harwood Street; the Dallas Museum of Art is at 1717 N. Harwood.

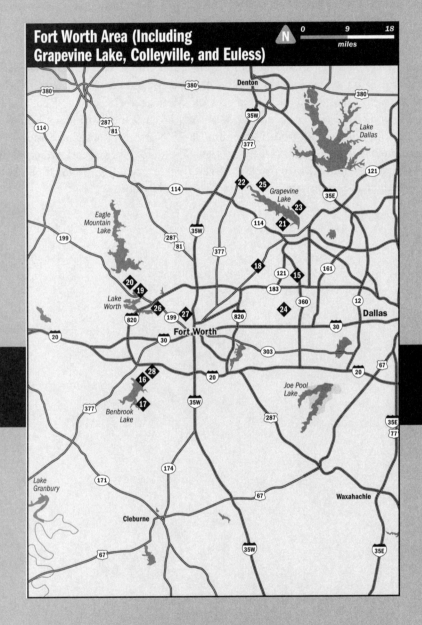

Fort Worth Area (Including Grapevine Lake, Colleyville, and Euless)

N 0 9 18
miles

Denton

380 380 380

114 287 81

35W

377

114 22 25 Grapevine Lake 121 Lake Dallas

Eagle Mountain Lake

199 114 35W 377 114 23 35E

287 81 21

Lake Worth 20 19 26 199 27 18 121 15 161 12

820 820 183 360 24 Dallas

20 30 Fort Worth 30

303

28 20 67

16 20 Joe Pool Lake 35E 77

377 17 Benbrook Lake 35W 287

174

Lake Granbury 171 67 Waxahachie

Cleburne 35W 35E

67

15 Bear Creek–Bob Eden Trail 80

16 Benbrook Dam Trail 84

17 Benbrook Lake Trail 88

18 Colleyville Nature Trail 92

19 Fort Worth Nature Center:
    Canyon Ridge Trail 96

20 Fort Worth Nature Center: Prairie Trail ... 100

21 Horseshoe Trail 104

22 Knob Hill Trail 108

23 Northshore Trail 112

24 River Legacy Trail 116

25 Rocky Point Trail 120

26 Sansom Park Trail 124

27 Trinity River Trail (Northside) 128

28 Trinity River Trail (Oakmont Park) 132

FORT WORTH AREA
(INCLUDING GRAPEVINE LAKE, COLLEYVILLE, AND EULESS)

15 BEAR CREEK-BOB EDEN TRAIL

KEY AT-A-GLANCE INFORMATION

LENGTH: 5.88 miles

CONFIGURATION: Out-and-back

DIFFICULTY: Easy

SCENERY: Creek, pond; woodland mixture of elms, oaks, and pecans; greenbelt

EXPOSURE: Partially sunny

TRAIL TRAFFIC: Heavy

TRAIL SURFACE: Paved

HIKING TIME: 2 hours

ACCESS: Free; open daily, 7 a.m.–11 p.m.

FACILITIES: Restrooms, water fountains, picnic tables

WHEELCHAIR TRAVERSABLE: Yes

SPECIAL COMMENTS: For a shorter hike, turn around at McCormick Park.

DRIVING DISTANCE FROM MAJOR INTERSECTION: 3.8 miles from TX 360 and TX 183

GPS TRAILHEAD COORDINATES

Latitude: N 32° 51' 42"
Longitude: W 97° 4' 1"

IN BRIEF

Leave your plant-identification guidebook at home on this scenic trail along Bear Creek, which winds through an undeveloped corridor linking three city parks. Plant markers, a bird-watching area, and well-maintained park areas make this an enjoyable year-round hike.

DESCRIPTION

As far as greenbelts go, this linear trail connecting Bear Creek Park with Bob Eden Park is one of the prettier ones in the Metroplex. It's a wild, green oasis, so inventively designed that you'll hardly notice the urban setting it slices through. The community surrounding the trailhead consists mostly of quiet, well-kept apartment complexes inhabited by young professionals. You're likely to encounter many of these folks on the trail, walking their dogs or jogging along with iPod buds in their ears. Midway along the trail, a small pond attracts parents looking to laze away the afternoon fishing with their kids.

Among the things I love most about this trail are the dozens of markers labeling the various plants, trees, and shrubs along its route. If you're like me, you enjoy examining the leaves, bark, and fruit of trees you're unfamiliar with; this trail really delivers on helping you identify them. If you've paid attention, after a few visits here you'll be able to pick out

----

Directions ———————————→

Take TX 183 (Airport Freeway) into Euless and turn north onto TX 360. Go about 0.7 mile, then turn left onto Harwood Road. Drive about 0.8 mile and take first right onto Bear Creek Parkway. Park in the lot on your right, in Bear Creek Park.

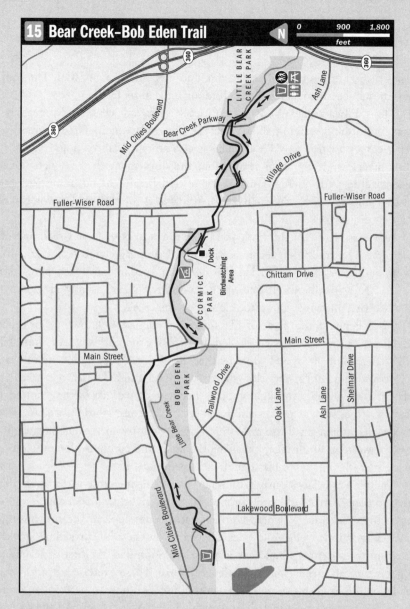

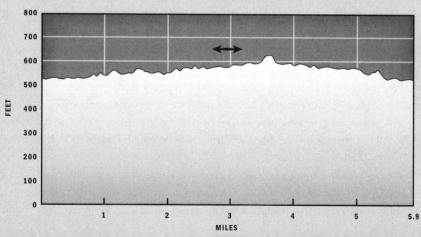

species such as chittamwood, cedar elm, and box elder on any trail. The trail has even fittingly been labeled a Texas Outdoor Education Trail.

The trailhead is in 40-acre Bear Creek Park, adjacent to the parking lot. Wear comfortable walking shoes, because the trail, which starts as fine gravel, later becomes a hard, paved path. This is also a great trail for dogs. Not only do fellow hikers welcome them readily, but the dogs themselves seem to love the shade-covered path—a few I passed even held firmly to souvenir sticks they'd picked up along the way. Waste bags are available at the trailhead so you can clean up after your pet.

As you start down the trail, you'll see the waters of Bear Creek just off to your right. The trail is shaded by a mixture of slippery elm, ash, Indian currant, eastern red cedar, box elder, black walnut, and cedar elm—each painstakingly marked. Occasionally you'll find BEAR CROSSING signs, usually in spots where the trees part, allowing you to look out over the creek.

Pass a bench in the shade of a Shumard red oak (a tree known for its beautiful fall foliage) before the trail curves left and crosses the parkway. For those hiking with younger kids, it's good to know that this is not a busy street: motorists pass only occasionally, and at very slow speeds. The road also has a clearly marked cross-walk. The trail winds through a nicely manicured, parklike setting dotted with deciduous trees such as pecans and hackberries. Benches, a little plaza, and shaded picnic tables atop a small rise make this a pretty spot for picnickers. Bear right and cross the wooden footbridge, bypassing the park, and continue along the creek. In the summer, the unmistakable song of cicadas fills the air.

The path continues purposefully northwest, staying close to the creek. Every now and then, narrow dirt trails branch off to the right, leading a couple of dozen feet to the creek's edge, where you can get a better look at the brownish-green water. A mixture of elms and pecans close in on the trail, providing shade and obscuring the apartment buildings to your left. Soon pass the first of several sign-posts for the Advanced Timber Challenge Course. These exercise stations, a few of which you'll find in this section, instruct trail users on how to perform an exercise, such as the alternate-toe touch or horizontal ladder. As you continue, the vegetation becomes thicker and wilder, and you'll soon find yourself walking through a lush green understory that thrives in the shade of the surrounding tall trees.

At 1.2 miles, come to a junction and bear left. You'll skirt the edges of a small sports field, then reach another junction a few hundred feet down, where you'll again bear left. Now hike under a low overpass. When you emerge into the sun on the other side, you'll find the path has changed, having become more like a green-belt, with grassy, neatly maintained slopes bordering the sunny paved path. In the spring, small clusters of bluebonnets and Indian paintbrush bloom in rich displays of color just off the trail.

The trail winds through a field dotted with trees, then reaches a junction where a bridge heads off to your left. The path continues straight; for a pleasant detour, however, cross the bridge. On the other side, you'll find a little pond

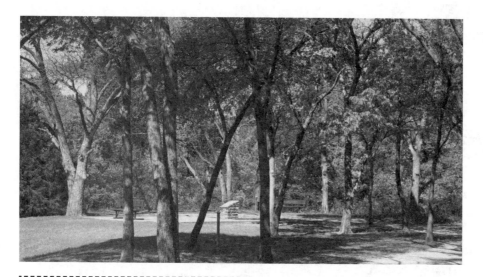

Markers identify trees and plants along the trail.

that's typically full of kids and parents fishing from a short dock. Just beyond the dock, to the right, is a designated bird-watching area, with a small wooden arbor amid a thick canopy of foliage adjacent to the creek. From here, retrace your steps across the bridge to the detour turnoff and continue on the trail, heading west. At the next turnoff, bear left onto Species Trail—a pretty section of shady gravel trail that traverses a wooded mixture of seep-willow, cedar elm, and bur oak. Sadly, severe erosion is causing this section of the creek's banks to deteriorate.

Soon reach a parking lot; at this point, you've entered McCormick Park, which was named after the McCormick family who, in the early 1900s, used the area as a 130-acre farm. From here, the trail reenters a manicured parklike setting, passing a playground on the left and a pretty gazebo on the right. Just beyond the park, the trail returns to greenbelt; you'll see little besides cactus and wildflowers along this long, sunny stretch of trail. A striped yellow line divides the trail in half here, hinting that bikers use this flat section; on my hike I saw only a few dog walkers. Briefly hike parallel to Mid Cities Boulevard before turning back south, crossing the creek, and reaching a sports field at Bob Eden Park. A few picnic tables provide a nice spot for lunching before you retrace your steps to the trailhead.

NEARBY ACTIVITIES

Baseball fans will enjoy a visit to Ameriquest Field in Arlington, home of the Texas Rangers. Check **texas.rangers.mlb.com** for ticket information during baseball season. Year-round you can visit the Legends of the Game Museum, also at the stadium; it has a huge collection from the National Baseball Hall of Fame. The ballpark is only about 9 miles away. To get there, go 6 miles south on TX 360 and take the Lamar Boulevard exit. Bear right onto Lamar and take a left onto Ballpark Way.

16 BENBROOK DAM TRAIL

KEY AT-A-GLANCE INFORMATION

LENGTH: 3.1 miles

CONFIGURATION: Out-and-back

DIFFICULTY: Easy

SCENERY: Lake

EXPOSURE: Sunny

TRAIL TRAFFIC: Light

TRAIL SURFACE: Paved/grassy

HIKING TIME: 1.5 hours

ACCESS: Daily; free

FACILITIES: Restrooms, picnic tables

WHEELCHAIR TRAVERSABLE: No

SPECIAL COMMENTS: After the hike, walk or drive south down the park road to the boat ramp for an up-close view of the water.

DRIVING DISTANCE FROM MAJOR INTERSECTION: 5.4 miles from I-820 and I-20

GPS TRAILHEAD COORDINATES

Latitude: N 32° 39' 1"

Longitude: W 97° 26' 45"

IN BRIEF

This trail runs along a grassy strip atop the Benbrook Dam and ends at the dam's spillway. Appealing for its unobstructed views of the lake and surrounding area, the flat, straight path is ideal for walkers and joggers.

DESCRIPTION

On the Clear Fork of the Trinity River just southwest of Fort Worth, Benbrook Lake offers impressive stretches of trail that extend for miles, affording hikers plenty of room to stretch their legs and roam around.

The lake, impounded in 1952, serves as a flood-control reservoir for the surrounding area. According to the Army Corps of Engineers, which operates the lake, it has served its purpose quite well, preventing flooding and destruction of populated areas during periods of severe rainfall, most notably in the early 1990s. The lake is also a popular spot for summer recreational activities and is lined with parks offering picnicking, swimming, fishing, camping, and hiking opportunities.

The trailhead is a short walk east of the roundabout, at the gated road. As you drive in, pass the gated road just to the right before you reach the parking lot. A tall locked metal gate deliberately blocks the road to car traffic;

Directions

Follow I-20 West toward Abilene and take Exit 434A toward Granbury Road/South Drive. Turn left onto Granbury Road and go about 3 miles, then turn right onto Dirks Road and travel 2 miles. Bear right onto Lakeside Drive and go 0.5 mile. The parking lot will be on the left, just past the lake office. Park near the roundabout, to the right.

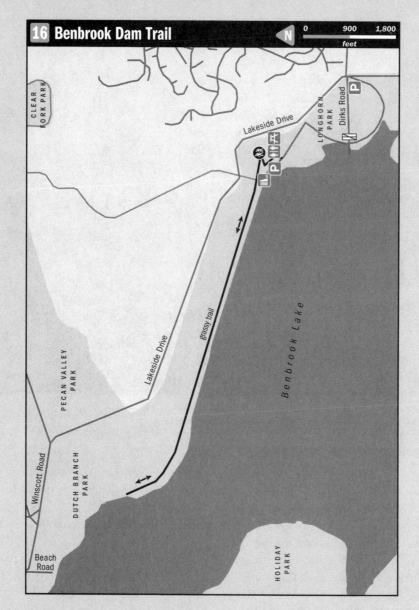

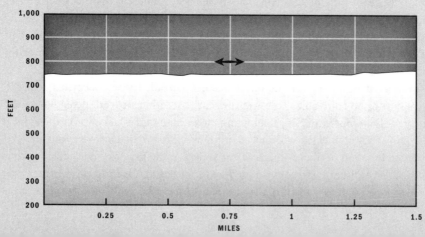

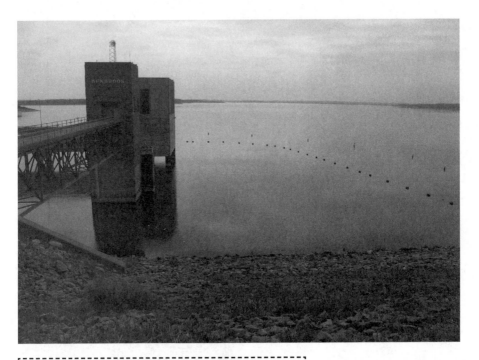

A windless day creates a mirrorlike surface on Benbrook Lake.

however, foot traffic is permitted. Although the latter was light on my visit due to overcast weather, the path is said to be especially popular with joggers. To access the area, you'll need to step over the low barrier adjacent to the gate. From here, head down the road toward the lake.

Yucca sprouts alongside the road, drinking in the sun on this exposed section of path. Continue west, following the road until you reach the lake. The trail surface changes from paved to partial grass as it keeps going west atop the crest of the dam, an earth-fill embankment that stretches 1.5 miles across the north end of the lake to a spillway at the western end. Steep, grassy slopes lead down to the lake level; you'll hike along the flat top. Be aware, however, that even though there is no fence restricting access to the dam's steep slopes, walking down or on them is strictly prohibited.

Because it was overcast the day I hiked this trail, I was concerned that the hike might not be enjoyable. To my surprise, the weather proved ideal. The cloud cover kept the temperature cool, allowing me to maintain a fast clip on the ridge's flat, even, exposed surface without even breaking a sweat. Lack of wind left the lake ripple-free and eerily still. The water reflected the gray sky perfectly, making it impossible to discern where sky ended and lake began. Overall, the weather was perfect. If you come on a sunny day, though, bring a hat and sunscreen, because there's no shade on this trail.

Regardless of the weather, your hike across the dam will afford fantastic views of the lake spreading below and to the left. To the right you'll enjoy a bird's-eye view of encroaching development to the north. You'll also be able to spot golf carts roaming the nearby Pecan Valley Municipal Golf Course, and you'll hear the rumble of cars as they barrel down Lakeside Drive.

As you hike, keep an eye out for birds flying low over the lake or standing along the shoreline. You're most likely to see waders and shorebirds such as herons, grebes, cormorants, ducks, and egrets. Bird-watchers have spotted more than 269 species in the area, so bring some binoculars.

As you approach the western side of the dam, you'll see a narrow road running down along the shoreline to your left and curling out to a small inlet. Unfortunately, the road starts on the opposite side of the lake and is inaccessible from this side of the dam.

A short walk farther and you'll have reached the spillway, where the path ends at a locked gate. Although the gate prohibits you from crossing to the other side of the lake, you'll find a nice overlook with views of the spillway. From here, just retrace your steps across the dam to the trailhead.

NEARBY ACTIVITIES

The Fort Worth Botanic Garden, at 3220 Botanic Garden Blvd., comprises 109 acres with more than 2,500 species of plant life, including a Japanese garden, rose garden, and fragrance garden. The grounds are open 8 a.m.–sunset; visit **fwbg.org** for specifics on fees and the hours of the on-site restaurant. Near the garden, Forest Park offers a few acres and the Log Cabin Village, a living-history museum featuring interpreters and demonstrators. For more information, visit **logcabin village.org**. To get to Forest Park from the trail, drive down Dirks Road and turn left onto Bryant Irvin Boulevard. After 6 miles, turn right onto Camp Bowie Boulevard. After 0.5 mile, bear right onto I-30 East; go 2 miles, then take Exit 12A onto West Rosedale Street toward University Drive. Bear right, heading south onto South University Drive; the Log Cabin Village is about 1 mile ahead on the right. To get to the garden from the intersection of I-30 and University Drive, go north on University Drive. The entrance is on the left.

17   BENBROOK LAKE TRAIL

KEY AT-A-GLANCE INFORMATION

LENGTH: 3 miles

CONFIGURATION: Out-and-back

DIFFICULTY: Easy

SCENERY: Lake views, woodlands

EXPOSURE: Partially shady–sunny

TRAIL TRAFFIC: Moderate

TRAIL SURFACE: Packed dirt

HIKING TIME: 1 hour

ACCESS: Open daily, sunrise–sunset

FACILITIES: None

WHEELCHAIR TRAVERSABLE: No

SPECIAL COMMENTS: This hike can easily be extended for many miles. Bring binoculars, sunscreen, and plenty of water, and spend the whole day exploring.

SUPPLEMENTAL MAPS: www.swf-wc.usace.army.mil/ benbrook/Information/Maps.asp

DRIVING DISTANCE FROM MAJOR INTERSECTION: 12 miles from I-20 and I-35W

GPS TRAILHEAD COORDINATES

Latitude: N 32° 36' 24"

Longitude: W 97° 27' 2"

IN BRIEF

This hike along the lake's edge yields scenic views and sections of wooded trail with plenty of opportunities to spot local wildlife. Bring your lunch to a tucked-away cove at the water's edge.

DESCRIPTION

On the Clear Fork of the Trinity River just southwest of Fort Worth, Benbrook Lake offers impressive stretches of trail that extend for miles, affording hikers plenty of room to stretch their legs and roam around.

The lake, impounded in 1952, serves as a flood-control reservoir for the surrounding area. According to the Army Corps of Engineers, which operates the lake, it has served its purpose quite well, preventing flooding and destruction of populated areas during periods of severe rainfall, most notably in the early 1990s. The lake is also a popular spot for summer recreational activities and is lined with parks offering picnicking, swimming, fishing, camping, and hiking opportunities.

Rocky Creek Park, on the eastern side of the lake, serves as the starting point for this hike. Find the trailhead just before you reach the gatehouse at the park entrance, off a small gravel parking lot to the right. You'll often

----

Directions

The trailhead is just outside Rocky Creek Park in Benbrook. From southwest Fort Worth, take I-20 West to Exit 434A onto Granbury Road. Turn right onto Sycamore School Road, which becomes Columbus Trail, then Old Granbury Road, to the park entrance. Alternatively, from FM 1902, take Old Granbury Road (CO 1902) 3 miles north to the park entrance.

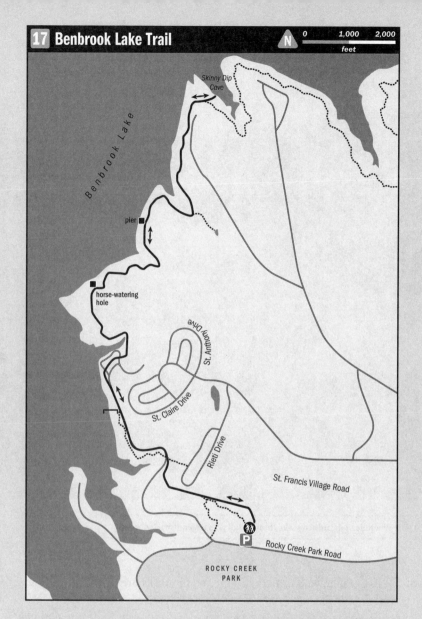

N

0   1,000   2,000
feet

Skinny Dip
Cove

Benbrook Lake

pier

horse-watering
hole

St. Anthony Drive

St. Claire Drive

Rield Drive

St. Francis Village Road

P

Rocky Creek Park Road

ROCKY CREEK
PARK

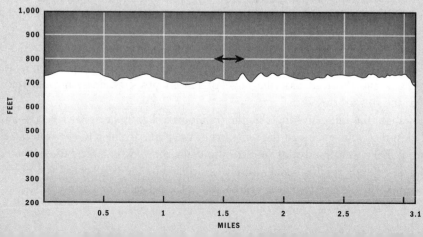

1,000
900
800
700
600
500
400
300
200

FEET

0.5   1   1.5   2   2.5   3.1

MILES

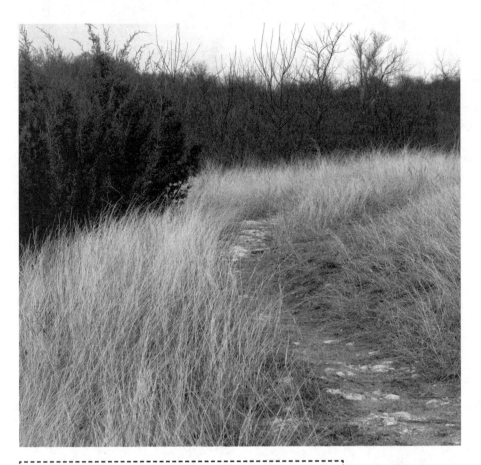

The trail winds alongside the lake through tall grasses and shaded woods.

spot a horse trailer or two parked here, as the trails are open not only to hikers but also to equestrians.

Before you start your hike, decide how long you want to be out, and plan your water and food needs accordingly. This hike covers only 3 miles of the Benbrook Lake Trail, but if you're interested in something a little lengthier, you can simply continue on at the turnaround point. The total trail length is about 10 miles.

Pick up the trail on the far side of the parking lot. At the first junction bear right, following the trail past the edge of fenced property lines, through tall grasses, and toward the lake.

At about 0.6 mile into the hike, the trail joins a slightly overgrown road—an indication that you've entered the outskirts of the park. To the left, the waters of Benbrook Lake welcome you. Don't stop to enjoy the view just yet, but continue on and at 0.9 mile reach a bench, ideally positioned by the Boy Scouts as a place to rest, take in the pretty views, search for gulls, pelicans, or cormorants, and enjoy the cooling breeze.

When you're ready, continue down the road and pick up the trail a couple hundred feet down, where it parallels the road along a grassy bank that yields pleasant lake views along the way. You're likely to pass not only the occasional hiker but the occasional equestrian—horseback riders favor the trail because of its length and location.

At 1 mile and 1.13 miles, you'll cross roads before leaving civilization and heading back into the brush, where the flatness of the trail starts to give way to a few small hills. Pass plenty of cactus (particularly beautiful in the spring), a creek crossing, and a few trail markers before you reach a horse watering hole at 1.6 miles. Views of the lake persist until the trail curves out of the sun and into a thick grove of trees. When you reach an old sign labeled PIER ONE, you're about 2.1 miles into the hike. In this area you'll stand a good chance of spotting wildlife: on a recent hike, I heard a rustling in the trees and sudden movement in the woods, which manifested as a couple of huge white-tailed deer. Upon realizing they'd been spotted, they bolted quickly out of view, only to reappear farther down the trail. Birders may be rewarded with sightings of painted buntings or, for the especially lucky, the Rio Grande turkey, which, according to the Texas Parks and Wildlife Department, can sometimes be spotted in this area very early in the morning.

At 2.5 miles, go left over a small brook, then left again at the next trail intersection. The trail winds back toward the lake and Skinny Dip Cove, an intriguing name for a pretty spot known as a horse-watering hole. Follow the trail another 150 feet toward the small cove, where the lake waters lap onto an intimate, rocky beach area. This is an ideal place to stop and enjoy lunch, after which you can examine the fossils embedded in the rocky bank or simply spend some time watching fishermen float quietly past you.

When you're ready, retrace your steps to the trailhead or return to the Skinny Dip Cove junction and hike on. The trail continues for about 7 more miles.

NEARBY ACTIVITIES

Adjacent to the trailhead, Rocky Creek Park ([817] 346-2199; **www.swf-wc.usace .army.mil/benbrook/Recreation/Parks/Corpsparks.asp**) provides primitive camping as well as opportunities for picnicking, fishing, and swimming. The admission fee is $3 per car for day-use activities and $10 per night for tent camping.

18   COLLEYVILLE NATURE TRAIL

KEY AT-A-GLANCE INFORMATION

LENGTH: 1.38 miles

CONFIGURATION: Loop

DIFFICULTY: Easy

SCENERY: Multiple ponds, ducks, geese

EXPOSURE: Sunny–shady

TRAIL TRAFFIC: Moderate

TRAIL SURFACE: Packed dirt, paved path

HIKING TIME: 35 minutes

ACCESS: Free; open daily, 30 minutes before sunrise–30 minutes after sunset

FACILITIES: Playground, picnic table

WHEELCHAIR TRAVERSABLE: No

SPECIAL COMMENTS: Identified by the Fort Worth Audubon Society as a great spot for birding; they suggest looking for warblers during the winter months.

DRIVING DISTANCE FROM MAJOR INTERSECTION: 5 miles from TX 183 and Northeast Loop 820

GPS TRAILHEAD COORDINATES

Latitude: N 32° 52' 35"

Longitude: W 97° 9' 58"

IN BRIEF

This hike starts on a paved trail through the woods, then heads off onto a dirt path that winds around some picturesque ponds, where you'll find ducks, geese, and folks fishing.

DESCRIPTION

Though small, the 46-acre Colleyville Nature Center is remarkably picturesque, boasting pretty nature trails that wind around nine different ponds. It's popular with both adults and kids, many of whom are drawn in by the charm of resident ducks and geese that move from pond to pond in a never-ending quest for food. Fishing is allowed, and on a sunny day you're likely to see parents with their kids on the banks of the ponds, casting lines and hoping for nibbles. Pets are allowed but must be leashed.

The trailhead is the paved path adjacent to the parking lot. Turn right, following the wide path toward the tree line. To your left you'll see a short trail leading to a small pond where a wooden pier overlooks the water. You can sometimes spot ducks huddled on the bank, in the shadow of the pier's wooden decking. To the left of the pond is a small pavilion with a picnic table, where I spotted a gaggle of geese congregating—likely hoping to get food left by a fellow hiker finishing his lunch.

The trail winds beneath some towering trees, then, at 0.13 mile, reaches a split where

Directions

Take TX 114 West toward Grapevine; exit onto TX 26 West/Ira E. Woods Avenue, and travel 5 miles. Turn right onto Glade Road and go 0.5 mile, then turn left onto Mill Creek Drive. Continue 0.3 mile to the Colleyville Nature Center entrance.

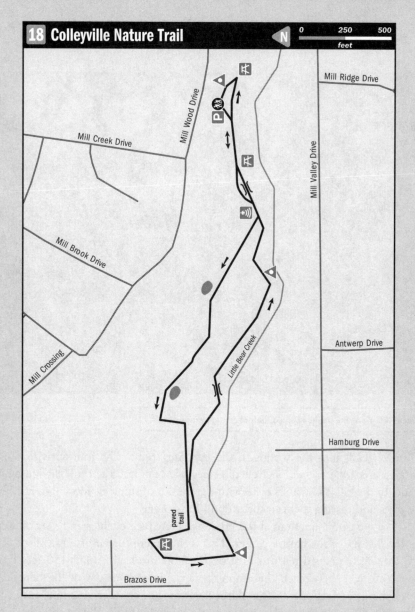

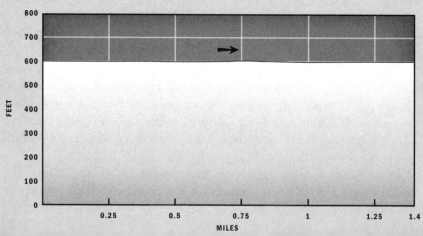

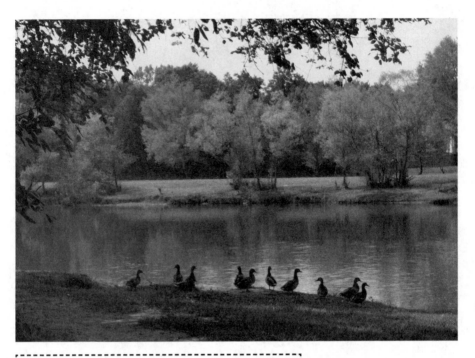

Ducks rest along the banks of one of nature center's many ponds.

a bridge heads into the woods to the left. Stay right. The trail curls through a wooded area where vines encircle tall trees that lean into the trail, shrouding it in shade. In the fall, the woods echo with the sounds of squirrels loosening nuts from the trees and tossing them to the ground for storage.

The next trail junction, at 0.2 mile, has some picnic tables and a sign describing the history of the nature center. This is the where the nature trail starts. Turn left, leaving the paved path to turn onto the nature trail. About 150 feet down, cross a bridge, then reach the amphitheater, an open area with log benches. A couple hundred feet past the amphitheater, come to another junction. Turn right, following the wide dirt trail northwest through the forest. Listen for the happy trills of warblers (small songbirds you may spot here).

A couple of interpretive signs are found along the trails. The first you'll come across is at 0.3 mile, at a turnoff to the right; it discusses the inhabitants of the surrounding forest. Continue straight west, bypassing the junction. The trail leaves the shelter of the trees and emerges onto a sunny, grassy lawn that abuts a small pond. Yellow wildflowers, berry-bearing bushes, and small bird boxes make for a charming scene. At 0.4 mile, another interpretive sign describes aerial residents you may spot here, including great blue herons and the smaller green herons, kingfishers, and flycatchers.

At 0.53 mile, reach another pond; two more are within sight to the west. The trail curves along the pond's edge and, at 0.65 mile, connects with a paved path that runs along a narrow bank between the ponds—turn left at this junction. You can sometimes catch sight of ducks waddling happily in straight lines out of one pond and into another. Keep an eye out for turtles, whose heads you'll catch popping in and out of the water if you look carefully, and small frogs, which quickly hop off the trail as you pass by.

A few hundred feet farther, the paved path ends, becoming gravel; take a right at the trail split. You'll see a pond to the right for a few more minutes before you're back in the shade of the forest. This section is fairly close to the nature center's boundaries. Though you'll briefly glimpse some houses to the right, the trail veers away from them and they're quickly hidden from view.

Continue on the gravel trail, bypassing any smaller turnoffs you see. At 0.85 mile, reach an overlook with a view of a small, babbling creek; shortly thereafter, bear right, off the gravel trail and back onto the paved path.

You'll soon find yourself back in the familiar territory near the ponds. Bear right to rejoin the dirt trail along the lake, then make another right to reenter the forest. Next, take the right-hand trail as it curves south around a large pit of dirt mounds.

The distinctive cacophony of cicadas drowns out the gurgling of the creek to your right as you continue through the forest. At 1 mile, cross a bridge. Continue another 0.1 mile to the next junction, where you'll turn right. You'll soon reach a sign, mounted on a stone pillar overlooking the water, that identifies the stream as Little Bear Creek. Watch for turtles lazing on its banks and small birds darting through the trees along its shore. Head right at the next split, at 1.2 miles. Pass some cedar trees to find yourself back at the amphitheater. From here, retrace your steps to the trailhead.

NEARBY ACTIVITIES

The popular North East Mall, with department stores such as Macy's, Nordstrom, and Sears and dozens of smaller specialty shops, is only 5 miles southwest of the Colleyville Nature Center. There is a wide selection of restaurants in and around the mall. To get there, head south on Colleyville Boulevard; turn left onto Precinct Line Road and go 1.5 miles, then make a right onto West Bedford and travel 0.6 mile before turning left onto Melbourne Road.

19 FORT WORTH NATURE CENTER:
Canyon Ridge Trail

KEY AT-A-GLANCE INFORMATION

LENGTH: 4.71 miles

CONFIGURATION: Loop

DIFFICULTY: Hard

SCENERY: Woodlands, canyon views, yucca

EXPOSURE: Partially shady–sunny

TRAIL TRAFFIC: Light

TRAIL SURFACE: Dirt

HIKING TIME: 2.5 hours

ACCESS: $5 adults, $2 children ages 3–12 (kids under age 3 free), $3 seniors (65+); summer: open weekdays 8 a.m.–7 p.m., weekends 7 a.m.–7p.m.; winter: open 7 days a week, 8 a.m.–5 p.m. Hardwicke Interpretive Center: open daily, 9 a.m.–4:30 p.m.

FACILITIES: Restrooms, water fountains, picnic tables

WHEELCHAIR TRAVERSABLE: No

SPECIAL COMMENTS: Bring repellent for spiders, gnats, and other flying insects. Pets are welcome but must be leashed. Because bicycles are prohibited on the trails, many cyclists take advantage of the slow and sparse traffic on the nature center's roads to ride around.

SUPPLEMENTAL MAPS: fwnc.org/docs/map/TrailMap11.pdf

DRIVING DISTANCE FROM MAJOR INTERSECTION: 3.5 miles from Jacksboro Highway and I-820

GPS TRAILHEAD COORDINATES

Latitude: N 32° 49' 28"

Longitude: W 97° 27' 35"

IN BRIEF

This rigorous trail climbs into the hills, winds through massive patches of yuccas, and provides scenic views of Lake Worth before descending back to lake level. Deer are abundant on this trail.

DESCRIPTION

One of the best spots in the Metroplex in which to spot wildlife while hiking is on a trail at the Fort Worth Nature Center and Refuge. The center's sprawling 3,600 acres compose one of the largest city-owned nature centers in the country and include miles of hiking trails covering a range of habitats, including woodlands, grasslands, and wetlands.

With such a wide range of habitats, it should come as no surprise that the area is abundantly full of wildlife, and visitors are almost guaranteed an animal sighting. If you don't spot something on the trail, you're almost certain to catch sight of something in the enclosed buffalo range, in the field housing the well-established prairie dog population, or on the boardwalk.

Although wildlife can be spotted at any time, you'll have a particularly good chance if you arrive early in the morning. Hikers have encountered everything from white-tailed deer,

----

Directions

Take Loop I-820 to Jacksboro Highway (TX 199). Go 4 miles west and exit at Confederate Park Road. Go about 0.5 mile and turn right onto Buffalo Road to reach the entrance to the Fort Worth Nature Center and Refuge. From the entrance, take a right at the first two forks to get to the trailhead. The road ends at the trailhead parking lot.

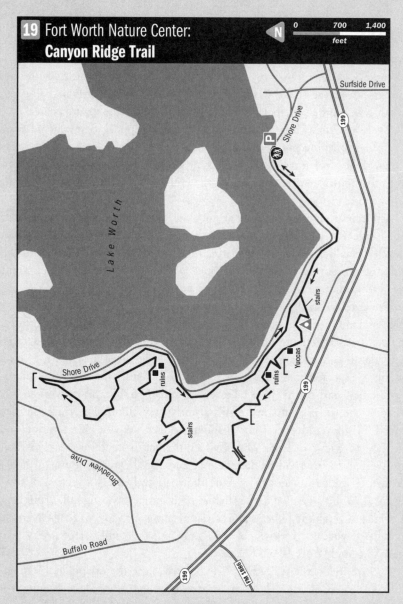

N

| 0 | 700 | 1,400 |

feet

Surfside Drive

Shore Drive

199

P

Lake Worth

stairs

Shore Drive

ruins

ruins

Yuccas

199

stairs

Broadview Drive

Buffalo Road

199

FM 1886

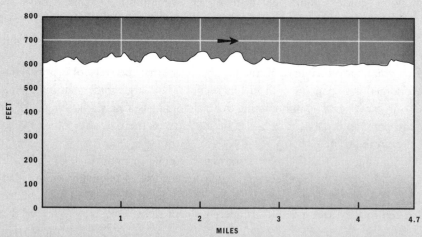

800			
700			
600			
500			
400			
300			
200			
100			
0			

FEET

| 1 | 2 | 3 | 4 | 4.7 |

MILES

wild turkeys, rabbits, possums, raccoons, and bobcats to alligators. More-obscure sightings include the "Lake Worth Monster"—a tall, hairy, half-man, half-goat creature last seen on the lake in 1969 but still celebrated by the nature center.

There's enough variety in the center's trails to appeal to anyone. Hikes climb the hillsides, offering pretty views, or meander lazily along the river bottom. Of the many hikes worth trying, I've selected two that will give you a good introduction to the nature center. (To explore the entire center, though, you'll need more than one visit.)

The center charges a small entrance fee, which goes toward improvements. In exchange for your fee, you'll receive a map of the park, which is worth a review, especially if you plan on visiting the Hardwicke Interpretive Center (in the middle of the nature center) or driving by the buffalo range. Water fountains, picnic areas, and restrooms can be found at the interpretive center.

To get to the trailhead from the entrance booth, take a right at the first intersection and another right at the next intersection. The road ends 1 mile down, at a small parking area—the trailhead is on the southwest side of the lot. The trail heads steeply uphill and is marked with the Canyon Ridge Trail insignia: a picture of a flowering yucca. Your map has a key to help you identify the other trail signs.

The first part of this hike takes you gradually uphill. Stairs worked into the hillside at the steep points make this a fairly easy climb. The trail continues up wooded hillsides and over some wooden bridges. As you gain altitude, look to your right for views of Lake Worth, which the nature center abuts. The trail runs fairly parallel to the road in this section, and you'll catch glimpses of it to your right before the path veers away from the road and enters a section of towering trees. At 0.73 mile, reach a long staircase built into a towering hill. From here, the trail winds through the hilltops after circumventing a couple of fields overtaken by hundreds of yucca. Overlooks at 0.83 mile and 0.98 mile offer pretty vistas of Lake Worth and Greer Island below.

At 1.08 miles, the trail splits. To your left, note the dilapidated remnants of an old bathroom. If you decide to explore, look out for spiders hanging from its entryway and corners. Ruins such as these, left over from the Civilian Conservation Corps' initial work in the area, can be found all along the trail.

The rocky trail climbs a little more through the wooded hillside and, at 1.4 miles, reaches a bench positioned to overlook the canyon—a nice spot to take a break. If you like to hike early in the day, be aware that the webs of orb-weaving spiders sometimes span the trail in this section. The large spiders sitting in the center of the webs can be intimidating to arachnophobes. Carry a walking stick to clear the path. Alternatively, consider hiking later in the day after other hikers have cleared the trail.

Continuing on, the trail passes through a couple of pretty fields filled with purple wildflowers—an excellent spot for sighting some of the many white-tailed deer that live here. I came upon a couple of groups of them that I was able to admire before they saw me and scampered out of sight. On my way out of the

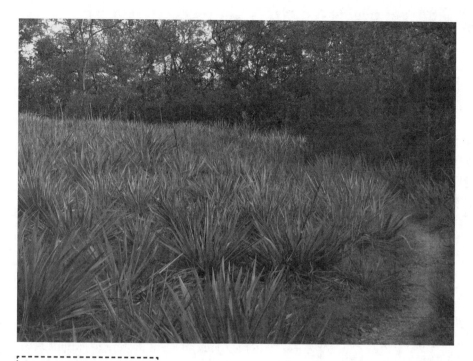

A hilltop overtaken by yucca

nature center, I spoke with a visitor who was equally impressed by the deer he had seen, having spotted both a ten-point stag and an eight-point stag bolting into the woods elsewhere in the park.

The trail continues past a couple bridges and starts a gradual descent past more old building remnants, including one at 2.61 miles that affords a beautiful view of Lake Worth. Just after the ruins, there are stairs built into the hillside. Descend these and you'll quickly spot the park road through the woods. At 3.11 miles, the trail intersects the road, then picks back up across the street, continuing as Riverbottom Trail. For this hike, turn right onto the road and follow it back to the trailhead.

NEARBY ACTIVITIES

The nature center offers monthly canoe tours down the West Fork of the Trinity River, along with a monthly canoe fest—for a small fee, you're provided with canoes, paddles, and life jackets and can float around Greer Island. Check **fwnaturecenter.org** for a calendar of events and fees.

Year-round, stop by downtown Fort Worth to visit Sundance Square, the city's entertainment and shopping district, with restored buildings housing museums, galleries, gift shops, and a diverse selection of restaurants covering everything from sandwiches to sushi to steaks.

20 FORT WORTH NATURE CENTER:
Prairie Trail

KEY AT-A-GLANCE INFORMATION

LENGTH: 1 mile

CONFIGURATION: Loop

DIFFICULTY: Easy

SCENERY: Prairies

EXPOSURE: Sunny

TRAIL TRAFFIC: Moderate

TRAIL SURFACE: Packed dirt

HIKING TIME: 25 minutes

ACCESS: $5 adults, $2 children ages 3–12 (kids under age 3 free), $3 seniors (65+); summer: open weekdays 8 a.m.–7 p.m., weekends 7 a.m.–7p.m.; winter: open 7 days a week, 8 a.m.–5 p.m. Hardwicke Interpretive Center: open daily, 9 a.m.–4:30 p.m.

FACILITIES: Restrooms, water fountains, picnic tables

WHEELCHAIR TRAVERSABLE: No

SPECIAL COMMENTS: This is a sun-drenched trail, so bring sunscreen and water. Binoculars are also useful—the prairie dogs are small and stay a few hundred feet behind a fence. Pets are allowed but must be leashed. Because bicycles are prohibited on the trails, many cyclists take advantage of the slow and sparse traffic on the nature center's roads.

SUPPLEMENTAL MAPS: fwnc.org/docs/map/TrailMap11.pdf

GPS TRAILHEAD COORDINATES

Latitude: N 32° 50' 30"

Longitude: W 97° 28' 42"

IN BRIEF

Children especially will love this flat trail that winds alongside a buffalo range and Prairie Dog Town, then through a wide prairie that offers excellent wildlife viewing.

DESCRIPTION

From the entrance, get to the trailhead by turning left at the first fork in the road. About 1 mile down, you'll see a small parking lot on the right with a huge BUFFALO RANGE sign; a smaller sign next to it announces PRAIRIE DOG TOWN. The trailhead is just to the right of the signs. A huge fenced-in prairie adjacent to the trailhead keeps the aforementioned buffaloes and prairie dogs separated from hikers so they can be viewed from a safe distance.

If you look closely at the prairie, you'll spot dozens of dirt mounds throughout it, marking prairie dog burrows. These small, squirrel-like rodents can be difficult to spot at first because their fur is so close to the color of the dirt. Look for the prairie dogs by their burrows; you'll see them bobbing up and down—and their high-pitched barks (which alert the colony to predators) are hard to miss.

You may or may not see the other prairie resident—the buffalo—in this area; the Buffalo Range is actually quite large, and the animals

Directions

Take Loop I-820 to Jacksboro Highway (TX 199). Go 4 miles west and exit at Confederate Park Road. Go about 0.5 mile and turn right onto Buffalo Road to the entrance of the Fort Worth Nature Center and Refuge. From the entrance, bear left at the fork in the road to get to the trailhead; you'll see a parking area about 1 mile ahead on the right.

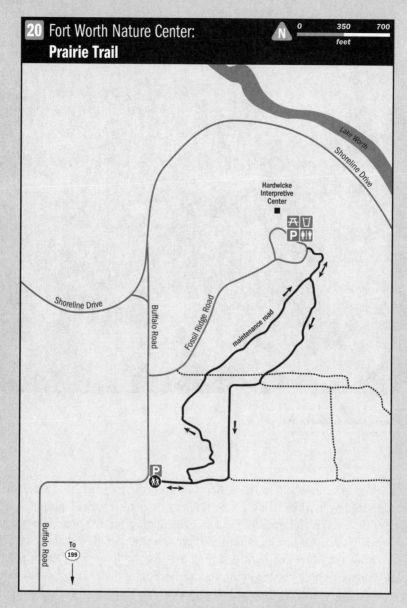

N

0	350	700

feet

Lake Worth

Shoreline Drive

Hardwicke
Interpretive
Center

Shoreline Drive

Buffalo Road

Fossil Ridge Road

maintenance road

Buffalo Road

To
199

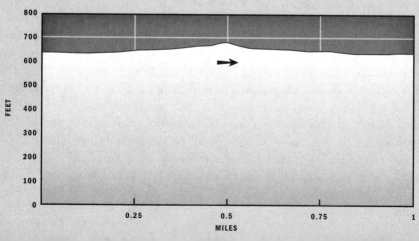

FEET			
800			
700			
600			
500			
400			
300			
200			
100			
0			

0.25	0.5	0.75	1

MILES

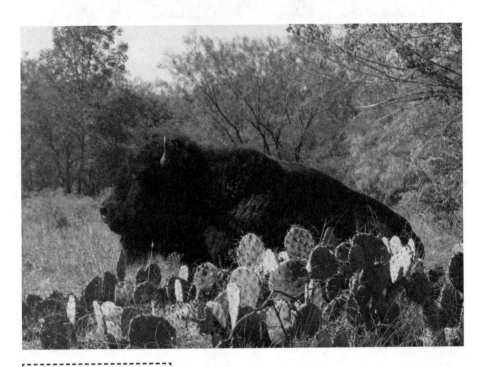

A resident of the Buffalo Range

have a lot of space in which to roam. Benches along the trail face the fence, offering a nice spot to linger while looking for wildlife. I stopped at various points along the fence, waiting with high hopes for even a single sighting, but the prairie dogs seemed to have taken over the entire prairie and there was not a single buffalo to be seen. I did not, however, leave the park disappointed—as we drove away from the trailhead, I spotted a whole herd roaming another section of their range, within a dozen feet of a fenced enclosure alongside the park road. Park staff at the interpretive center or the gate entrance can often tell you where the herd is.

The trail follows the fence east. At about 400 feet, bear left (north), away from the Buffalo Range and through some brush. Keep an eye out for the variety of birds that migrate through the refuge. The Fort Worth Audubon Society lists the refuge as good for bird-watching and notes that in the summer you'll find a variety of hummingbirds, whereas in winter sightings include the yellow-bellied sapsucker, purple finch, and blue warbler.

At 0.25 mile, the trail crosses a grassy maintenance road and continues northeast into a huge, sunny prairie filled with tall grasses and small red and purple flowers; this is a good spot for sighting some of the many white-tailed deer that live here. The prairie buzzes with the pleasant hum of grasshoppers, crickets, and the occasional flying insect, so it's a good idea to apply insect repellent before your hike.

Reach a split at 0.45 mile. Bear right to loop back south through the prairie. Heading left would take you to the Hardwicke Interpretive Center, which has refuge information and exhibits, including a reclusive bobcat that can sometimes be seen in his outdoor enclosure. The center is also adjacent to an interesting short trail along a fossil-shell outcrop.

Continue straight, following the trail until you reach the Buffalo Range again at 0.7 mile; turn left. The trail splits again at 0.9 mile. Following the left trail takes you alongside the Buffalo Range another 500 feet until you're back at the trailhead. On my visit, I noticed that at least one trail in this area had been blocked off and marked with an EARTH HEALING sign—encourage children to stay on the trails to minimize visitor impact to the refuge.

NEARBY ACTIVITIES

The nature center offers monthly canoe tours down the West Fork of the Trinity River, along with a monthly canoe fest—for a small fee, you're provided with canoes, paddles, and life jackets and can float around Greer Island. Check **fwnature center.org** for a calendar of events and fees.

Year-round, stop by downtown Fort Worth to visit Sundance Square, the city's entertainment and shopping district, with restored buildings housing museums, galleries, gift shops, and a diverse selection of restaurants covering everything from sandwiches to sushi to steaks.

21 HORSESHOE TRAIL

KEY AT-A-GLANCE INFORMATION

LENGTH: 4.08 miles

CONFIGURATION: Out-and-back

DIFFICULTY: Easy

SCENERY: Lake, woods

EXPOSURE: Sunny

TRAIL TRAFFIC: Heavy

TRAIL SURFACE: Paved

HIKING TIME: 1.5 hours

ACCESS: Daily; free

FACILITIES: Restrooms, picnic tables, benches

WHEELCHAIR TRAVERSABLE: Yes

SPECIAL COMMENTS: Dogs are welcome on this lively trail.

DRIVING DISTANCE FROM MAJOR INTERSECTION: 6 miles from TX 121 South and TX 114 West

GPS TRAILHEAD COORDINATES

Latitude: N 32° 57' 49"
Longitude: W 97° 5' 39"

IN BRIEF

A very popular spot with locals, Horseshoe Trail offers a lively hike along a paved path circling the a small section of Lake Grapevine's southern edge. Dog walkers, hikers, joggers, and bikers. You also have the opportunity to hike some dirt paths if you're so inclined.

DESCRIPTION

Horseshoe Trail is inside Oak Grove Park, which sits on the southern shoreline of Grapevine Lake, very close to downtown Grapevine. When you enter the park, turn left at the park sign and park by the restrooms, a short drive down on the right.

The trailhead is on the pathway across the road from the restrooms. To your left, the paved pathway has a yellow stripe down its center; to your right, you'll see an old park road just beyond a gate blocking auto traffic. A marker adjacent to the gate identifies the road as Horseshoe Trail. Take a right here. Small brush and trees adjacent to the trail conceal the lake (which is off to the right) as you make your way southwest. Train your eyes upward for brilliant red cardinals.

This is not a trail for those looking to be alone with their thoughts—to the contrary, it's almost always bubbling with the infectious cheer of fellow outdoors sorts. Folks wave or

- -

Directions

From Dallas, take TX 114 West toward Grapevine and exit at TX 26/TX 114 Business, turning right onto Texan Trail. From here, turn left onto Northwest Highway, pass Main Street, and turn right onto North Dove Road (which becomes Dove Loop Road), heading north into Oak Grove Park.

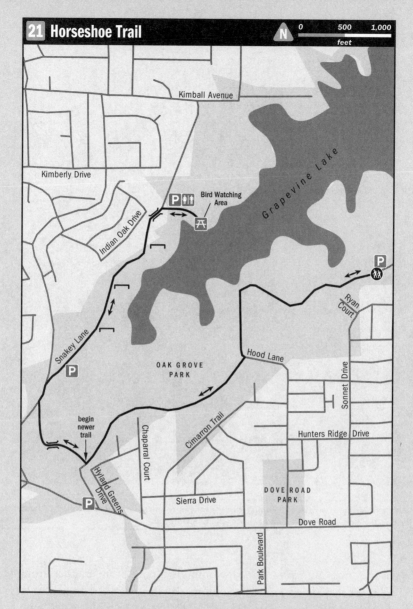

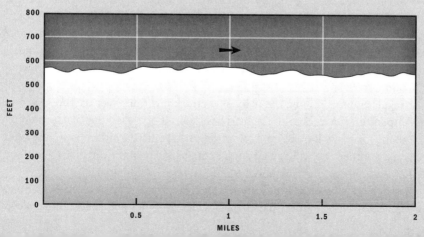

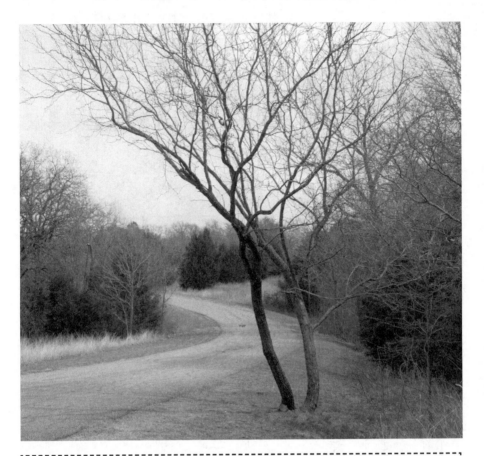

Don't let this photo fool you—the trail is hardly ever empty unless it's cold and overcast. The sunnier the day, the more people you'll find enjoying the trail with you.

smile as they pass by, giving you a few minutes alone before another group passes by. Trail users include everyone from inline skaters and bikers to dog walkers and joggers to those just looking to get outside. Unlike other trails, which can become popular with a certain niche, folks on this trail seem to include every age group. I've spotted every demographic, from young families out for the day to older couples out for a stroll to teenagers and 20-somethings out for some sun. Once I spotted a group of Boy Scouts marching happily along an adjacent path, following their Scoutmaster.

At regular intervals along the path, singletrack dirt trails veer off the road and disappear beneath the trees to the right. These trails loop out to the lake, providing a nice detour for those looking to explore the woods. If you miss a path, just keep walking and another one will appear soon enough. Many of the dirt trails you'll see to the left lead only to the back porches of local residents' houses.

The road curls southwest past more thickets and scrubby trees. At 0.55 mile, reach a junction with another park road, which is gated and inaccessible; keep straight. You'll come upon the intersection of Horseshoe Trail and Colt Road 0.1 mile later. Near the intersection is a solitary bench. It may have served a purpose at some time, but it now sits almost inaccessible amid a small patch of grassland at the junction of two roads open only to foot traffic. Continue straight on Horseshoe Trail. A short trek later, come to a junction with Bronco Drive. Again, continue straight along the trail.

On the left, the backyards and back porches of houses abutting the trail spring into view. A short distance farther, reach another junction. At this point, the trail changes from old paved road to a narrower paved path with a yellow dividing line down its center. To the left, you'll see an alternate trailhead and parking lot with a plastic-bag dispenser for cleaning up after your dog. This is a busy access point, and the parking lot is often quite full. To the right, the trail continues northwest. Bear right and follow the trail downhill past much of the same scenery: trees and underbrush. The trail follows the shoreline, making its way around the end of the lake.

As you round a bend of the lake the foliage clears, and you find yourself sandwiched between a road to the left and the lake to your right. Thankfully, the roadway is slightly raised above the trail and mostly blocked from view, so you won't find the car traffic distracting. At 1.23 miles, cross a bridge. Just 0.25 mile farther, a parking lot on the left marks another trail entrance. To the right, you have a clear view of the end of the lake—a barren expanse of marshland. A sign adjacent to the trail indicates that this section is part of a Blue Bonnet Naturalization Eagle Scout Project.

At 1.93 miles, cross another bridge before reaching yet another parking area at 2 miles. Just beyond the lot and to the right, find a bird-watching area dotted with a few picnic tables. My favorite spot is at the back of the picnic area, where one table has been placed on the edge of the outcrop to overlook the lake. This is the perfect spot to have lunch and scan for herons and egrets in the shallow waters and along the sandy shore below. From here, turn back and retrace your steps to the trailhead.

NEARBY ACTIVITIES

Head into downtown Grapevine and take a ride on the Grapevine Vintage Railroad. The steam locomotive and open-air coaches head down the Cotton Belt Route into Stockyards Station in Fort Worth. The train runs only on the weekends; for schedules and fees, visit **grapevinesteamrailroad.com**. The depot is at 707 S. Main St. in Grapevine, just off Northwest Highway.

22 KNOB HILL TRAIL

KEY AT-A-GLANCE INFORMATION

LENGTH: 6.96 miles

CONFIGURATION: Out-and-back

DIFFICULTY: Moderate with some strenuous sections

SCENERY: Cactus, wildflowers, woods, hilly meadow

EXPOSURE: Mix of sun and shade

TRAIL TRAFFIC: Moderate

TRAIL SURFACE: Packed dirt

HIKING TIME: 3 hours

ACCESS: Free; closed when muddy

FACILITIES: No restrooms or water

WHEELCHAIR TRAVERSABLE: No

SPECIAL COMMENTS: The trail can take some time to dry out after a rainstorm, so check dorba.org/trail/knob-hills before you visit to see if the trail is open.

DRIVING DISTANCE FROM MAJOR INTERSECTION: 13 miles from the I-35E–I-35W split

GPS TRAILHEAD COORDINATES

Latitude: N 33° 02' 41"
Longitude: W 97° 12' 26"

IN BRIEF

West of Grapevine Lake, this trail roughly traces Denton Creek on a pleasant trek through impressive stands of cactus and wildflowers. A bench atop a wildflower-covered hill awaits you at its end.

DESCRIPTION

This unexpectedly scenic trail lies just west of Grapevine Lake. From the trailhead, the path makes a roundabout loop toward the lake. In the spring, when the cactus flowers are blooming and the hills are green and dotted with wildflowers, the trail inspires a sense of renewal.

Maintained by the Dallas Off-Road Bicycle Association (DORBA), this trail sees its fair share of mountain bikers, who love it for its initial steep, winding sections. Though bike traffic can be moderate on the weekends, bikers pass by quickly, intent on doing the full 9-mile-plus round-trip in an hour, which makes traffic feel much lighter. Because the trail is winding and some parts are also narrow, allowing for only single-file walking, you'll need to let others know bikers are

---

Directions ———————————————➤

Take TX 114 West to FM 377 North. About 1.3 miles down, just after you cross Denton Creek, you'll see the trailhead and a small dirt parking lot just off FM 377 to the right. Don't let the trailhead's highway-adjacent location scare you: this is a secondary rural highway, and the parking area is sufficiently large and acceptably safe. When visiting for the first time, keep an eye out for the dirt parking lot, which often has at least a few cars in it—if you whiz down FM 377 too fast, you may miss it.

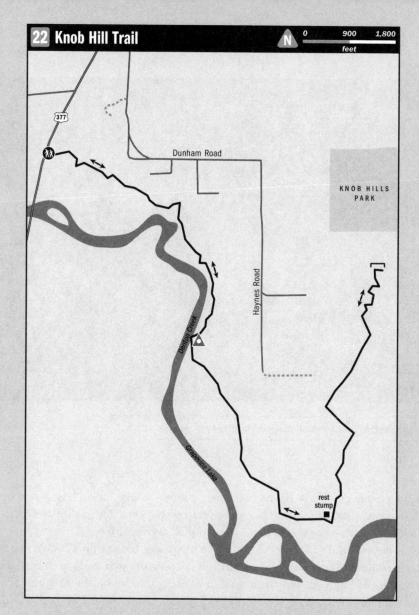

N 0   900   1,800
feet

377

Dunham Road

KNOB HILLS
PARK

Haynes Road

Denton Creek

Grapevine Lake

rest
stump

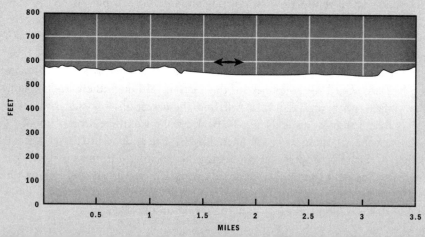

800
700
600
500
400
300
200
100
0

FEET

0.5   1   1.5   2   2.5   3   3.5
MILES

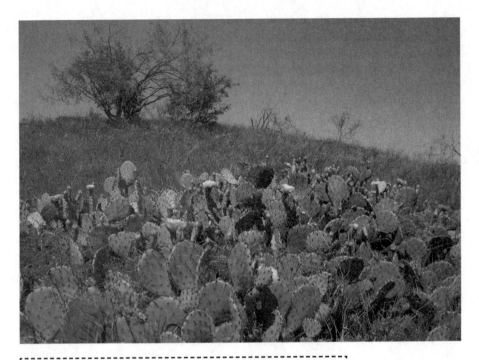

In the spring, cactus and wildflowers bloom in force alongside the trail.

approaching, especially if you're bringing kids. Yelling "Bike!" as a signal for everyone to step to the same side of the trail works best. The trail is closed when muddy, so if it's just rained, you'll have to pick another hike.

The trailhead is almost adjacent to the highway, but within a couple hundred feet the sounds of cars are replaced by the chirping of birds as the trail curls away from the road and around some small hills. The hillsides on the first half of this trail are blanketed with hundreds of prickly pear cacti. In the spring, they bloom with large, beautiful yellow flowers, creating an impressive display. Even the remnants of an old abandoned road have been taken over by the wild-cactus garden.

The trail winds gently downhill into a small section of woods, where the path has a few short, steep drops—a favorite section of mountain bikers. On my hike, helmet fragments littered a portion of the trail, evidence that some unfortunate person had misjudged the roughness of this section. Although there are a couple of steep, slick spots, careful hikers will find these sections of wide and easily maneuverable. The most difficult spot—a neck-breaking clifflike drop of about 12 feet—has a gently sloping footpath encircling it. The trail soon crosses a small creek littered with horse apples (also known as hedge apples) from a nearby Osage orange tree. The path soon reaches a small opening in the brush overlooking the muddy, slow-moving waters of Denton Creek. Although the trail loosely follows the creek, this is the only glimpse of it you'll find on the hike.

From here, the trail's terrain quickly changes as you leave the woods and head into a sunny, flat section that leads through a large field of tall reeds. A little farther down the trail and just past the billowing, fluffy seed-clouds of a cotton-wood tree, look for a large log, which marks the outbound midpoint and serves as an excellent place to take a break.

From here, the surrounding terrain changes yet again as the trail turns north through dense green foliage, where hundreds of delicate purple wildflowers do their best to flourish in patches of sun. If you listen beyond the cicadas, crickets, and birds, you're likely to hear the moos of nearby cows. As you emerge into an area open to the sky, the path soon changes from hard-packed brown dirt to packed red clay. Ahead, the trail curls through a rolling meadow dotted with Indian paintbrush and other wildflowers. The nearby mooing perfects the restful country feeling. Although I didn't see any cattle, I did see a couple of cow patties on the trail, so you may have company in the vicinity.

Where the path forks, choose the left branch for a longer walk; this spur winds around the hill before rejoining the main path. At the next fork, turn right to find a lonely bench surrounded by wildflowers atop a small hill. Take in the view before heading back. To extend the hike, turn left at the previous fork. The trail winds downhill, continuing on toward the lake for another couple miles. The path eventually reaches a fork that leads to Dunham Trail. Staying on the main trail, you'll reach a bridge and eventually the end of the trail at Pocahontas Road, near Grapevine Lake.

NEARBY ACTIVITIES

If you're a NASCAR fan, the Texas Motor Speedway is just 6 miles away. For a schedule of race events, visit **texasmotorspeedway.com.** To get to the speedway, go south on FM 377 for about 1.2 miles and turn right onto TX 144 West. Go 3.8 miles and turn right on Allison Avenue.

23 NORTHSHORE TRAIL

KEY AT-A-GLANCE INFORMATION

LENGTH: 8.96 miles

CONFIGURATION: Out-and-back

DIFFICULTY: Easy–moderate

SCENERY: Lake views from bluffs, hardwood forest, birds

EXPOSURE: Mix of sun and shade

TRAIL TRAFFIC: Heavy

TRAIL SURFACE: Packed dirt

HIKING TIME: 4.5 hours

ACCESS: $5 per vehicle, $1 per pedestrian or cyclist; April 1–September 30: Sunday–Thursday, 9 a.m.–sunset, Friday and Saturday, 8 a.m.–sunset; October 1–March 31: daily, 9 a.m.–sunset

FACILITIES: Restrooms, picnic area

SPECIAL COMMENTS: Very popular with mountain bikers and joggers in addition to hikers, this trail is especially busy on weekends and holidays.

SUPPLEMENTAL MAPS: www.swf-wc.usace.army.mil/grapevine/PDF/Northshore.pdf

DRIVING DISTANCE FROM MAJOR INTERSECTION: 4.2 miles from I-635 and TX 121

GPS TRAILHEAD COORDINATES

Latitude: N 32° 58' 58"

Longitude: W 97° 4' 4"

IN BRIEF

Nice views from the bluffs overlooking the lake dominate the first half of this popular trail. The second half is less busy because it twists and turns through the hardwood forest just out of view of the lake.

DESCRIPTION

Dammed in the 1950s, Grapevine Lake is a very popular reservoir just north of Dallas–Fort Worth International Airport. The lake gets very busy on weekends with families who come to enjoy camping, boating, fishing, and picnicking, and miles of multiuse trails. Northshore Trail, certified as a National Recreation Trail in 1991, is one of the most popular trails on the lake and arguably the most popular in the area. A deserved favorite thanks to its accessibility, length, and scenic lake views, the trail sees a high volume of hikers, joggers, and bikers.

As its name indicates, the trail is on the north side of the lake in Rockledge Park. In years past, the trail was notorious for being incredibly crowded. More recently, the City of Grapevine began managing the park and started charging an admission fee. As a result, the massive number of visitors who once crowded the trailhead has decreased. On nice

----

Directions

From I-635 West, take Exit 36B, Bass Pro Drive. Go 0.5 mile and turn left on Bass Pro, then go about 0.6 mile and turn left onto TX 26. Continue about 0.5 mile and turn right on FM 2499 (Fairway Drive). Cross the dam and turn left into Rockledge Park. Stay to the right; the road dead-ends at the parking lot.

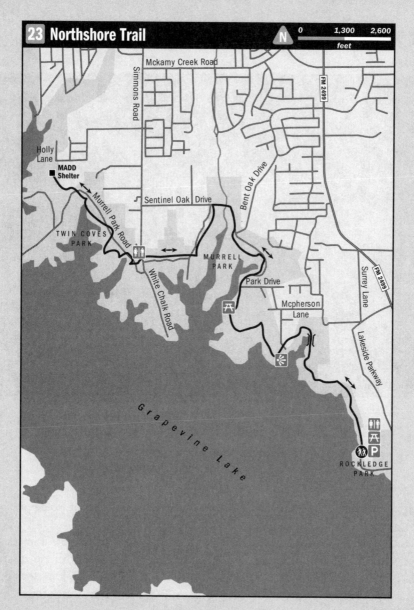

N

0   1,300   2,600
feet

Mckamy Creek Road

Simmons Road

FM 2499

Holly Lane

MADD Shelter

Murrell Park Road

Sentinel Oak Drive

Bent Oak Drive

TWIN COVES PARK

MURRELL PARK

White Chalk Road

Park Drive

Mcpherson Lane

Surrey Lane

FM 2499

Lakeside Parkway

G r a p e v i n e   L a k e

ROCKLEDGE PARK

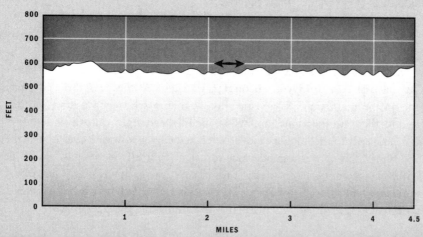

FEET

800
700
600
500
400
300
200
100
0

1   2   3   4   4.5

MILES

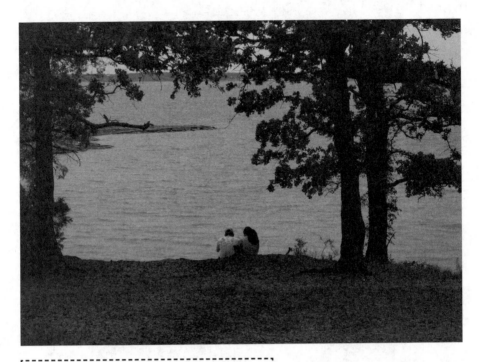

A couple enjoys a view of the lake on a rocky outcrop.

days, however, the small admission fee isn't much of a deterrent, so be prepared for plenty of company along the trail.

The trailhead is tucked in the back corner of the parking lot. Immediately pass a small rock-strewn beach, which dog owners and amateur fishermen scramble down to access the lake. Continue on the trail as it winds along the top of some small, rocky cliffs that hug the shoreline. On sunny days, watch for sailboats gliding past as they circle around the lake.

The path then climbs uphill and meanders around some of the large rocks (which help give the park its name) before flattening and heading slightly away from the shoreline and among tall trees with an understory of dense brush. The path parallels the water slightly inland, offering occasional glimpses of the lake.

At the first two forks you encounter, go right. At the next fork, continue straight on the main trail. As you near the 1-mile mark, reach a long wooden bridge and then another junction, where you'll head right onto a wider trail. About 1.2 miles into the hike, gaze over the lake below at a scenic overlook at the top of a bluff. This spot is a good place to orient yourself. To the left, you'll see the 1,500-plus-room Gaylord Texan, a resort and convention center. The airport is also nearby, and though for the most part air traffic is not overly noticeable, you'll probably have already seen a plane or two making their approach.

More interesting than airplanes, fossils have also been found nearby. Recent record heat has left the lake level substantially below normal, exposing million-year-old dinosaur tracks embedded in sandstone along the shoreline on this side of the lake. Unfortunately, visitors are prohibited from viewing the tracks because vandals destroyed a couple of them, prompting the lake's controlling authority, the Army Corps of Engineers, to block access and cover the tracks until the water levels rise enough to hide them again.

Continuing along the trail, head through grasslands and, at 1.6 miles, come to an old road. Cross the road and pick up the trail on the far side, continuing until you reach a clearing at about 1.8 miles. This area, which is virtually always empty, has a vacant parking lot and about a half-dozen old picnic tables tucked under the trees. Probably attracted by the solitude, the birds here are loud and abundant. On my hike, I was able to spot only the most obvious—cardinals, whose telltale bright-red plumage makes them easy to pick out, and a vulture that slowly circled nearby. If you want to shorten this hike, this is a good spot to turn around.

Pick up the trail as it enters a patch of forest on the opposite side of the parking lot. At 2.2 miles, come to a small bridge and, shortly thereafter, cross an old gravel road. At 2.5 miles, reach another road where you'll hang a left, following the road until it deteriorates into a dirt path and then rejoins a paved road. When you reach a spot where the road forks, turn left and, at the next fork, at 3.1 miles, bear right. You'll eventually reach another road where you'll cross and pick up the trail on the opposite side. For the next mile, the trail twists and turns through the trees, more of a thrill for mountain bikers. The trail comes out at the trailhead by the MADD Shelter at Murrell Park.

NEARBY ACTIVITIES

After the first half of your hike, while you're still at the Murrell Park trailhead, walk over to the marina for a bite to eat at Little Pete's, where you can sit on the patio overlooking the water and the boats and munch on comfort food such as burgers or chicken-fried steak. In the evenings, there's typically entertainment such as karaoke or poker. Visit **littlepeteslakegrapevine.com** for more information.

The Gaylord Texan, which sits on Grapevine Lake, is another fun place to stop after your hike. This huge resort has a 4.5-acre atrium, each section of which represents a different part of Texas. A short stroll takes you to the Hill Country, Palo Duro Canyon, and the San Antonio Riverwalk, where there are plenty of spots for grabbing a cold drink and some hot food. For more information, visit **gaylordhotels.com/texan-home.html**.

24 RIVER LEGACY TRAIL

 KEY AT-A-GLANCE INFORMATION

LENGTH: 5.46 miles

CONFIGURATION: Out-and-back

DIFFICULTY: Easy

SCENERY: Woods, river

EXPOSURE: Shady

TRAIL TRAFFIC: Moderate–heavy

TRAIL SURFACE: Paved path

HIKING TIME: 1.5 hours

ACCESS: Free; open daily, 5 a.m.–10 p.m.

FACILITIES: Water fountain

WHEELCHAIR TRAVERSABLE: Yes

SPECIAL COMMENTS: Presentations and festivals are among the events at the Living Science Center; check the calendar at riverlegacy.org.

SUPPLEMENTAL MAPS: riverlegacy .org/images/pdfs/river-legacy -park-aerial-map-090110.pdf

DRIVING DISTANCE FROM MAJOR INTERSECTION: 4 miles from I-30 and TX 360

GPS TRAILHEAD COORDINATES

Latitude: N 32° 47' 20"

Longitude: W 97° 5' 56"

IN BRIEF

This lengthy paved trail stretches alongside the river, offering a few good overlooks for bird-watching.

DESCRIPTION

River Legacy Parks' 1,300 acres and 8 miles of trails are a popular attraction in Arlington, drawing hikers, bikers, joggers, and dog walkers. A few different access points to the parks' recreational trails help spread the visitors throughout. The parks' name originates from the River Legacy Foundation's vision of preserving a "living legacy for future generations."

Trail maps and park information are available a short drive from the trailhead at the River Legacy Living Science Center. The center's unique design was inspired by a children's fort built of sticks and leaves, a picture of which can be found at the center's website. According to the website, the center is not only designed to be part of its natural surroundings, but its construction included trees salvaged from a city project, and its maintenance relies on recycled gray water for landscaping. Another reason to stop by the center is its large exhibit hall and pretty observation decks. A short trail winds through the grounds surrounding the center. To get to the trailhead for this hike, however, you'll have to drive a few blocks to the lengthier paved sections of the parks.

Directions _____

Follow I-30 toward Arlington, take Exit 28, and turn left onto FM 157. The entrance to River Legacy Parks is 0.6 mile down Collins Street on the left, at 3020 N. Collins. Park in the first parking area.

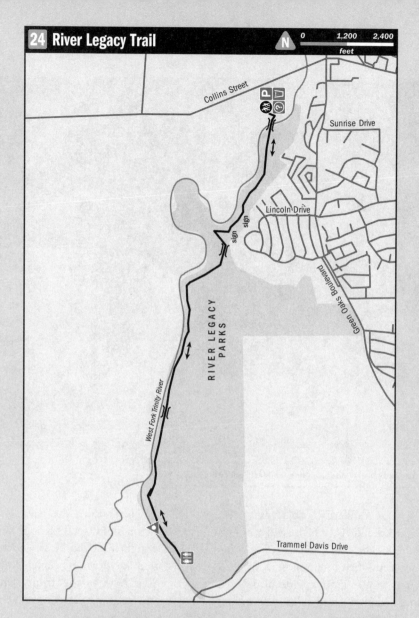

N

0   1,200   2,400
feet

Collins Street

Sunrise Drive

Lincoln Drive

Green Oaks Boulevard

RIVER LEGACY
PARKS

West Fork Trinity River

sign   sign

Trammel Davis Drive

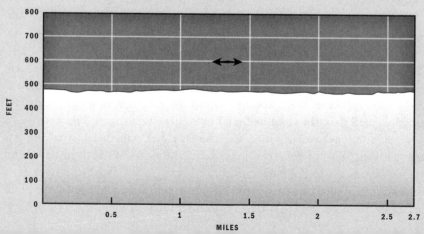

800
700
600
500
400
300
200
100
0

FEET

0.5   1   1.5   2   2.5   2.7

MILES

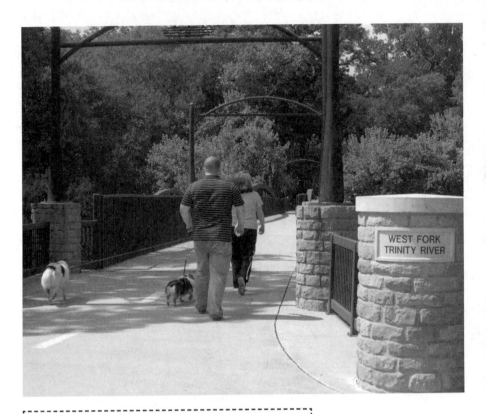

The busy trail winds alongside the West Fork of the Trinity River.

The trailhead is adjacent to the parking lot. Head down the paved path toward the kiosk, which is adjacent to a water fountain and displays a huge aerial photo of the area. After getting oriented, head straight past the kiosk and turn right at the first junction onto the path with a dotted line down its center. Immediately come upon a wide bridge spanning the West Fork of the Trinity River. You're likely to find folks at its railings enjoying the relaxing views of its green, slow-moving waters.

The trail continues through the woods along the river. The route is mostly shaded, making it a good hike for a hot day. At 0.17 mile, bear right at the junction onto the path with a red-dotted stripe down its center.

A couple of interpretive signs along the trail provide information on local wildlife. You'll pass one of these signs on the left; it tells about raccoons: the small masked creatures, commonly associated with trash cans and late-night raids, are nocturnal animals that can often be found in hollowed-out tree trunks.

As you continue, you'll notice some smaller dirt trails heading to the left toward the river. Some of these overlooks offer nice views of the river. Be careful not to step too close to the edge, which is slightly raised above the river. The banks easily erode and can cause you to slide right in. Farther down the trail, structured overlooks complete with benches offer safer viewing.

At 0.6 mile, reach another display on the left, describing an insect commonly found here—the wolf spider. These large brown spiders, which can grow to more than an inch long, are typically spotted scurrying along the ground as opposed to hanging in webs.

At 0.88 mile, reach a long wooden bridge across a narrow river. The path continues with woods on both sides until it forks at 0.92 mile; here, bear right onto a path with a blue line. In another couple hundred feet, come to another trail split. To the right, the trail terminates at a bench set alongside the river—a good spot for a quick break. The initials of two lovers are carved into a tall tree at this pretty spot.

When you've rested, continue on the path, staying to the right. The trail reaches a break in the trees, where, to the left, you'll see a large pavilion across a field. From here you'll pass a few more overlooks, which provide opportunities to scan for turtles and birds, before reaching 1.34 miles; at this point head right, following the yellow-striped path. The trail straightens here; among the few distractions are folks jogging with their dogs and others cruising on their bikes toward the end of the trail. I was even passed by a fellow in his wheelchair, sailing along toward the turnaround just a little more than a mile down.

Pass a circular stone bench, to the right, at 1.82 miles, before reaching a wooden deck overlooking the river at 2.47 miles. The deck has high wooden railings, providing adequate cover for bird-watchers discreetly scoping the river. The trail continues another 0.26 mile to a dead end, where you'll find trees and a ring of seats. Retrace your steps to the trailhead.

NEARBY ACTIVITIES

Baseball fans will enjoy a visit to Ameriquest Field in Arlington, home of the Texas Rangers. Check **texas.rangers.mlb.com** for ticket information during baseball season. Year-round you can visit the Legends of the Game Museum, which is on the same site and has a huge collection from the National Baseball Hall of Fame. To get to the ballpark, go south on North Collins Street and turn left onto Northeast Green Oaks Boulevard. Continue 1.4 miles, then turn right onto Ballpark Way. The baseball stadium is 2 miles down.

25 ROCKY POINT TRAIL

KEY AT-A-GLANCE INFORMATION

LENGTH: 3.84 miles

CONFIGURATION: Out-and-back

DIFFICULTY: A couple of rough patches in the beginning

SCENERY: Creek, woods, lake beach

EXPOSURE: Partially shady–sunny

TRAIL TRAFFIC: Light

TRAIL SURFACE: Dirt, sand

HIKING TIME: 1.75 hours

ACCESS: Free; open daily

FACILITIES: None

WHEELCHAIR TRAVERSABLE: No

SPECIAL COMMENTS: Bring a bag to carry the goodies you collect while beachcombing.

DRIVING DISTANCE FROM MAJOR INTERSECTION: 14 miles from I-35E and TX 121

GPS TRAILHEAD COORDINATES

Latitude: N 33° 2' 1"
Longitude: W 97° 9' 0"

IN BRIEF

This peaceful trek descends a rocky hill and follows alongside a wooded creek toward Grapevine Lake. When you near the lake, the path changes from dirt to soft sand as it leads onto the lake's beach.

DESCRIPTION

This rocky trail is one of Grapevine Lake's less frequented paths, often overlooked in favor of other, more popular trails such as Northshore Trail (see page 112). Its small parking area—which holds maybe a half-dozen cars—is just off the shoulder of a secondary residential road and marked by nothing more than a small trail sign. If you're not paying attention, you're likely to drive past before you realize there's actually a trail here. You'll therefore be fairly surprised when you step onto the trail and discover a lovely tree-covered path following a creek. It's a great choice if you're looking for a winter hike; the cooler weather will allow you to spend as much time as you want beachcombing the long, sandy lakeshore at its end.

The trail heads east into a narrow, grassy, tree-covered strip of land sandwiched between private homes. The path parallels the boundary fence of a private driveway. After a few hundred feet, it starts to descend, becoming steep and rocky as it makes its way to a creek. If you have a hiking stick, bring it along—most

----

Directions

Take FM 1171 (Cross Timbers Road) west from I-35E in Lewisville or east from I-35W in Justin. Turn south onto High Road. There is a small parking area on the left, about 0.5 mile down, between Stallion Circle and Sunnyview Lane.

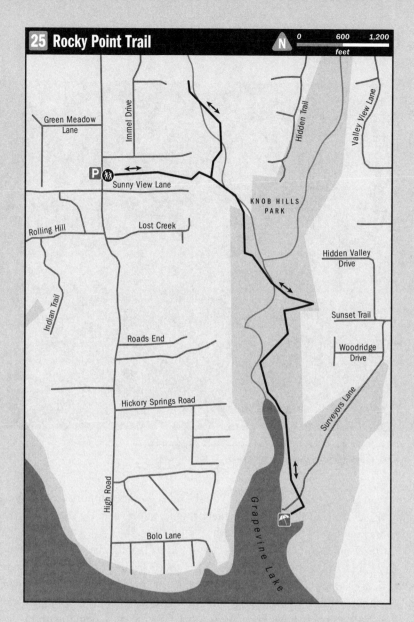

N

| 0 | 600 | 1,200 |

feet

Green Meadow Lane

Immel Drive

P

Sunny View Lane

KNOB HILLS PARK

Hidden Trail

Valley View Lane

Lost Creek

Rolling Hill

Hidden Valley Drive

Indian Trail

Sunset Trail

Roads End

Woodridge Drive

Hickory Springs Road

Surveyors Lane

High Road

Bolo Lane

Grapevine Lake

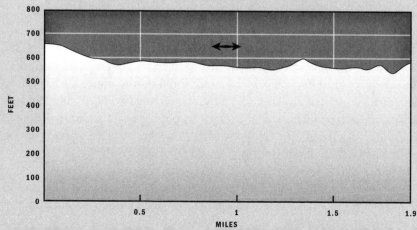

FEET				
800				
700				
600				
500				
400				
300				
200				
100				
0	0.5	1	1.5	1.9

MILES

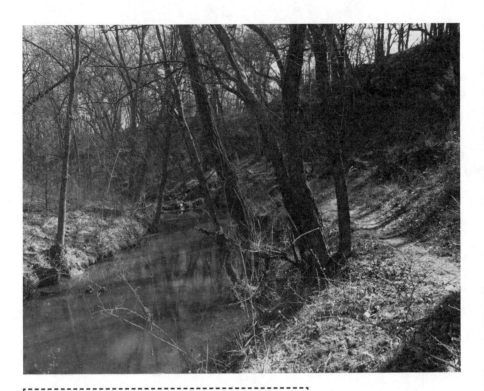

The trail follows the creek as it heads toward Grapevine Lake.

of the trail is only slightly hilly, but you'll find the extra support useful for navigating the descent in this section, which, though short, is fairly steep, with rocks and roots making for uneven footing.

At 0.33 mile, come to the creek. Here the path splits, heading north toward FM 1171 and south toward the lake. Turn south (right). Lush green vegetation grows richly along the creek's banks, and unlike many streams, which stagnate in murky puddles, this one's waters flow briskly over the rocks, providing a pleasant gurgling backdrop for your hike. After a brief flat stretch, climb gently through wooded terrain, away from the creek. Bear right at the junction at 0.73 mile, and round a small pond decorated with bird boxes.

If you could see an aerial view of the trail, you'd realize that you're actually winding around the outskirts of a residential neighborhood on a small point that juts into the lake. Just after you pass the pond, you'll start to notice the backyards of some of these residences. They are, however, set amid wooded hilly lots and widely spaced; as a result, they don't feel overly obtrusive and are easily ignored. The trail curls back toward the creek—which by now has widened to the width of a river. It peeks in and out of view to your right and stays within sight the rest of the way to the lake.

You'll soon see Grapevine Lake ahead of you in the distance. The lake is popular, and if it's nice out you'll likely spot motorboats chugging to and from the more than half a dozen boat ramps along its shores. The trail progresses steadily toward the water, passing through a small stand of eastern red cedars, before emerging into the sun. To your left, huge houses sit atop a small hill, their backyards overlooking the lake.

With the lake only a short distance away, the trail becomes sandy and the trees fall back, leaving you in full sun. To your right, the river, which had been gradually widening, is now a couple hundred feet across. During droughts, the part nearest the lake dries out, forming a long, brown beach where the water should be. During my visit, the water was so low that an entire dock was stranded on the dry banks.

You'll soon reach a trail split; keep straight, heading up a short, rocky hill. A few hundred feet farther, reach a detour; going left will take you out to Rocky Point, whereas if you go right you'll reach the beach, where you can spend some time walking the soft, sandy lakeshore. When the lake is low and the water has receded, shells, old driftwood, and all manner of other interesting artifacts are exposed, making it a fun spot to explore. If it's a sunny day, you're likely to spot kids playing in the water and folks with towels and beach chairs soaking up the rays. It's easy to lose track of time lazing around the shore, making this a good spot to have a picnic lunch on the beach before retracing your steps to the trailhead. If you'd like to keep going, just go back to the turnoff and bear left; the trail continues around Rocky Point.

NEARBY ACTIVITIES

The huge Grapevine Mills Mall—with more than 190 shops and a 30-screen AMC movie theater—is only a short drive away. You'll also find a selection of restaurants both within and around the mall. To get there, turn right onto FM 1171 (Cross Timbers Road) and go about 5 miles. Turn right onto FM 2499 south (Long Prairie Road) and drive 5.6 miles. The mall is on your left.

26 SANSOM PARK TRAIL

KEY AT-A-GLANCE INFORMATION

LENGTH: 2.24 miles

CONFIGURATION: Loop

DIFFICULTY: Hard

SCENERY: Lake

EXPOSURE: Partially shady–sunny

TRAIL TRAFFIC: Heavy on weekends

TRAIL SURFACE: Dirt

HIKING TIME: 55 minutes

ACCESS: Free; open daily

FACILITIES: Picnic table

WHEELCHAIR TRAVERSABLE: No

SPECIAL COMMENTS: A lot of winding and twisting back and forth, but it's rugged and fun.

DRIVING DISTANCE FROM MAJOR INTERSECTION: 1 mile from Jacksboro Highway and Northwest Loop 820

GPS TRAILHEAD COORDINATES

Latitude: N 32° 47' 44"

Longitude: W 97° 24' 47"

IN BRIEF

Rough, rocky trail dominates the first half of this hike, which winds down a bluff and along the southeastern edge of Lake Worth before circling back on a flatter route. Fossils can easily be spotted in the path's rocky sediment.

DESCRIPTION

Thanks to the efforts of the Fort Worth Mountain Bikers' Association (FWMBA), Marion Sansom Park offers good hiking on hike-bike trails built along Lake Worth's shoreline. Although it looks fairly small from the park, which is on the lake's southeastern tip, the lake continues around to the north. An impoundment of the West Fork of the Trinity River, the lake was created in 1914. Parks, including the huge Fort Worth Nature Center and Refuge, abound along the lake's shoreline, offering plenty of recreation for locals. Fishing is a popular activity, and you're likely to see anglers searching for white crappie, large mouth bass, and catfish.

This city park has little by way of amenities, except for a couple of picnic tables and the trails; however, this doesn't deter visitors, and you'll often find at least a few cars in the large parking lot. Most of the visitors are bikers drawn in by FWMBA's efforts to build the trails, but the 5 or so miles of trails accommodate both hikers and bikers, so you won't feel overrun. Sections of

----

Directions

Take Jacksboro Highway/TX 199 West. Turn left onto Biway Street, then right onto Roberts Cut Off Road and into Marion Sansom Park.

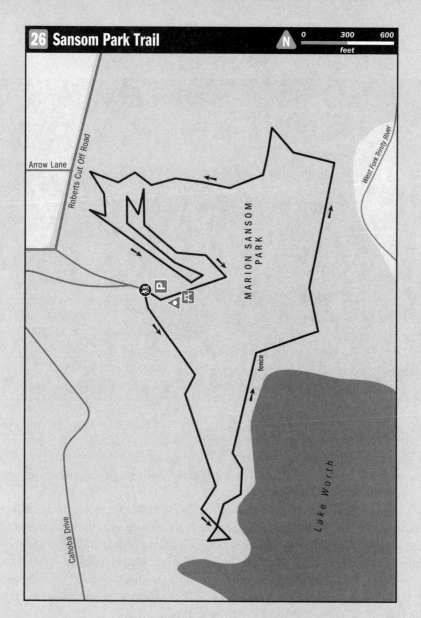

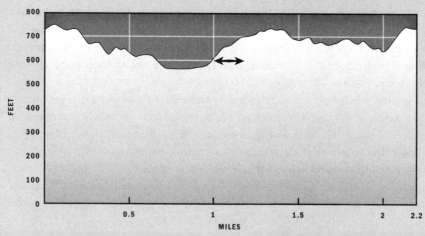

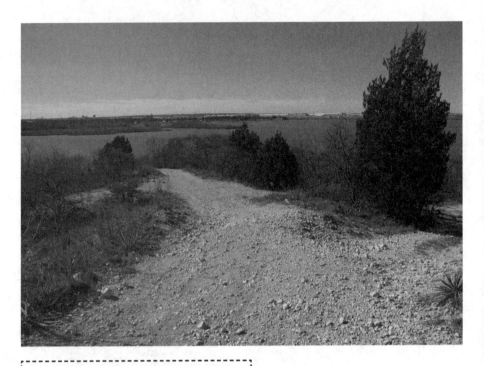

The rocky trail offers some nice vistas of the lake.

the trail are fairly rugged, so come prepared with sturdy hiking shoes and a walking stick.

Just to the south of the parking lot, find a scenic overlook for viewing the southeastern end of the lake. A table here is an ideal spot to have lunch after the hike. Continue to the trailhead by walking down the wide, rutted dirt path to the right of the overlook. At 0.2 mile, bear left, continuing steeply downhill. Ignore any smaller side trails and stay on the wide dirt lane, following it downhill toward the lake. To the left, glimpse a rolled-earth dam abutting the southeastern edge of the lake. Cacti and small shrubs dot the trailside.

The trail winds parallel to the lake and west through steep, rocky terrain. Stay to the left at the junction at 0.3 mile, then follow the path as it swings left onto a narrow singletrack trail heading back southeast. (If you were to continue heading straight downhill toward the lake, the path would loop back to your present location after a few hundred feet.)

The trail winds uphill through scrubby trees and follows the shoreline, below and to your right. As you hike, keep an eye to the ground for fossils from millions of years ago when this area was under water. Without much effort, it's easy to find shells and imprints from ancient ammonites—extinct mollusks distinguishable by their spiral shape—in the trail's rocky sediment.

Yucca and juniper encroach upon the trail as you continue east. The lake stays almost constantly within view to your right. The gentle lapping of its waters on the shoreline below remind you it's there even when it briefly disappears from sight. The trail starts a brief, rocky descent as it continues winding through the brush, then climbs a small hill, exposing the rocky wall of the outcrop from which you've just descended. Just beyond, pass the dam, which is surrounded by a chain-link fence with a NO TRESPASSING sign.

The narrow dirt path winds around the fence and continues briefly through the woods before merging with an old road. Follow the road past an overlook with a view of the blue-green waters of an inlet of the lake on the right. The Fort Worth Fish Hatchery is just to the south. Continuing down the trail, at 0.95 mile, bear left back onto a narrow dirt path that heads steeply up an uneven, rocky hillside. When you reach the summit, enjoy the bird's-eye view of the lake below, then bear left to return.

At the next two junctions, keep left. Compared with what you've done already, this last half of the trail is relatively flat. Wind over a hill to make your way back to the trailhead. At 1.13 miles, reach a junction, with another trail to your right; keep following your trail to the left. Wind through more wooded terrain and bear left yet again a few hundred feet down, following the green arrow on the rock. The green trail is the easy one for mountain bikers, so you're likely to encounter a little traffic here. Continue, staying to the left at the next junction. Finally, at 1.33 miles, bear right, following the blue arrow. Take a right at the next junction, at 2 miles. At this point, you're in the home stretch. Continue straight through the next junction and finish the final uphill stretch back to the overlook and parking area.

NEARBY ACTIVITIES

Head over to Exchange Avenue to see cowboys and cowgirls drive Texas long-horn steers down Exchange Avenue through Stockyard Station. The cattle drive happens twice daily, at 11:30 a.m. and 4 p.m. To get there from Sansom Park, turn right onto Jacksboro Highway (TX 199) and go about 1.5 miles, then turn left onto TX 183 North. Go 2 miles, turn right onto Main Street, then turn left onto Exchange Avenue.

27 TRINITY RIVER TRAIL (Northside)

KEY AT-A-GLANCE INFORMATION

LENGTH: 3.9 miles

CONFIGURATION: Out-and-back

DIFFICULTY: Easy

SCENERY: River

EXPOSURE: Sunny

TRAIL TRAFFIC: Light

TRAIL SURFACE: Paved

HIKING TIME: 1.5 hours

ACCESS: Daily; free

FACILITIES: Benches

WHEELCHAIR TRAVERSABLE: Yes

SPECIAL COMMENTS: The entire Trinity River Trail network is extensive and will take you many days to thoroughly explore; visit trinitytrails.org for a complete map of the system.

SUPPLEMENTAL MAPS: trinitytrails .org/maps.html

DRIVING DISTANCE FROM MAJOR INTERSECTION: 4 miles from I-30 West and I-35W

GPS TRAILHEAD COORDINATES

Latitude: N 32° 46' 42"

Longitude: W 97° 20' 27"

IN BRIEF

Views of the skyscrapers in downtown Fort Worth dominate the skyline of this flat, sunny trail that winds alongside the West Fork of the Trinity River.

DESCRIPTION

Fort Worth's Trinity Trail system comprises about 40 miles of hike-bike trails along the Trinity River. It is readily accessible and is bordered by a number of city parks, including downtown Fort Worth's Heritage Park. The trail has a few different legs, which all meet in or around the park, making it a popular starting point for newcomers to the trail system. Bikers, inline skaters, joggers, and walkers all frequent the trail, attracted by the paved surface. Trinity Park, the Fort Worth Zoo, and the Fort Worth Botanic Garden also border sections of the trail.

This trail covers a short section of one of the northern legs of the trail network. Although the Northside and Heritage Park trailheads allow you to start from either direction, I've found that the trail is best started from the

---

Directions

Start this trail at the Northside Drive trailhead of the Trinity River Trails, at 600 E. Northside Dr. To get there, follow I-35W north and take Exit 53 to Northside Drive; then turn left onto East Northside and go 1.5 miles. The trailhead is below the bridge. Alternatively, you can start the hike from the other end, at Heritage Park, on Congress Street on the northeast side of downtown Fort Worth. To get there, follow I-30 West toward Abilene and take Exit 13B. Turn right on Henderson Street, then right again on Congress to reach the parking lot. Feed the meters weekdays 8 a.m.–6 p.m.

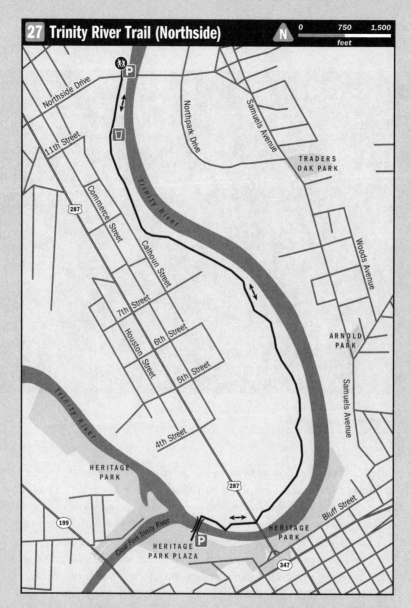

N

0   750   1,500
feet

Northside Drive

11th Street

Commerce Street

287

Calhoun Street

7th Street

Houston Street

6th Street

5th Street

4th Street

Trinity River

Northpark Drive

Samuels Avenue

TRADERS OAK PARK

Woods Avenue

ARNOLD PARK

Samuels Avenue

287

Trinity River

HERITAGE PARK

199

Clear Fork Trinity River

HERITAGE PARK PLAZA

P

HERITAGE PARK

Bluff Street

347

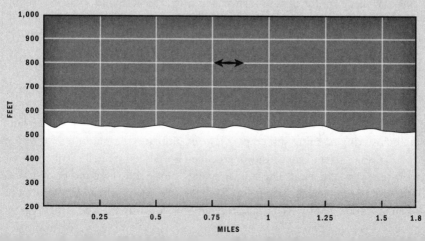

1,000
900
800
700
600
500
400
300
200

FEET

0.25   0.5   0.75   1   1.25   1.5   1.8

MILES

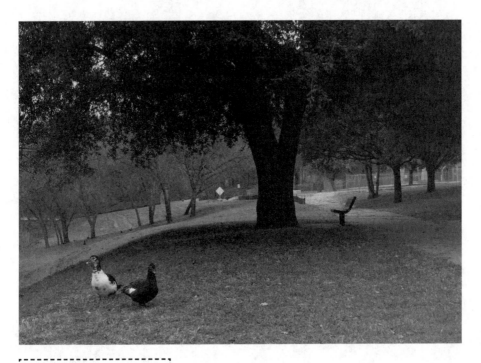

A peaceful day in Heritage Park

Northside trailhead, heading south toward downtown Fort Worth. Starting at this end, you'll have a fantastic view of the Fort Worth skyline to motivate you throughout the hike. The skyscrapers—which are just a small grouping on the horizon at the start of the hike—will loom larger and more massive with your every step, until you finally reach Heritage Park, which sits just in their shadow.

Bring your own water and wear plenty of sunscreen—this hike is completely exposed. There's a water fountain just beyond the trailhead, but on my visit it wasn't working.

The Northside trailhead is at a small parking area with a kiosk and benches just at the base of the Northside Drive Bridge. The trail itself is very clean and well maintained. You'll also find the parking lots on both ends of the trail to be safe and secure. To see a good map of the entire Trinity Trail network, visit **trinitytrails.org** before you leave home.

The trail curls away both to the north and to the south, following the curve of the Trinity River. Turn right onto the trail, passing under the bridge and down the paved path. The downtown skyline is on the horizon ahead and to the left; this small clustering of shiny skyscrapers is your ultimate destination.

The flat, smooth trail runs inside a greenbelt bordered by small earth embankments on the west and east. The embankments block the surrounding city and neighborhoods from view, isolating you from the stresses of urban life. Within the embankments is the Trinity River, just to your left. A neatly mowed strip of grass reaches toward the embankment to the right. Trees and benches, placed carefully at regular intervals along the trail, complete the parklike setting.

At 0.6 mile, reach a junction where the main path continues straight and a spur splinters left, crosses the river, and continues along the opposite bank. Continue straight along the main trail, bypassing the river crossing. As you hike, you'll pass a few rocks with plaques describing the history and significance of portions of the trail.

With little to block the scenery ahead, you'll have charming views of the upcoming sections of trail snaking off into the distance before they disappear around the bends of the river. Downtown is always within tantalizing view. Although the embankment to your right blocks almost everything in that direction, you'll soon start to see houses and businesses sitting atop the embankment on the opposite side of the river to your left, signaling that you're approaching downtown. Soon you're within the shadows of the buildings you had admired from afar. Cross under a bridge where ducks and geese can regularly be seen resting in the shade. Finally, following a last sharp curve, find yourself at a bridge spanning the river. The path crosses the bridge, delivering you into Heritage Park. From here, the trail branches in several directions, allowing you to continue the hike if you're not yet ready to turn back. Ducks and geese are likely to come up to greet you in their never-ending quest for food. Visit with them a bit before retracing your steps to the trailhead.

NEARBY ACTIVITIES

Only 8 miles away, the Fort Worth Zoo is a great spot to explore; its residents include raptors, primates, cheetahs, and Komodo dragons. The zoo also has a petting corral and a rock-climbing wall. Visit **fortworthzoo.com** for information on entrance fees and hours. To get there, take I-35W south to I-30 West toward Abilene. Take the University Drive exit and head south on University Drive 1 mile, then turn left onto Colonial Parkway.

28 TRINITY RIVER TRAIL (Oakmont Park)

KEY AT-A-GLANCE INFORMATION

LENGTH: 3.36 miles

CONFIGURATION: Out-and-back

DIFFICULTY: Easy

SCENERY: Woods, champion oak tree

EXPOSURE: Partially shady

TRAIL TRAFFIC: Light–moderate

TRAIL SURFACE: Paved path and short, dirt trail

HIKING TIME: 1.25 hours

ACCESS: Free; daily

FACILITIES: Picnic tables

WHEELCHAIR TRAVERSABLE: On the paved portion

SPECIAL COMMENTS: The trail has only a few river overlooks, but they're great for birders nevertheless. Bring binoculars.

SUPPLEMENTAL MAPS: trinitytrails .org/maps.html

DRIVING DISTANCE FROM MAJOR INTERSECTION: 6 miles from the I-20–I-820 merge

GPS TRAILHEAD COORDINATES

Latitude: N 32° 40' 13"

Longitude: W 97° 25' 52"

IN BRIEF

A paved section of the Trinity River system, this pleasant trail is popular with bicyclists and dog walkers. The trail winds through the woods between two parks. A turnoff near the park at the other end takes you down a dirt trail to the huge state-champion bur oak tree.

DESCRIPTION

Part of the Trinity River Trail system—a network that spreads spiderlike for a total of 30 miles through Fort Worth—this paved trail follows the Clear Fork River (a branch of the Trinity River) southwest from Oakmont Park to Pecan Valley Park. The trail is popular with bikers, joggers, and walkers because it is level, with only gentle turns. Hikers will find the trail, which curls through the woods, a nice escape from the bustle of the nearby city. The Texas Parks and Wildlife Department recently listed Oakmont Park among its suggested routes for hikes in the Prairies and Pineywoods areas.

The small parking area at the trailhead fills up quickly on pretty days; arrive early to secure a spot. If the parking lot is full, you can do the hike in reverse, starting from Pecan Valley Park, which has much more parking.

The trailhead is marked by a couple of picnic tables. Follow the trail over a bridge spanning a small creek. Pass the park's playground,

----

Directions ⎯⎯⎯⎯⎯⎯⎯⎯⎯⎯⎯⟶

Take I-20 West toward Abilene to Exit 431, and turn left onto Bryant Irvin Boulevard, heading southwest. Turn right onto Oakmont Boulevard and go about 0.5 mile to Bellaire Drive South; then turn right again to Oakmont Park. Parking is on the left.

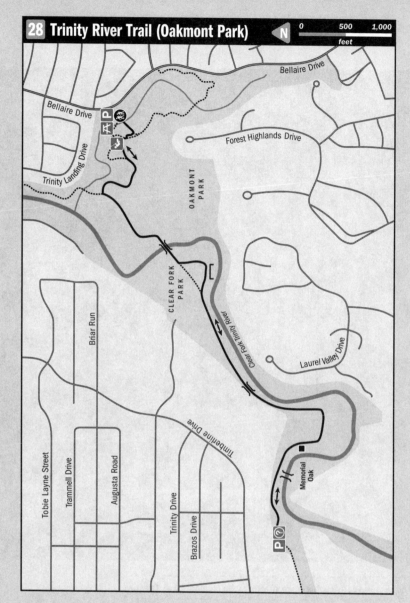

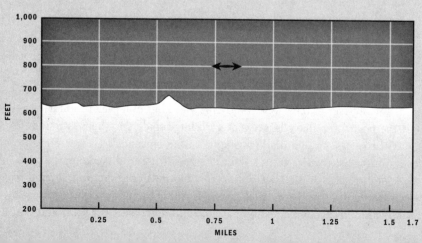

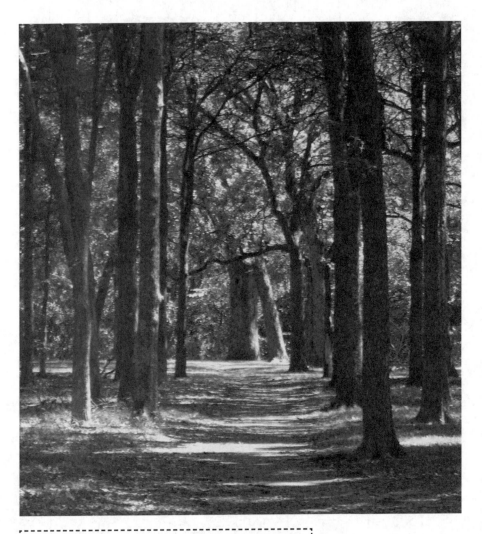

The path winds through a grove straight to the Memorial Oak Tree.

then hike through a wide field dotted with trees. The trail then curls downhill, crosses a dried-up gully, and passes another field, this one dotted with purple wildflowers, bright-yellow sunflowers, and trees such as mesquite and oak.

Turn left at the junction, at 0.28 mile. Continue until you reach a bridge spanning a wide river at 0.63 mile. Enjoy the view, but don't lean too far into the railing—the posts often have large webs with huge spiders in them awaiting prey. Signs just across the bridge mark this spot as the entrance to Clear Fork Park. Continue southwest. Native trees line both sides of the trail, keeping the path in partial shade for most of the hike. Sunflowers bloom alongside the trail, and butterflies flutter across the path. Trail traffic is light, though cyclists occasionally pass. Many are kids accompanied by parents, and all respect the signs and cruise at low speeds. Once they've disappeared around the bend, you may find yourself completely alone again, with only the chirping of birds for company. Just when you've begun to wonder where the trail is going, pass a sign indicating that a rest area is 1 mile farther up the trail. The trail winds slowly here, passing more oak trees and wildflowers.

At 0.63 mile, cross a bridge. Continuing straight, the trail passes a ranch on the right, where donkeys and horses sometimes linger by the fence. At 1.58 miles, you'll see a footbridge off to the left. Turn left and cross the bridge. (If you were to continue straight, you'd reach the Pecan Valley Park parking area, just 0.1 mile farther down the trail. In front of the parking lot there, you'll find a kiosk with a detailed map of the entire trail network.)

The small bridge spans a wide creek with pretty green water. As I crossed the bridge, I spotted a beautiful great blue heron perched on a log downstream stalking fish. Wishing I had brought my binoculars, I watched him for a few minutes, until the huge bird spread his wings and took off with a few elegant strokes. I later found out from the Texas Parks and Wildlife website that several herons nest in the area, and it is not unusual to see them.

Across the bridge are a few narrow posts and a gate. Walk through the gate and onto the dirt trail. Within a few steps, reach a junction; take the trail to your left, which runs closest to the creek. Ahead, you'll see a lovely grove of tall trees, so unexpectedly picturesque that you'll feel as if you've just crossed a bridge into another world. After passing through the grove, you'll see a small fence to the right marking the boundary of a golf course. About 300 feet down the dirt trail, find the Memorial Oak, a huge bur oak tree. Listed on the Texas Big Tree Registry, sponsored by the Texas Forest Service, this tree boasts recorded dimensions of 81 feet tall by 18 feet around. After you're done admiring the tree, have lunch at the picnic tables a couple hundred feet farther up the trail, behind the grove. Then retrace your steps to the trailhead.

NEARBY ACTIVITIES

The Fort Worth Zoo, which is home to primates, cheetahs, and the Komodo dragon, among other species, is only 8 miles away. Check **fortworthzoo.com** for special events and hours. To get there, take Oakmont Boulevard east 2 miles, then turn left onto South Hulen Street and drive 3 miles. Turn right onto Bellaire Drive South, which becomes West Berry Street. Turn left onto South University Drive and bear right onto Colonial Parkway.

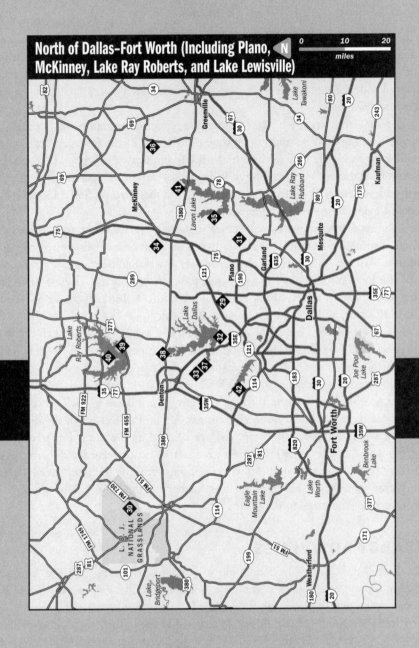

North of Dallas–Fort Worth (Including Plano, McKinney, Lake Ray Roberts, and Lake Lewisville)

29 Arbor Hills Loop 139

30 Black Creek–Cottonwood Hiking Trail 143

31 Breckenridge Park Trail 147

32 Cicada–Cottonwood Loop 151

33 Elm Fork Trail 155

34 Erwin Park Loop 159

35 Lavon Lake: Trinity Trail 163

36 Parkhill Prairie Trail 167

37 Pilot Knoll Trail 171

38 Ray Roberts Greenbelt 175

39 Ray Roberts Lake State Park, Isle du Bois Unit:
    Lost Pines Trail 179

40 Ray Roberts Lake State Park, Johnson Branch
    Unit: Johnson Branch Trail 183

41 Sister Grove Loop 187

42 Walnut Grove Trail 191

NORTH OF DALLAS-FORT WORTH
(INCLUDING PLANO, McKINNEY, LAKE RAY ROBERTS, AND LAKE LEWISVILLE)

29 ARBOR HILLS LOOP

KEY AT-A-GLANCE INFORMATION

LENGTH: 2.3 miles

CONFIGURATION: Loop

DIFFICULTY: Easy–moderate

SCENERY: Blackland prairie, riparian forest, upland forest

EXPOSURE: Partially shady

TRAIL TRAFFIC: Heavy

TRAIL SURFACE: Paved path

HIKING TIME: 55 minutes

ACCESS: Free; open daily, 5 a.m.–11 p.m.

FACILITIES: Restrooms, water fountains, picnic tables, playground

WHEELCHAIR TRAVERSABLE: Yes

SPECIAL COMMENTS: Dogs are allowed but must be leashed.

SUPPLEMENTAL MAPS: pdf.plano .gov/parks/AHNPPedestrian NaturalSurfaceTrailSystem.pdf

DRIVING DISTANCE FROM MAJOR INTERSECTION: 2 miles from Plano Parkway and Midway Road

GPS TRAILHEAD COORDINATES

Latitude: N 33° 2' 51"
Longitude: W 96° 50' 55"

IN BRIEF

Popular with young families, this trail winds its way slowly uphill, moving from wetland to prairie to forest before looping back to the beginning. On any sunny weekend, you'll find the trails bustling with families.

DESCRIPTION

In West Plano, the 200-acre Arbor Hills Nature Preserve is laid out in three sections: Blackland Prairie, Upland Forest, and Riparian Forest. On any given weekend you'll find the parking lot busy. Most visitors—young parents strapping their kids into strollers and young professionals leashing their dogs—are regulars who live in the area, already have their favorite routes in mind, and disappear down the trail within seconds. For newcomers, a map at the trailhead describes the three zones, offering a wealth of information for the nature maven, including the types of trees and animals you can find in each zone, and displays a map of the entire trail network. In addition to the paved trail, Arbor Hills boasts some primitive nature trails. These dirt trails are unstructured and their access points unmarked, disappearing into the woods at various spots along the main paved trail.

The trailhead is inside the pavilion and picnic shelter adjacent to the parking lot. Follow the paved trail south through the pavilion and past the playground toward West Parker Road. The trail quickly loops back north, head-

- -

Directions —————————————————➤

Take the Dallas Tollway north to the Parker Road exit. Turn left onto West Parker Road. Arbor Hill Nature Preserve is a mile ahead on the right, just past Midway Road.

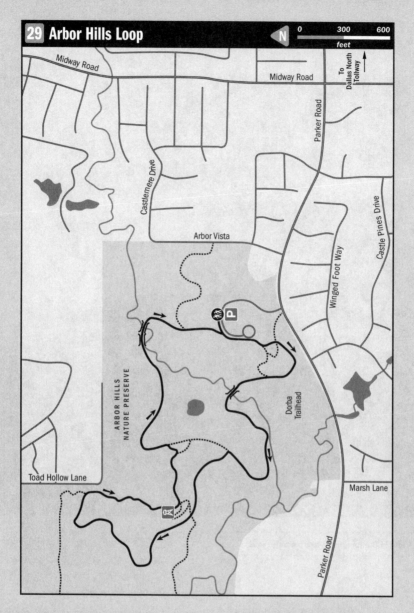

N

0   300   600
feet

Midway Road

Midway Road

To Dallas North Tollway

Parker Road

Castlemere Drive

Castle Pines Drive

Arbor Vista

Winged Foot Way

ARBOR HILLS NATURE PRESERVE

Dorba Trailhead

Toad Hollow Lane

Marsh Lane

Parker Road

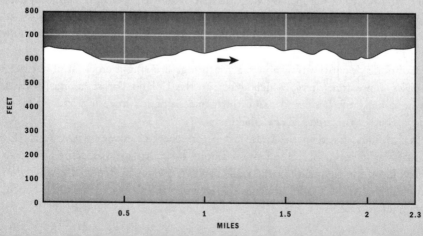

FEET

800
700
600
500
400
300
200
100
0

0.5   1   1.5   2   2.3

MILES

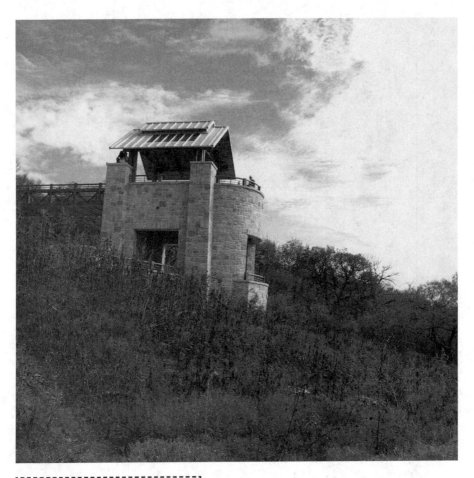

View of the lookout tower from the trail

ing into the Riparian Forest habitat. Mountain bikers are welcome here, but they do not pose a nuisance—most head straight for the DORBA (Dallas Off-Road Bicycle Association) trail. At about 0.2 mile, pass that trailhead, which diverges into the brush to the left.

Continue down the trail and reach a bridge crossing a creek at about 0.35 mile. The dense trees here, which make up the Upland Forest habitat, form a relaxing canopy of shade and make this a nice spot for lingering and trying to identify some of the area's avian inhabitants.

A little farther down the trail, just before the tree cover gives way to sky, you'll pass a huge bur oak tree nestled among other hardwoods. Keep an eye to the ground on the right side of the trail. You'll know you've reached it when you see its golf-ball-sized acorns littering the ground; if you reach the stone bench, you've gone too far.

As you continue, the trees thin and the trail winds into the Blackland Prairie zone. This type of prairie, which is quickly disappearing because of urbanization, takes its name from its rich black clay soils. The prairie consists of tall grasses such as little bluestem, a bunchgrass that grows 2–4 feet tall. Wildflowers, such as Mexican hat, a pretty red wildflower with a distinctive long, cone-shaped head; black-eyed Susan, a sunny yellow wildflower with a domelike head; and the blue-bonnet, Texas's state flower, abound. In the fall, when the flowers aren't in bloom, the prairie is a dark mass of brittle yellow grasses that look black from a distance, thanks in part to the hundreds of spent flower heads. Visitors can often be seen here wandering the trails, entranced by the rippling of the tall grasses in the wind. The sun in this exposed area can be brutal in the summer, but you soon reenter forest just up the trail.

At 0.68 mile, you'll reach a junction where you should turn left, heading uphill alongside the prairie. Another junction, at 0.83 mile, leads to a tower over-looking the preserve; the trail you're on climbs to the tower the back way, so continue on this path, bypassing the turnoff. The trail continues, leaving the prairie behind as it heads slightly uphill, past wildflowers and into a forest of tall trees. To the right in the distance, you'll see apartment complexes abutting the edge of the preserve.

At 1.5 miles, reach the lookout tower. You'll usually find a few people at its railings enjoying the breeze and the views of the landscape. You'll also have a bird's-eye view of the trail you just came up.

Back on the trail, you'll head through the forest, following the path as it winds slowly downhill. The trail easily accommodates wheelchairs, and alongside the hikers, dog walkers, and joggers, I encountered a couple of folks in wheel-chairs, happily enjoying the outdoors. I also couldn't help but notice that the preserve's smooth, gentle slopes lured a surprising number of new and young parents, who were enjoying a nature walk and a workout as they pulled toddlers in little red wagons uphill or pushed strollers and baby carriages downhill.

At 1.63 miles, you'll find a wheelchair-access point. Head left, following the trail another 100 feet to a turnoff, on which you should again head left. Cross a couple of bridges, then, at 1.98 miles, come to a trail split where you'll bear right. Heading south now, reach the parking lot and trailhead from the other end.

NEARBY ACTIVITIES

Southfork Ranch, made famous on the TV show *Dallas,* lies just to the west of Plano. Its magnificent white mansion served as the home of the show's infamous J. R. Ewing from 1978 to 1991. The ranch was opened to the public in 1985 and continues to offer daily tours of the mansion and grounds. Visit **southfork.com** for more information. To get there from Arbor Hills, go east 15 miles down Parker Road toward Lavon Lake. Turn right onto Hogge Road.

30 BLACK CREEK-COTTONWOOD HIKING TRAIL

KEY AT-A-GLANCE INFORMATION

LENGTH: 9.58 miles

CONFIGURATION: Out-and-back

DIFFICULTY: Moderate

SCENERY: Grasslands, woodlands, small lakes

EXPOSURE: Partially sunny

TRAIL TRAFFIC: Light

TRAIL SURFACE: Dirt

HIKING TIME: 4.5 hours

ACCESS: $2 day-use fee; open daily

FACILITIES: Pit toilet, picnic tables

WHEELCHAIR TRAVERSABLE: No

SPECIAL COMMENTS: There is no water at either recreation area. Pack a lunch, plenty of water, and insect repellent.

SUPPLEMENTAL MAPS: fs.usda.gov/Internet/FSE_DOCUMENTS/stelprdb5302850.pdf

DRIVING DISTANCE FROM MAJOR INTERSECTION: 34 miles from the I-35W–I-35E split

GPS TRAILHEAD COORDINATES

Latitude: N 33° 20' 42"
Longitude: W 97° 35' 42"

IN BRIEF

This long day hike explores the wild, grassy woodlands between the small Black Creek and Cottonwood lakes of the LBJ National Grasslands. Although the bulk of the trail is open woodland, you will pass through many small pockets of sunny grassland as you make your way north.

DESCRIPTION

One of only 20 national grasslands in the country managed by the USDA Forest Service, the Caddo–Lyndon B. Johnson (LBJ) National Grasslands consists of close to 40,000 acres of land. The grasslands are divided into two sections: the Caddo section, northeast of the Metroplex, and the LBJ section, northwest of the Metroplex.

The Caddo is slightly smaller than the LBJ and comprises a few recreational areas at Lake Coffee Mill and Lake Davy Crockett—small lakes built in the 1930s, when the land for the preserve was acquired. Its trails are popular with equestrians. The LBJ is a hiking hub. Not only does it have a 75-mile multiuse trail system accessible from its main campsite, TADRA Point, it also has a 4-mile hiking trail

---

Directions

From Decatur, take US 287/TX 81 North and turn right at the rest area onto County Road 2175, heading east. Cross the railroad tracks and turn left, heading north on Old Decatur Road. After about 4 miles, turn right onto CR 2372, heading east. Turn left, heading north on CR 2461, then make another left onto FS 902, following it to the entrance of the Black Creek Recreational Area. Parking is on the left, adjacent to the lake.

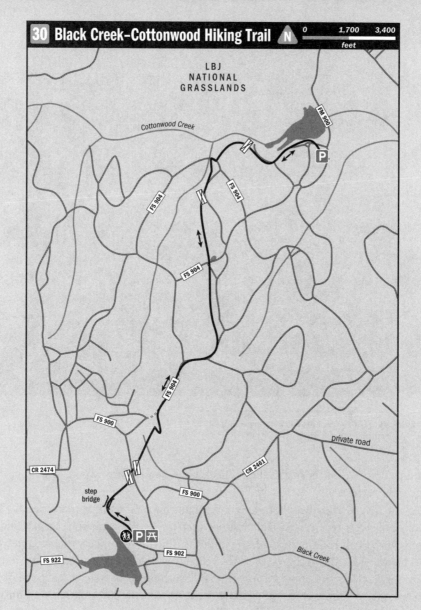

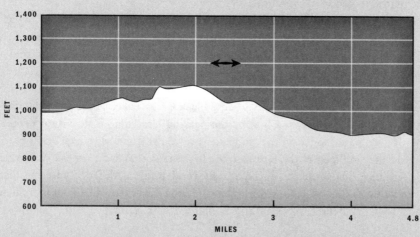

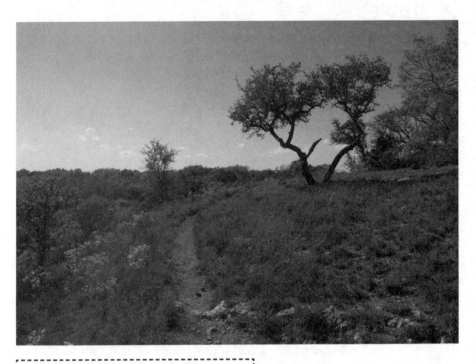

Enjoy stunning views of the surrounding countryside.

connecting two of its small lakes—Black Creek and Cottonwood. This hike features the latter trail.

Be aware that there are designated hunting seasons in the grasslands. The trail, however, receives enough visitors that, as long as you stay on designated trails and aren't rooting through the underbrush, you're unlikely to encounter any problems. The USDA Forest Service recommends that if you're hiking during hunting season, you should wear colorful clothing to be safe. Check the Texas Parks and Wildlife website (**tpwd.state.tx.us**) for specific information on hunting-season dates, which vary by animal.

It's a long drive down a remote, primarily gravel road to the trailhead, which is in the Black Creek Recreational Area. Although you'll feel like you're driving to a secluded, little-visited place, if you visit on a weekend you'll be surprised to find a fair number of folks at the rec area, which attracts a lively mixture of hikers, equestrians, hunters, and campers. I also noticed quite a few local teenagers who drove up for the day to splash around the 30-acre Black Creek Lake. There is a small day-use fee; drop your money in a box by the parking lot. There is no visitor center, office, or even park ranger on site, so make sure you've come with exact change.

Find the trailhead at the entrance to the recreational area, on the right side of the entrance road and just behind a large wooden sign with faded lettering that identifies this as Black Creek–Cottonwood Hiking Trail 901. The trail is hidden in the shrubbery behind the sign and is marked with a smaller "901" signpost.

There are markers at regular intervals along the trail, so if you're ever in doubt at a junction, look for that number to get you back on the right track.

The trail heads northwest through thickets and shrubbery occasionally interspersed with small, sunny clearings filled with prairie grasses. On this hike, you won't find the expansive grasslands you might envision when you hear the term "national grassland." Instead, this trail traverses a number of small clearings with tall grasses that harbor butterflies, crickets, and dragonflies, all of which emerge to greet you as you pass.

At 0.35 mile, reach a split where you'll bear right. The trail becomes rough, with a couple of short, steep, rocky grades before it reaches another junction. Bear right and cross the barbed-wire fence by going over the small step bridge intended to keep horseback riders out of the developed recreational area. At 0.75 mile, bear left. The trail becomes wider, following an old, partially overgrown park road enclosed by light woodlands. Pass through a few small patches of grassland that are quietly being overtaken by shrubs and small trees. White-tailed deer, cottontail rabbits, wild turkeys, and coyotes are all commonly found here. If you're not lucky enough to catch sight of these creatures, you're likely to spot their tracks in the loose dirt of the trail.

As you hike, you'll find a series of metal gates along the trail, separating tracts of land. Pass the first of these at 0.95 mile, where you bear right to head north just after you go through the gate. Bypass the next gate, keeping straight. At 1.35 miles, bear right and climb the steep grade to the top of the hill; the trail here has been severely eroded, so a hiking stick would be useful. This is one of the highest points on the trail, and at the top you'll find a pleasant breeze and a nice view. The path rounds the ridge, then emerges onto the hilltop—a grassy plain with a dirt park road passing through it. The road is used but not busy; this is the route you'd take if you were to drive to Cottonwood Lake. It's also the hiking route, and as you walk along you'll see the "901" trail markers.

Head straight (north) on the dirt road, then turn right onto the gravel road at 1.55 miles. It's sunny and hot in this section, but a cool breeze and the flat road make for fast, easy hiking. Bypass a small half-loop in the road where you may see campers or RVers; turn left at 2.3 miles. A few trails join in this section, and it can be hard to figure out which one you should take—just stay on the road until you see the dirt trail just off the road to the left at 2.45 miles; the "901" signpost marks it. Turn onto the dirt path and then bear right at the next junction.

At 3 miles, turn left onto a wide, flat trail. TADRA Point, which has a huge multiuse trail system popular with equestrians, is just to your right. (TADRA stands for the Texas Arabian Distance Riders Association, a horse club that worked closely with the Forest Service to develop the campsite and trail system.) The trails are color-coded, and as you hike you'll see signs pointing the way to the Blue, Yellow, and Red trails. Bypass all turnoffs, cross the road, and pass through another metal gate at 3.45 miles. Bear right, descending through cactus and shrubs, then turn left through a wide grassland. At the next junction, bear right again.

Pass through another gate at 4.1 miles. Here the trail winds through a thicker mixture of trees and underbrush before finally emerging at Cottonwood Lake. Although the lake is only 40 acres, you'll still see a fair amount of activity, including ducks and egrets along its marshy edges, fishermen settled onto its sandy banks, and possibly a boat or two sitting quietly on the lake's edge. Walk along the shoreline until you reach the shady parking area. If you're planning to eat lunch here, make sure you've brought along a picnic blanket to lay out on the grassy banks of the lake—besides the boat launch and parking area, you won't find any picnic tables or other facilities at this end of the trail. From here, retrace your steps to the trailhead.

NEARBY ACTIVITIES

Head 10 miles south to Decatur for a burger at the Whistle Stop Cafe, a lunchroom dating to 1929. It's part of the Texas Tourist Camp Complex, designated a Texas Historical Landmark in 1995. The complex also includes the Petrified Wood Gas Station and some cabins that, until the 1960s, were popular among travelers. There are even unsubstantiated rumors that Bonnie and Clyde may have stayed here. To reach the complex, take US 287/81 South back into Decatur and turn left on US 380 Business. The cafe is about 0.5 mile ahead on the right.

BRECKENRIDGE PARK TRAIL

IN BRIEF

This scenic trail winds through a beautiful city park and offers excellent birding, a picturesque lake, and innumerable scenic spots where you can stop and enjoy a picnic lunch.

DESCRIPTION

As far as paved trails go, this one, at Breckenridge Park in Richardson, is one of my favorites. It offers something new around every turn, has tons of birdlife, and offers surprisingly scenic paths. The trails are meticulously maintained and landscaped to preserve a wild and natural feel. For example, instead of planting one small tree for shade, the park plants many trees in natural clusters and groves. In the springtime, instead of putting in rows of planted flowers, sections of grass alongside the trail are left unmowed to allow colorful wildflowers to sprout. The cumulative result is that when you hike here, you feel one step removed from the stresses of urban life—and yet not so removed that you'll have to do anything other than slip on a pair of comfortable shoes.

The 417-acre park consists of a small lake, pavilions, a playground, and 12 (yes, 12)

KEY AT-A-GLANCE INFORMATION

LENGTH: 3.27 miles

CONFIGURATION: Loop

DIFFICULTY: Easy

SCENERY: Creek, lawns, lake, woodlands, birds

EXPOSURE: Partially shaded–sunny

TRAIL TRAFFIC: Moderate

TRAIL SURFACE: Paved

HIKING TIME: 1.5 hours

ACCESS: Free

FACILITIES: Toilets, picnic tables, water fountains, playground

WHEELCHAIR TRAVERSABLE: Yes

SPECIAL COMMENTS: Great option for those with younger kids

DRIVING DISTANCE FROM MAJOR INTERSECTION: 5.2 miles from TX 190 and US 75

Directions

The park is at 3300 Brand Rd. in Richardson. To get there, follow US 75 North and take Exit 28B (President George Bush Turnpike). Go 1.8 miles to the Renner Road exit, and turn left onto East Renner Road. Go 3 miles, then turn right onto Brand Road. Follow the signs to Breckenridge Park Parking Lot A. Park on the northern side of the soccer fields, in the lot adjacent to the toilets. (The entrance to the soccer field is down a one-way road; you'll see the parking area and toilets just in front of it, on your left).

GPS TRAILHEAD COORDINATES

Latitude: N 32° 59' 51"

Longitude: W 96° 37' 44"

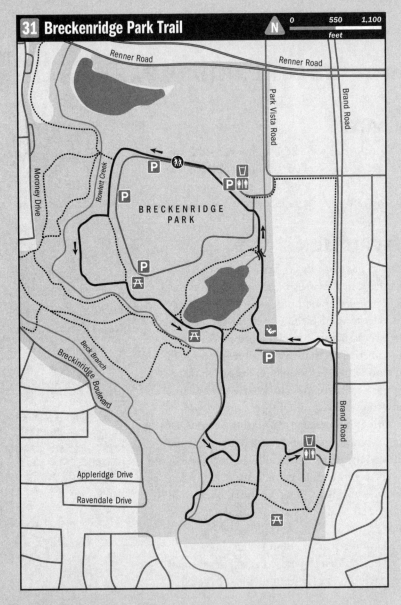

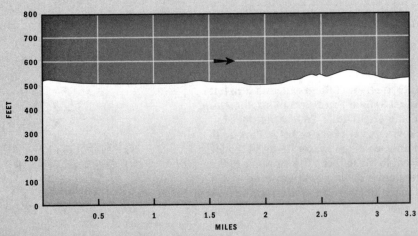

soccer fields—although you won't see much of them, except at the very beginning and end of the hike. The trails are popular with bikers, hikers, and explorers of all ages. The park is also well known throughout Richardson as the site of its annual Fourth of July celebration.

Pick up the trail just across the road from the restrooms and parking area. The trail descends gently, just low enough that the soccer fields to your left are blocked by a grassy hillside. Bypass the first turnoff, where you'll see a bridge to your right, and continue straight until you reach the turnoff at 0.33 mile. Turn right at this junction and follow the trail as it makes a half-loop detour into the woodlands bordering Rowlett Creek. When you turn down the path, you'll see the creek just to your right, its waters rushing and gurgling loudly as it cuts a wide swath through a pretty rock bank. The dense foliage in this loop keeps the temperature a few degrees cooler than the rest of the trail and attracts not only hikers but also birds, who chirp and whistle loudly in the surrounding trees. As you near the end of the half-loop, you'll pass a picturesque picnic area beneath a grove of tall trees on your left.

Back on the trail, turn right, heading southeast. The open path winds ahead of you, offering a clear view straight ahead to the central part of the park, where you'll see crisp, green, neatly mowed lawns punctuated by clumps of trees. To your right are the thick woodlands surrounding the creek that abuts the western edge of the park; they have been left undeveloped, and you can see lots of birds along this stretch. Bring binoculars so you'll have an easier time identifying them.

To your left is the mowed, grassy slope that hides the soccer fields above. As you pass the southern edge of the soccer fields, the park's small lake comes into view ahead of you. A green expanse of lawn leads down to its grassy shore—an ideal spot for laying out a blanket for a picnic. Across the water are a pavilion, a small bridge, and a thick grove of trees. Benches along the trail allow you to relax and enjoy the beauty of this scenic spot.

The path turns slightly southeast. Stay to the right at each trail junction you pass in order to get into the very southern portion of the park. On your way, the trail curls lazily through a beautiful, open, parklike setting. When you enter a huge grove of tall trees dotted with picnic tables and benches, you'll know you're nearing the park's southern boundary. The trail then loops back east and north alongside the grove. Again, stay to the right at any trail junctions you pass.

The path then takes you uphill and past a pavilion and parking area. Follow the route past the restrooms, and you'll soon find yourself atop a rise overlooking the park. For the first time on the hike, you have a glimpse of the soccer fields as the trail traverses the eastern edge of the southern field grouping before it cuts west, past another parking area, and heads back downhill toward the lake and playground. Stay to the right at each junction, passing the pavilion and crossing the bridge. On the other side, bear right; the trail winds around a final curve, then presents you with the northern section of soccer fields where you started the hike.

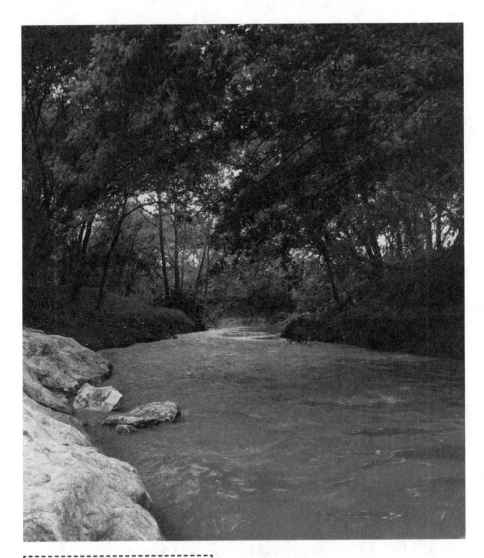

Rowlett Creek rushes past a rocky bank.

Follow the trail to the 3-mile point and turn left onto the redbrick path, which will take you back to the parking area.

NEARBY ACTIVITIES

If you feel like shopping, don't miss the popular Allen Premium Outlet Mall—a collection of about 100 upscale retail outlet stores, including Eddie Bauer, Kenneth Cole, Anne Klein, DKNY, and Tommy Hilfiger. The mall is only 13 miles away in nearby Allen. To get there, head north on US 75 and take Exit 37 toward Stacy Road, where you'll turn left and see the mall.

CICADA-COTTONWOOD LOOP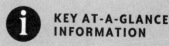

IN BRIEF

Hike through the woods to an overlook with a view of the wetlands, where a camouflaged blind allows for bird-watching. The trail's highlight is a restored pioneer cabin from the 1850s, complete with period furnishings.

DESCRIPTION

The 2,000-acre Lewisville Lake Environmental Learning Area (LLELA) is adjacent to the southern shore of Lewisville Lake, opposite the lake's dam. A Federal Wildlife Management Area, LLELA offers a variety of activities, including primitive camping, canoeing, kayaking, fishing, and hiking. The area also offers guided tours of its bison herd on the last Sunday of the month for an additional $2; if you're interested, call ahead at (972) 219-3930 or (972) 219-7980 to confirm tour times. The bison are in a separate enclosure, so there is no worry of being confronted by an errant bull while hiking.

Operated by a consortium of local universities, the city of Lewisville, and the Lewisville Independent School District, LLELA is involved in ongoing research and education programs, including prairie restoration, wetland research, and water retention. A number of graduate theses and dissertations have also focused on the habitat and ecology of LLELA and the surrounding lake area.

Directions

Follow I-35E north toward Denton and take Exit 454A toward 407/Justin. Turn right onto East Jones Street. The LLELA entrance is at the end of Jones, at the intersection with North Kealy Street. To get to the trailhead, follow the road from the entrance booth to the first parking area on your right.

KEY AT-A-GLANCE INFORMATION

LENGTH: 1.7 miles

CONFIGURATION: Loop

DIFFICULTY: Easy

SCENERY: Woods, wetlands, interpretive signs, pioneer log cabin

EXPOSURE: Shady–sunny

TRAIL TRAFFIC: Light

TRAIL SURFACE: Packed dirt

HIKING TIME: 45 minutes

ACCESS: $5 per person, cash only; children under age 5 free; November 1–March 1: Friday–Sunday, 7 a.m.–5 p.m.; March 2–October 31: Friday–Sunday, 7 a.m.–7 p.m.

FACILITIES: Toilet, picnic tables, benches

WHEELCHAIR TRAVERSABLE: No

SPECIAL COMMENTS: Bring binoculars and spend some time scoping the wetlands.

SUPPLEMENTAL MAPS: ias.unt.edu/llela/assets/documents/trail_brochure.pdf

DRIVING DISTANCE FROM MAJOR INTERSECTION: 8 miles from I-35E and TX 121

GPS TRAILHEAD COORDINATES

Latitude: N 33° 3' 56"

Longitude: W 96° 58' 31"

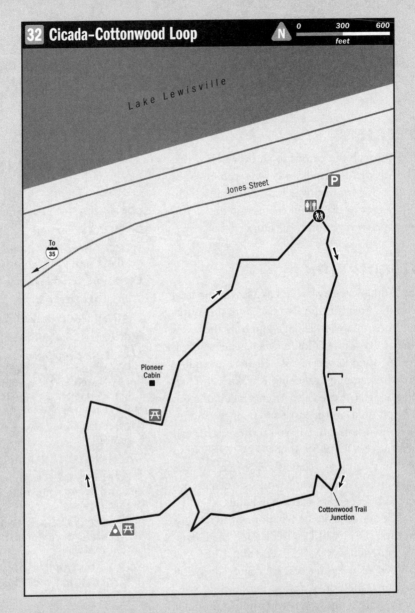

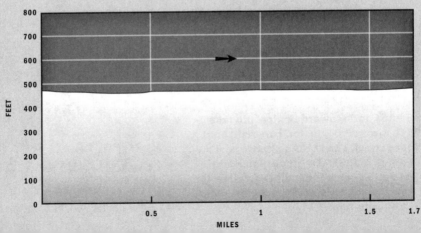

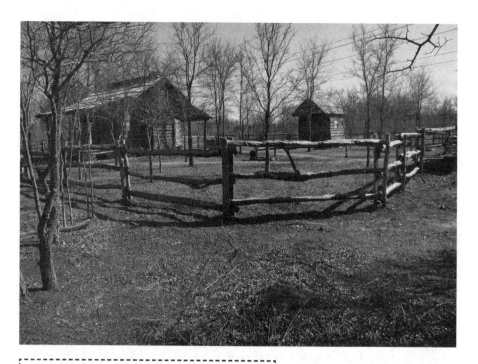

A restored pioneer cabin from the 1850s abuts the trail.

At the LLELA entrance, someone in the small booth will collect your admission fee and give you a pamphlet that includes a small map of the grounds. The hike starts on Cicada Trail, just to the south of the parking area and behind the Cicada Pavilion picnic tables. A small sign marks the trailhead.

Cicada Trail is a self-guided nature trail that meanders south through the woods and past signs describing the foliage, including cedar elm, coralberry, elderberry, and bois d'arc. The signs are actually quite descriptive, so plan on setting aside extra time along this section if you intend to read each marker.

Turn left at the trail junction at 0.33 mile. To the left, catch glimpses through the trees of a river that helps make the path a good place to spot birds. Year-round birds such as the red-winged blackbird, the northern cardinal, and the Carolina chickadee are regularly spotted in the area.

At 0.4 mile, bear right at the split. Pass another interpretive sign; just beyond this, the trail splits. To the left, the trail ends at a lookout over a gully. Bear right and follow the trail downhill. It emerges from woods, then joins the wide Cottonwood Trail. Head right to take Cottonwood Trail, following the road as it heads west.

Pass a group of picnic tables abutting a narrow creek at 0.83 mile. Snakes such as the southern copperhead and the western cottonmouth are commonly spotted in the surrounding habitat. Although I haven't seen any, remind younger hikers to be cautious when traipsing off-trail through tall grass or dense underbrush.

Continuing down the road, reach a camouflaged lookout over the surrounding wetlands. The pavilion is nicely shielded, allowing you to view the wetland wildlife unnoticed. A peek through the netting on my hike revealed dozens of ducks resting peacefully on the calm waters. Keep an eye out for other common birds, including the great blue heron, the great egret, and the smaller snowy egret.

Heading back down the trail, the marsh stays within sight to the left, with small trees and shrubs to the right. You're likely to spot gulls, turkey vultures, and red-tailed hawks circling overhead. Power lines briefly cross the path, reminding you of civilization. Just a few feet past the towers, however, the present is forgotten and you're instantly transported into the past as an old log cabin comes into view amid woods on your right. The cabin is surrounded by a few other log buildings and suggests what life must have been like on the North Texas prairie in the pioneer days. A log fence encloses the complex.

The cabin, built in the 1850s, originally belonged to a local resident. It was donated and transported to LLELA, where it has since been carefully restored to create a pioneer setting. The house sports original period furnishings and has a separate garden and smokehouse out back. The buildings are all made of logs and insulated with packed mud. As you explore, don't be surprised if you see the remnants of ashes in the pit of the smokehouse—it has even been put to use to roast a pig at a recent LLELA event! From here, head 0.3 mile back down the road to finish the trail loop and reach the trailhead.

NEARBY ACTIVITIES

If you're looking for a change of pace after the hike, stop by Vista Ridge Mall, only 6 miles away. It has a few large department stores, such as Macy's, Sears, Dillard's, JCPenney, and dozens of smaller gift shops and boutiques. There are also a number of eateries in and around the mall. To get there, follow I-35E south 3.5 miles, and take Exit 448B. Turn left onto East Round Grove Road.

ELM FORK TRAIL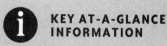

IN BRIEF

Explore a historic bridge associated with tales of spooky hauntings, then enjoy a pleasant hike through the woods.

DESCRIPTION

The trailhead for this hike is in Old Alton Bridge Park, just outside Denton near the town of Copper Canyon. The park houses the historic Old Alton Bridge—not only well known for its historical importance but also notorious for its much-researched paranormal activity.

The bridge is just west of the parking lot. Built in 1884, it was added to the National Register of Historic Places in July 1988. More recently, Denton's population growth has prompted the creation of a new bridge for motor traffic; this new route bypasses the narrow, iron-truss, one-lane, wood-planked Old Alton Bridge, which is now open only to pedestrian and equestrian traffic.

From the parking lot, the trail splits, heading southeast (left) and southwest (right). If you go right, you'll cross the bridge and head south, eventually joining Pilot Knoll Trail, which descends toward Pilot Knoll Park. The hike described here does not cross the bridge in that direction, but rather follows the trail on the left. But before heading down the trail, take a detour to check out the bridge. Local legend holds that it's haunted, and it has

KEY AT-A-GLANCE INFORMATION

LENGTH: 3.8 miles

CONFIGURATION: Out-and-back

DIFFICULTY: Moderate

SCENERY: Historic bridge, marshy banks of lake, woods

EXPOSURE: Partially shady–sunny

TRAIL TRAFFIC: Moderate

TRAIL SURFACE: Dirt

HIKING TIME: 1.5 hours

ACCESS: Daily; free

FACILITIES: Picnic tables

WHEELCHAIR TRAVERSABLE: No

SPECIAL COMMENTS: Bring water; there are no drinking fountains. Avoid this trail after rainstorms, as the latter portion of the trail can stay muddy for days.

SUPPLEMENTAL MAPS: www.swf-wc.usace.army.mil/ lewisville/images/Elm_Fork_Pilot _Knoll_Public_Map1.pdf

DRIVING DISTANCE FROM MAJOR INTERSECTION: 8 miles from the I-35E–I-35W split

Directions

From I-35E, exit onto Swisher Road and head west about 3 miles. Just after Swisher Road becomes Teasley Road/FM 2181, turn left onto Old Alton Road. The entrance to Old Alton Bridge Park is down a steep driveway to your left, just before you cross the bridge.

GPS TRAILHEAD COORDINATES

Latitude: N 33° 7' 46"

Longitude: W 97° 6' 14"

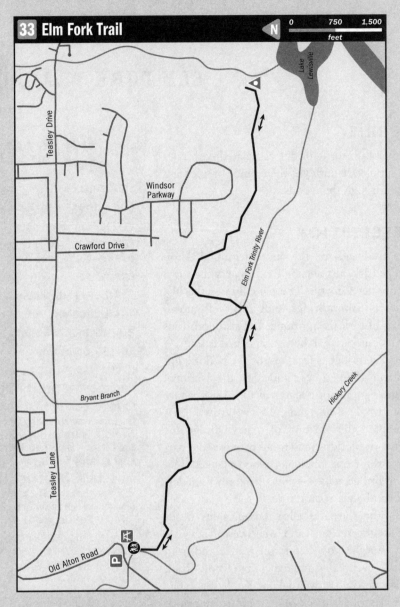

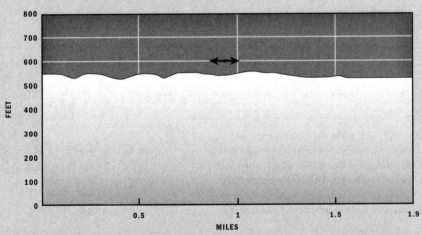

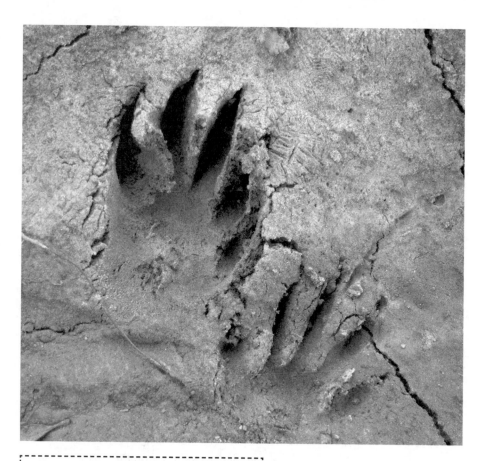

Evidence of wildlife is easily visible after a rainstorm.

become a favorite spot for thrill-seekers, especially at Halloween. Those who know the legends will sometimes refer to it as Goatman's Bridge. There are several versions of the story, but essentially they all involve a man who was killed on the bridge and comes back as a creature that is half-man and half-goat. Some accounts say he was a goatherd; others say the man lost his head and now has to wear a goat's. Most accounts say that if you honk your horn two or three times (depending on the story), you'll see the goat-man in the distance. The legends attract not only local kids but also paranormal investigators, many of whom have posted photos and reports of their investigations online.

When you're done checking out the bridge, go back to the parking lot and then left down Elm Fork Trail. The wide path travels south through an open grassy plain toward a wood on the horizon, then turns east. Butterflies, dragon-flies, and crickets buzz past, hopping and flying out of your path. A few narrow trails branch off the main trail to your right, leading to fishing spots at the creek's edge. Stay on the main trail, bypassing all turnoffs. The trail eventually reaches the trees and cuts a wide path through them, keeping you clear of any shade they might cast. To your left, a wire fence partially hidden beneath vines and mesquite trees marks the outer perimeter of a ranch where cows graze lazily in their sunny pasture, watching you as you pass. You'll traverse more grassland, which is punctuated by thin groves of short trees, before reaching a creek crossing. The trail stewards have layered blocks along the creek's banks here to prevent erosion and allow hikers to step across easily without getting their feet wet.

On the other side of the creek, you'll find less grass and more trees growing closer to the trail. A lush green understory provides dense pockets of shade. Birds are much more prevalent on this side of the creek as well, and you'll hear them whistling and chirping in the background, though spotting them in the trees is fairly difficult.

The flatness of the first half of the trail is soon replaced by slight hills, and the trees give way to shrubby grassland dotted with junipers before you finally reach another creek. Continue past it and you'll soon start to hear the sounds of civilization; then, with some abruptness, the trail is interrupted by new road and bridge construction. At the time I hiked, the trail was still open at this point, offering access to the sandy lakeshore under the new bridge, where you can take in the views and the breezes before retracing your steps to the trailhead. Before you visit, note that access here may be limited due to the ongoing construction, but don't let that discourage you from this trail—it's a pleasant outing and hike, regardless of whether or not you can actually reach the lake.

NEARBY ACTIVITIES

Visit Denton's historic town square, where you can often find musicians performing. The square's focal point is the old County Courthouse, which dates back to 1896. Restaurants, art galleries, boutiques, and other retail shops offer shopping and dining. To get there, take I-35E south about 1.5 miles, exit at US 377/Fort Worth Drive, and then turn right onto West Hickory Street.

ERWIN PARK LOOP

IN BRIEF

This easy trail leads you through open meadows as it loops in and out of the woods and
through the preserve. Enjoy colorful wildflower displays in the spring and a variety of
birdlife year-round.

DESCRIPTION

The 212-acre Erwin Park is a McKinney city
park in a somewhat rural area surrounded by
ranchlands, just north of Dallas–Fort Worth.
Donated in 1971 to the Texas Conservation
Foundation by the Erwin family, the land has
belonged to the city of McKinney since 1973
and has been developed into a large park with
much of its natural area preserved. It even
offers overnight camping; call (972) 547-2690
to make reservations.

The park's trails, maintained by the Dallas Off-Road Bicycle Association (DORBA),
include about 8 miles of path through meadows and woodlands. The trails are narrow,
and you'll have to step aside to let bikers pass;
however, a lot of this hike travels through
open, tree-studded meadows, and you'll have
no problem seeing the bikers as they approach.
The trail traffic varies, and there are times

Directions ⟶

Follow US 75 north toward McKinney. Take
Exit 41 toward US 380/Greenville/Denton.
Turn left onto West University Drive/US 380E
and go 2.5 miles, then turn right onto FM 1461
and travel 2 miles. Turn right onto CR 164, go
about 1 mile, then turn left onto CR 1006. The
entrance to Erwin Park is on the right. Inside
the park, turn left at the end of the road and
park in the second lot, next to the pavilion
and picnic area. The trailhead, on the right, is
marked by a kiosk.

KEY AT-A-GLANCE INFORMATION

LENGTH: 2.6 miles

CONFIGURATION: Loop

DIFFICULTY: Easy

SCENERY: Meadows, woodlands

EXPOSURE: Partially shady–sunny

TRAIL TRAFFIC: Moderate

TRAIL SURFACE: Dirt

HIKING TIME: 1 hour

ACCESS: Free; open daily,
8 a.m.–10 p.m.

FACILITIES: Toilet (closed in winter),
picnic tables, water fountain

WHEELCHAIR TRAVERSABLE: No

SPECIAL COMMENTS: This hike can
easily be extended with a second
loop.

**DRIVING DISTANCE FROM MAJOR
INTERSECTION:** 6 miles from
North Central Expressway and
West University Drive

GPS TRAILHEAD COORDINATES

Latitude: N 33° 15' 19"

Longitude: W 96° 39' 18"

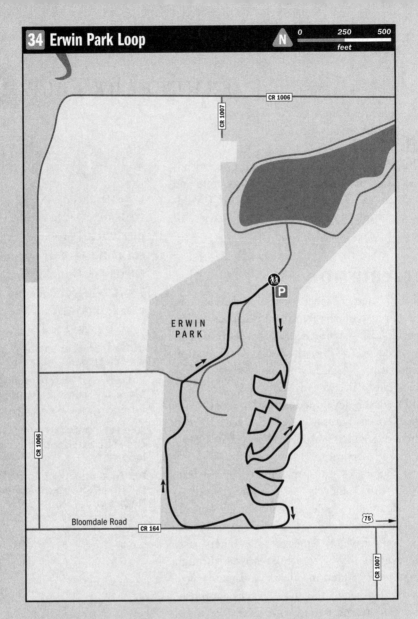

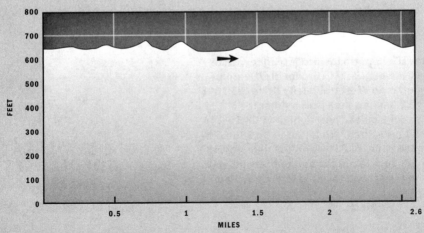

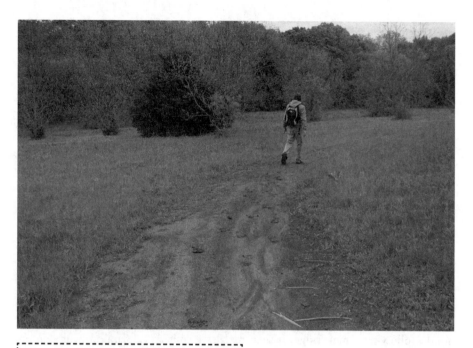

A hiker makes his way through a sunny meadow.

when you can come here and find no one else on the trail at all. I visited on a slightly overcast weekend morning to find the pavilion and playground full of picnickers but the trail empty except for one other hiker. Prettier days bring more bikers.

At the trailhead, you have two options: west (right) and south (left). The entire trail is actually one huge loop, and if you wanted to you could start on one side and come out 8 miles later at the other. For those wanting something a bit more manageable, there are turnaround spots that make the trail shorter, and I took advantage of that on my visit. This hike covers the southeastern corner of the park; you'll loop back to the trailhead before the turnoff into the western and northern sides of the park.

To start the hike, turn onto the trail heading left. You'll immediately find yourself hiking through an expansive meadow, which in the spring is blanketed with tiny yellow wildflowers. The terrain is not completely flat but instead dotted with gentle hills that expand to a tree line in the distance ahead of you. As you leave the vicinity of the picnic area, the sounds of folks laughing and kids playing will fade into the background and be replaced by other sounds echoing through the open clearing—woodpeckers rat-a-tatting in the woodlands up ahead and cows mooing somewhere nearby (don't worry, they're actually in an adjacent enclosed property, and you won't come face-to-face with any on the hike).

Continue toward the woods in the distance, bypassing other trails that join the one you're on. At the tree line, the path dives into the woods—a shady mixture of old and new growth, with thick vines climbing up the trees' trunks and branches. Small dips and tight twists intended to spice up bikers' rides also add interest to your trek. You'll briefly emerge into another smaller meadow before you're again enclosed by woodland.

At 0.43 mile, round a small pond hidden in the heart of the woods—one of two ponds you'll discover along the hike. If it's recently rained, the shallow dips in the path just around it can sometimes pool with water, creating mud pockets, even though the rest of the trail might be dry. They're easy to navigate unless it's rained heavily recently—in which case you might emerge a bit messier than when you entered.

A few hundred feet farther, bear left and head down a short, steep slope, where you'll find yourself walking atop a ridge beside a creek along the eastern side of the park. Stay straight at the next two four-way junctions, at 0.6 mile. The trail briefly merges with the overgrown remains of an old gravel road that passes through another open, grassy clearing dotted with red, blue, yellow, and purple wildflowers. Head slightly downhill, winding through open grassland for quite a while before roots start breaking up the path and the woodlands once again enclose you. Just beyond the tree line, you'll find the second pond at 1 mile. From here, the trail heads northeast, meets back up with the creek, then heads south, following a high ridge. It then reaches a split at 1.28 miles. Bear right at the junction, bypassing a steep dip and climb intended for mountain bikers; a few of these bike dips punctuate the trail, but most have turnoffs just before them, allowing hikers to circumvent them.

The trail then winds back east, passes the other side of the pond, and curls back out into an open, grassy field as it heads south. After some sun-drenched hiking through the grass, you'll spot the park road ahead of you. Meet the road at 2.3 miles and rejoin the trail just across it. Follow the trail as it heads north alongside the road. At 2.43 miles, stay to the left to enter a final bit of woods. Through the trees to your right, you'll spot the pavilion; a few hundred feet later, a narrow dirt path bears right, leading you back out and up through the picnic area and back to your car.

NEARBY ACTIVITIES

The Heard Natural Science Museum and Wildlife Sanctuary is only 10 miles away, just to the southeast. It features plant gardens, nature exhibits, and a wildlife sanctuary with hiking trails. The Heard is open Monday–Saturday from 9 a.m. to 5 p.m., and on Sunday from 1 p.m. to 5 p.m. Admission is $8 for adults and $5 for children ages 3–12. To get there, head south on US 75. After 3.7 miles, take Exit 38A onto TX 121 South toward Fort Worth. Make a U-turn onto Spur 399 North toward McKinney, then turn right onto TX 5 South toward Fairview. Go about 0.7 mile, then turn left onto FM 1378 and pass the country club to reach the entrance.

LAVON LAKE: Trinity Trail 35

IN BRIEF

This multiuse hiking and equestrian trail skirts the edge of Lake Lavon, offering scenic views as it makes its way through open woodlands and prairie. The entire trail is 9 miles long and can be extended to any hiker's content.

DESCRIPTION

With an impressive 25.5 miles of trail, the Trinity Trail on Lake Lavon is long enough to challenge even the hardiest of hikers. With trailheads along the western side of the lake at Brockdale Park, East Fork, and Highland Park, plenty of options exist for adventurers who want to explore its different sections. This hike starts at the Brockdale Park trailhead and heads south, loosely following the shoreline as it traverses open woodlands and prairie. It's the perfect choice for someone interested in seeing the flora and fauna of the lake. The trail is also a good option for hikers who want a trek they can extend—the portion of trail I've mapped here is only a small segment of the 9 miles along this section of the Trinity Trail.

Once you've hiked this trail, check out other sections of the Trinity Trail. In particular, the ambitious hiker might consider visiting the Highland Park trailhead to hike the Giant Sycamore Loop Trail, a trek of about 5 miles

----

Directions ————————————————➤

Take US 75 North and exit onto Bethany Drive in Allen. Turn right, heading east about 6 miles on Bethany (which becomes Lucas Road). At the stoplight next to Lucas Food Mart, turn left onto FM 3286. After 0.8 mile, turn right onto Brockdale Park Road. The gravel parking lot is about a mile down on the right, just before the boat ramp.

KEY AT-A-GLANCE INFORMATION

LENGTH: 3.2 miles

CONFIGURATION: Out-and-back

DIFFICULTY: Moderate

SCENERY: Lake, shorebirds, grasslands, open woodlands

EXPOSURE: Partially shady–sunny

TRAIL TRAFFIC: Moderate

TRAIL SURFACE: Dirt

HIKING TIME: 1.5 hours

ACCESS: Daily; free

FACILITIES: Restrooms

WHEELCHAIR TRAVERSABLE: No

SPECIAL COMMENTS: Hike this sunny trail in spring or fall; it heats up quickly in the summer.

SUPPLEMENTAL MAPS: www.swf-wc.usace.army.mil/ lavon/Information/Lavon Lake Map Final.pdf

DRIVING DISTANCE FROM MAJOR INTERSECTION: 12 miles from TX 121 and US 75

GPS TRAILHEAD COORDINATES

Latitude: N 33° 4' 23"

Longitude: W 96° 32' 57"

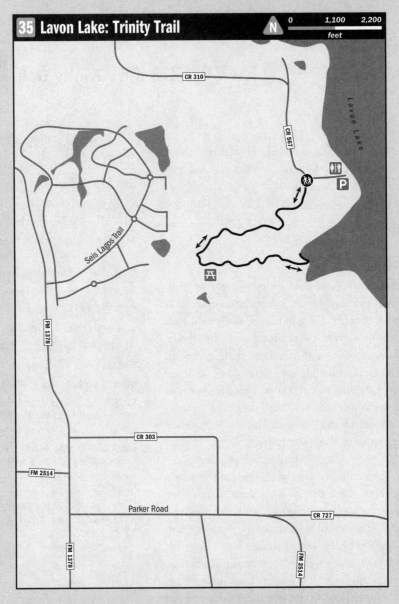

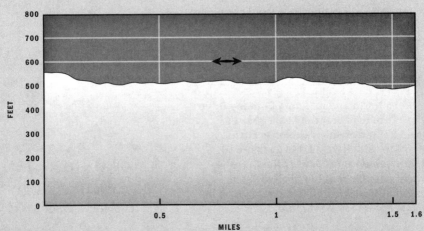

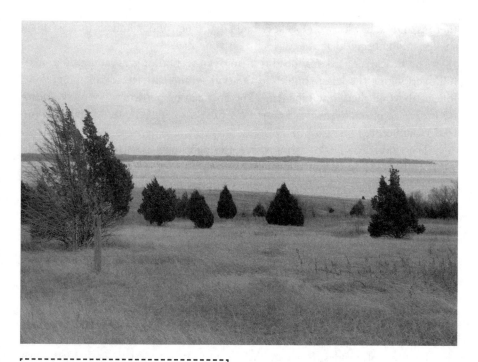

The trail offers excellent views of Lavon Lake.

out to a giant sycamore tree believed to be the largest tree in Texas. The tree stands 101 feet tall and measures 25.5 feet around. If you do consider this hike, leave early and bring plenty of water and snacks, as you'll be hiking about 10 miles round-trip.

Built in the early 1950s primarily for flood control, the 21,400-acre lake is on the East Fork of the Trinity River, northeast of Dallas near the town of Wylie. Some 20 parks along the lake offer myriad activities for fans of the outdoors, including bird-watching, boating, swimming, horseback riding, and camping. Lavon Lake has a reputation among anglers as an especially good spot for crappie fishing, and in the winter you'll see boats scoping the deeper waters in search of them. Hikers visiting any section of the lake would be well advised to check the U.S. Army Corps of Engineers' website (**www.swf-wc.usace.army.mil/lavon**) for park-closure information before visiting. Flooding, construction, and maintenance can sometimes affect operating dates and times for the lake's facilities.

Open to both equestrians and hikers, the Trinity Trail is maintained by the Trinity Trail Preservation Association, a volunteer equestrian organization that has nurtured and developed the trail into a treasure loved and frequented by not just riders but also by day hikers, photographers, walkers, and joggers. The Texas Parks and Wildlife Department has helped promote the trail as well, listing it among its Prairies and Pineywoods Wildlife Trails because of the variety of birds (herons, ducks, hawks, woodpeckers, and kingfishers) and mammals (prairie dogs, snakes, and bobcats) that you may spot on your visit.

The Brockdale Park trailhead is in an open section of grassland atop a small hill overlooking the lake; you'll find the trail on the eastern side of the parking lot, just beyond the white pipe gate. The area can be particularly muddy after a rainstorm, so check to see if it's rained recently; if so, give the trail plenty of time to dry out before you visit.

The trail starts out as a sunny trek through open grassland with easy lake views before curling away from the lake and into the woodlands, loosely following the shoreline as it heads southwest. The trees frame but do not envelop the trail, so it's only partially shaded. In the patches of sun that reach through and between the trees, clumps of grass grow freely, presenting you with a primarily open woodland free of dense underbrush and thickets. Bird boxes placed along the trail attract many colorful residents. Keep an eye out for small brown creepers camouflaged among the tree trunks and for other more colorful birds, such as bluebirds and common yellowthroats.

At 0.9 mile, reach a picnic area complete with picnic tables nestled in a grove of trees just off the path to your right. Continue heading straight, past the picnic area, and past a couple of little trails that branch off toward the lake.

Finally, at 1.6 miles, reach another turnoff toward the lake on the left. Turn onto the trail for a short hike to the lake's edge, where you can refresh yourself with the cool breezes sweeping off the water, enjoy full lake views, and start some impromptu beachcombing. When you've finished exploring the lake, you must decide if you'd like to continue outbound or complete the hike by retracing your steps to the trailhead. If you opt to keep going, the trail heads southeast, curving through the woodlands and teasing you with intermittent glimpses of the lake. The trail continues for miles, first passing Collin Park, with picnic tables for the weary traveler, before eventually ending at the southern trailhead in East Fork Park, 9 miles from the Brockdale trailhead.

NEARBY ACTIVITIES

Southfork Ranch, made famous on the TV show *Dallas,* lies just to the west of Plano. Its magnificent white mansion served as the home of the show's infamous J. R. Ewing from 1978 to 1991. The ranch was opened to the public in 1985 and continues to offer daily tours of the mansion and grounds. Visit **southfork.com** for more information. To get there from the trailhead, go back to the light at the Lucas Food Mart, and turn left onto FM 1378 (Southview Drive). After about 2.3 miles, turn right onto FM 2514 (Parker Road) and drive 2.5 miles. Turn left onto FM 2551 (Hogge Road/Murphy Road) The entrance is about 0.5 mile down on the left.

PARKHILL PRAIRIE TRAIL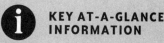

IN BRIEF

This reconstructed and restored native prairie is inspiring in the spring, when the wildflowers bloom.

DESCRIPTION

If you're familiar with the opening sequence of the old TV series *Little House on the Prairie*—in which the Ingalls girls skip and frolic through a wide, open field dotted with flowers—then you'll have a good idea of what the Parkhill Prairie Preserve is like. The beautiful 436-acre preserve is very similar to the scenery in that unforgettable shot, offering a gently rolling, sunny, grassland that is at its best in the spring, when the wildflowers bloom. The colorful display begins with prairie flowers, such as the bright-red Indian paintbrush and the violet-colored wine cup; late spring brings the wild petunia and Mexican hat; and late summer and fall see the bright-yellow goldenrod and the soft hues of the purple coneflower. The preserve has a remnant tract of blackland prairie, most of which is disappearing throughout the country as wild lands are converted to farmland.

The prairie is 60 miles northeast of Dallas in Collin County, making it one of this book's farthest hikes from the city, but it's certainly worth a visit for anyone seeking something a little different. It's fairly remote, set in

KEY AT-A-GLANCE INFORMATION

LENGTH: 1.88 miles

CONFIGURATION: Loop

DIFFICULTY: Easy

SCENERY: Prairie, wildflowers

EXPOSURE: Sunny

TRAIL TRAFFIC: Light

TRAIL SURFACE: Grass

HIKING TIME: 40 minutes

ACCESS: Free; open daily, sunrise–sunset

FACILITIES: Toilets, picnic tables, water fountain

WHEELCHAIR TRAVERSABLE: No

SPECIAL COMMENTS: Wear long pants and insect repellent if you visit in the summer—ticks love the long prairie grasses.

DRIVING DISTANCE FROM MAJOR INTERSECTION: 32 miles from US 75 and US 380 in McKinney

---

Directions

From McKinney, take US 380 East toward Farmersville, then turn north onto TX 78 and go about 9.4 miles toward Blue Ridge. At CR 825, turn right and drive 4.4 miles, then turn left onto CR 668. The entrance to Parkhill Prairie is about 2 miles down on the left. Park in the second parking area.

GPS TRAILHEAD COORDINATES

Latitude: N 33° 16' 19"

Longitude: W 96° 17' 58"

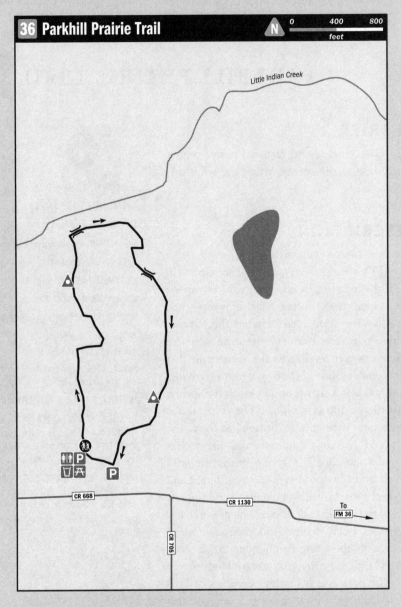

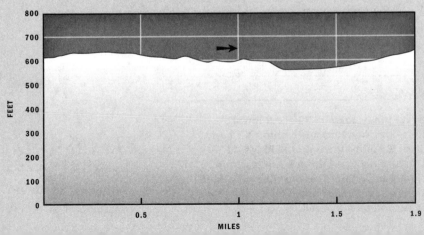

36 **Parkhill Prairie Trail**

N

| 0 | 400 | 800 |

feet

Little Indian Creek

CR 668

CR 1130

To
FM 36

CR 705

FEET

800
700
600
500
400
300
200
100
0

0.5   1   1.5   1.9

MILES

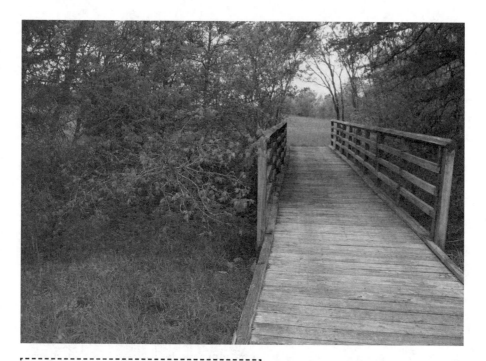

A bridge connecting to a section of secluded prairie

the country just north of Farmersville with few other houses around. From a rocky outcropping along the trail, you'll have fantastic views of the surrounding countryside, which consists primarily of gently rolling hills dotted with trees; the view is especially beautiful in the fall, when the leaves change colors.

Each season, after the spring wildflowers and grasses come in, the trail is mowed back into the prairie. You can hike here year-round, but be advised that if you come before mowing season, you're likely to only see faint hints of the trail and you'll have to navigate an overgrown path. Spikes mark the trail route at regular intervals, so even if the trail isn't mowed, you'll be able to find your way. Take care to avoid twisting your foot or stepping on snakes in the deep grass. Ideally, plan to visit after the trail has been mowed, which happens sometime after Mother's Day.

Collin County has been working with The Nature Conservancy to restore the prairie. Some of these efforts include undertaking prescribed burns—these help control intrusive nonnative plants, which can take over the prairie if left unchecked. Recent drought conditions have limited the number of burns allowed here; as conditions improve, however, more burns are planned. On your hike, you're likely to notice the charred remains of trees and shrubs.

Park in the spaces in front of the restrooms; the trailhead is opposite them and is marked by a kiosk. At the time of my visit, everything had been removed from the kiosk because the preserve was in the middle of an improvement project. Follow the mowed lane north past the kiosk, straight through the open prairie land. It's a gentle walk up and down some rolling hills, over a long wooden bridge, and through some shrubby tree growth to reach the overlook at 0.9 mile. A half-circle stone wall marks the spot atop a small rise and frames a lovely view of the rural countryside stretching out toward the horizon to the north and west.

Get back on the trail and follow it north. As you enter the northern section of the preserve, you'll notice clusters of shrubs and trees encroaching upon the prairie; you may also spot burn marks from the efforts to keep them from invading completely.

The path skirts the northern edge of the preserve. At 1.4 miles, bear left and enter a smaller section surrounded by trees. At the marker, turn left and cross the bridge to enter another small section of grassland screened by trees. Pass through a tree line and into yet another natural enclosure, which abuts the eastern edge of the preserve. To your left, a fence marks the preserve's boundaries; just beyond it, you can sometimes spot Black Angus peering curiously at you as you pass. Much to my surprise, just beside the trail here, I also encountered the skeletal remains of what appeared to be one of their herd members. How it got where I found it remains a mystery to me. Don't worry, though—you won't encounter any live steer on the trail.

You'll soon traverse the tree-lined meadow and be back on the open prairie. From here, it's a short hike uphill to the eastern rock-wall overlook, which offers picturesque views of the prairie to the north and west. From here, hike back 0.35 mile to the trailhead. You'll emerge from the prairie at a kiosk and parking area just up the road from where you parked. The parking lot and restrooms are within easy view down the road, a couple of hundred feet to your right.

NEARBY ACTIVITIES

Enjoy a picnic at Caddo Park on Lavon Lake after the hike. A day-use-only park 17 miles away, it offers more than a dozen picnic sites, a handicap-accessible fishing pond, and a boat ramp. To get there, turn left onto CR 668, which becomes CR 1130. Go 1 mile and turn right onto FM 36. Head south 3.8 miles, then turn right onto FM 2194 and travel 6.3 miles. Bear right onto TX 78 Business, then turn left onto TX 78. Turn left onto US 380. The park is about 2 miles ahead on your right.

PILOT KNOLL TRAIL 37

IN BRIEF

This trail, which winds alongside Lewisville Lake, is not the most scenic, but during hot, dry summers, the lake waters recede, leaving a marsh and exposing gnarled trees favored by vultures. Birds dominate the woodlands adjacent to the trail. Be aware that construction of FM 2499 may reroute portions of this trail.

DESCRIPTION

Lewisville Lake is very popular and is often referred to as Dallas's "party" lake. Like many of north-central Texas's artificial lakes, Lewisville functions primarily as a flood control and water supply, but it's also well known for its recreational opportunities. In the summer, Jet Skiers, boaters, and fishermen fill the waters, while the shores overflow with swimmers, picnickers, and campers. Because of its popularity, the lake is frequently in the news for its rowdiness, including boating accidents. Occasionally, alligator sightings prompt even more coverage. Game wardens advise that the gators' origins can be traced to the Trinity River. At any rate, alligators are a rarity here.

The lake dates back to the late 1920s, when the Elm Fork of the Trinity River was first dammed, creating the reservoir known as

KEY AT-A-GLANCE INFORMATION

LENGTH: 2.55 miles

CONFIGURATION: Balloon

DIFFICULTY: Easy

SCENERY: Lake, woods, birds

EXPOSURE: Partially shady

TRAIL TRAFFIC: Light

TRAIL SURFACE: Packed dirt

HIKING TIME: 45 minutes

ACCESS: Free; open daily

FACILITIES: Available in Pilot Knoll Park

WHEELCHAIR TRAVERSABLE: No

SPECIAL COMMENTS: This trail can be messy after a rainstorm.

SUPPLEMENTAL MAPS: www
.swf-wc.usace.army.mil/lewisville/
images/Elm_Fork_Pilot_Knoll
_Public_Map1.pdf

DRIVING DISTANCE FROM MAJOR INTERSECTION: 10 miles from the I-35W–I-35E split

Directions

Take I-35E and turn left (west) onto FM 407/Justin Road. Go about 4.5 miles to Chin Chapel Road, then turn north (right). Make a right turn to head east on Orchard Hill Road, which dead-ends at Pilot Knoll Park. Parking is available just outside the park gate.

GPS TRAILHEAD COORDINATES

Latitude: N 33° 6' 31"

Longitude: W 97° 4' 39"

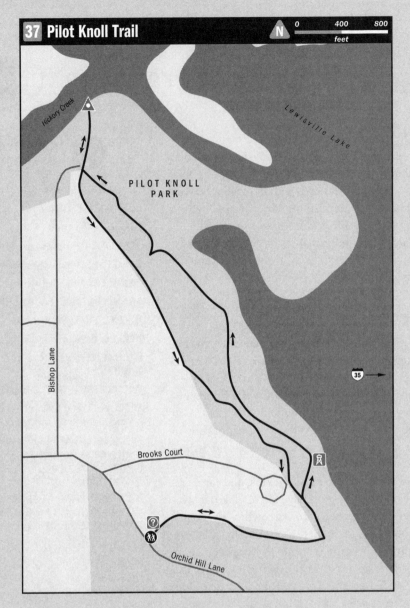

N

0   400   800
feet

Hickory Creek

Lewisville Lake

PILOT KNOLL
PARK

Bishop Lane

Brooks Court

35

Orchid Hill Lane

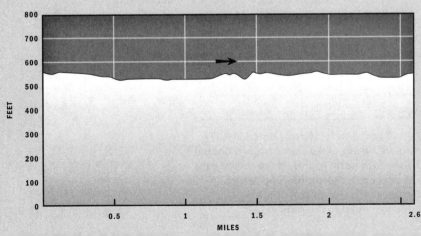

800
700
600
500
400
300
200
100
0

FEET

0.5   1   1.5   2   2.6

MILES

Lake Dallas. The lake was considerably smaller than today's Lewisville Lake, about a quarter of the current size. In the late 1940s, amid concerns for flood control, a new impoundment, the Garza–Little Elm Reservoir, was created nearby by damming a number of creeks. About a decade later, Lake Dallas and the Garza–Little Elm Reservoir were combined to form the huge reservoir of today, named Lewisville Lake in the 1970s.

The trailhead for this hike is just outside Pilot Knoll Park on the east side of the parking lot, just behind the map kiosk. There is a day-use fee for the immaculately maintained park, but because the trail is not maintained by the park, you can park your car or hike the trail at no cost. A sign for Hickory Creek Trail is next to the trailhead.

The wide trail winds east through the woods, following a small access road and passing RV campsites on the right and huge private homes on the left. About 0.3 mile down the trail, reach a fork in the path and bear right, heading north down Lake Shore Trail. The trail winds through a wooded area of tangled trees before reaching another split. Head right at this second junction, passing through more woods. The trail is also open to equestrian traffic—although I didn't see any riders on my hike—so keep an eye to the ground for the occasional horse dropping.

At about 0.48 mile, a break in the trees affords an unobstructed view of the lake on the right. When water levels are low, a wide expanse of sandy beach, dotted with old, twisted tree trunks, rims the deathly-still lake. On my hike, I counted at least a dozen huge turkey vultures perched at the water's edge, surveying the watery landscape.

The trail continues, with the lake coming in and out of view on the right and a dense wood on the left. In addition to the mess of vulture feathers I found strewn across the trail, other signs of wildlife along the path are abundant, including what appeared to be deer tracks in the trail's soft dirt, and a brief glimpse of a small animal scurrying off under the trees—a raccoon, judging from the tracks. At the next junction, 1.15 miles into the hike, take the right-hand fork to head north. Go straight past another junction, and at 1.2 miles find yourself at a junction where a wide road heads toward an overlook to the right. On the left is the parking area at the end of Bishop Road, which serves as a public entrance to this overlook.

At this point, if you turn right the trail goes about 0.1 mile and then reaches the overlook—a small hill overlooking the lake (or, on a dry summer hike, the remnants of the lake). The lake's party reputation is most evident at public-access points such as these. In other words, the better the access to the lake, the more likely you are to see evidence of late-night partying.

If you've ventured to the overlook, retrace your steps (or turn left if you didn't) to the Bishop Road parking area. You'll reach a junction with signs indicating that Hickory Trail is to the right and Lakeshore Trail is to the left. Go right onto Hickory Trail, heading south. The trail narrows and winds through woods. Look out for interesting birds, including some brilliant red ones that flitted across the trail continually during my hike. At 1.78 miles, a trail heads to the right, eventually fading out behind some private homes. Hang a left and follow the trail an additional 0.61 mile to close the loop. From here, turn left, retracing your steps 0.33 mile to the trailhead.

NEARBY ACTIVITIES

Pilot Knoll Park is a nice place to have a picnic lunch; its immaculate picnic area sits right on the lake's edge, yielding outstanding views of the lake. Just to the southwest, Rockledge Park at Grapevine Lake also offers picnicking, swimming, and sunning options.

RAY ROBERTS GREENBELT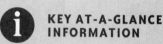

IN BRIEF

Thick woods loom over this wide, charming trail that winds north from Lewisville Lake to Ray Roberts Lake. It's a great, kid-friendly hike.

DESCRIPTION

The Ray Roberts Lake–Lewisville Lake Greenbelt Corridor extends about 10 miles through a wooded section of land between the two lakes. Officially part of the state-park system, the corridor requires no entry fee from those who have a state-park pass. There are three trailheads along the greenbelt: one at the southern end, on US 380; one at the northern end, on FM 455; and one halfway through the corridor, on FM 428.

This trail starts at the southern end of the corridor, near the northern side of Lewisville Lake. Watch for the brown state-park sign identifying the greenbelt.

The greenbelt originally offered two parallel trails: a dirt path for equestrians and a hard-surface multiuse trail for hikers. Recently, however, the entire section of equestrian trail south of FM 455 to Highway 380 has been closed due to erosion. According to the Texas Parks and Wildlife Department, it will not reopen in the near future; rather, proposed changes are in the works to relocate the equestrian trail to the same side of the river as the

KEY AT-A-GLANCE INFORMATION

LENGTH: 5 miles

CONFIGURATION: Out-and-back

DIFFICULTY: Easy

SCENERY: Dense woods

EXPOSURE: Partially shady

TRAIL TRAFFIC: Moderate–heavy

TRAIL SURFACE: Packed gravel

HIKING TIME: 1.75 hours

ACCESS: $5 per person; open daily until 10 p.m.

FACILITIES: Recycling toilet

WHEELCHAIR TRAVERSABLE: No

SPECIAL COMMENTS: Many miles of trail let you extend this hike for as long as desired.

SUPPLEMENTAL MAPS: tpwd.state .tx.us/publications/pwdpubs/ media/park_maps/pwd_mp _p4503_176a.pdf

DRIVING DISTANCE FROM MAJOR INTERSECTION: 9 miles from the I-35E–I-35W split

---

Directions

Follow I-35E north toward Denton and take Exit 463. Turn right onto TX 288 Loop and go about 3.5 miles. Turn right onto East University Drive. The trailhead is about 3 miles ahead on the left; keep an eye out for the brown RAY ROBERTS STATE PARK sign.

GPS TRAILHEAD COORDINATES

Latitude: N 33° 14' 26"

Longitude: W 97° 2' 30"

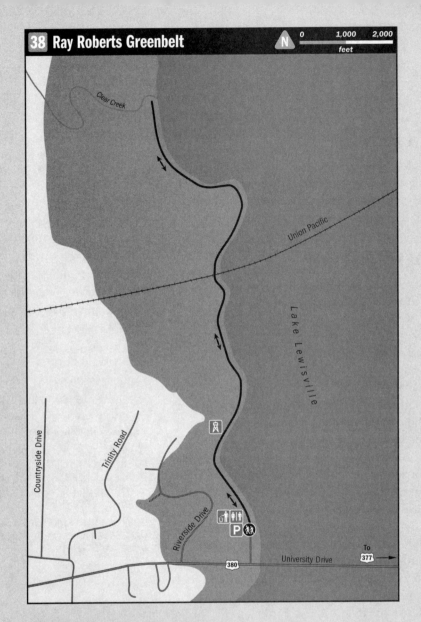

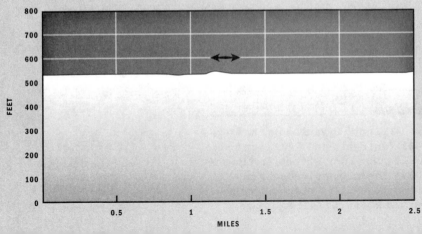

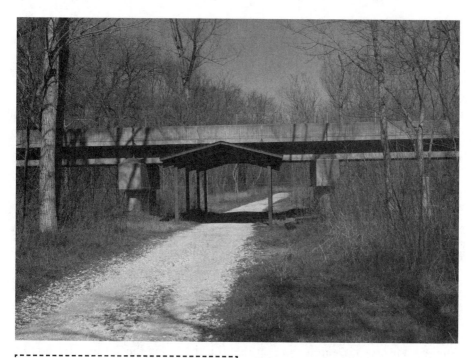

Railway tracks emerge briefly from the woods.

multiuse hiking trail. In the meantime, the hard-surface trail remains open and accessible to hikers.

The trailhead for this hike is in front of the gravel path next to the kiosk, on the north side of the parking lot. A self-pay booth at the trailhead allows you to deposit the small trail-use fee if you don't have a park pass. This is a great trail for youngsters because it's wide and partially shaded, has plenty of straight stretches to keep all members of the family within easy view, and is completely removed from potentially dangerous streets and highways. Encourage younger hikers to use the restrooms at the trailhead before you get under way—the other restrooms are 6.5 miles out at the FM 428 trailhead. Note also that there is no water along the trail, so make sure you've brought some, especially if it's a hot day.

I was actually much more impressed with this trail than I expected I would be. There's something special about it that's hard to put a finger on. It might be that it feels much wilder than the typical greenbelt. The land has been left in its natural state, and as you hike along, the elegance of the trees towering above and looming around you transports you into a different world. Ahead and behind you, the trail curves gently out of sight beneath the trees as it winds lazily north through the dense woods. Another part of its magic is that it's far removed from the ever-present hum of civilization. Deep within the greenbelt, you'll clearly hear the rustling of leaves and the creaking of limbs in the wind. The only sounds louder than these are the clear trills, whistles, and songs of birds watching you walk by. Surprisingly, the relaxing, peaceful atmosphere of the trail is not marred by the frequency of hikers, joggers, and dog walkers on the path. Most folks walk or jog quietly by, drinking in the calmness of the woods.

At 0.43 mile, pass an overlook to your left that offers a nice view of the Elm Fork of the Trinity River, which stays hidden from view for most of the hike. The trail follows the river as it heads north toward Ray Roberts Lake. Occasionally, signs of civilization do temporarily invade the beauty of the greenbelt—at 1 mile in, some power lines cross the path. Just beyond, at 1.15 miles, a railway line crosses the trail, creating another brief break in the otherwise continuous belt of woods.

The trail continues for much longer than you'll probably be willing or able to hike—10 miles in one direction. On most days, the trail is clear and quiet for as long as you're willing to walk. This trail can therefore be extended to just about any length you're comfortable with. When you're ready to head back, just retrace your steps. Reserve enough energy to make it back to the trailhead—if you're not paying attention, you could easily hike farther than you intended.

NEARBY ACTIVITIES

Stop by downtown Denton and visit the Courthouse-on-the-Square Museum, in the historic Denton County Courthouse at 110 W. Hickory St. Exhibits focus on African American Families of Denton County, Hispanic Families of Denton County, and Special Collections, such as Indian pottery, thimbles, and quilts. To get there, head back 5 miles down University Drive into downtown Denton, and turn left onto North Elm Street. Turn left onto West Hickory Street. You might also want to check out the nearby Golden Triangle Mall, with department stores, gift shops, and the Silver Cinema Theater, where you can see movies for $2.

RAY ROBERTS LAKE STATE PARK, ISLE DU BOIS UNIT: Lost Pines Trail 39

IN BRIEF

This pretty trek through hardwoods stops at interpretive signs identifying flora and leads to a pretty grove of pine trees. A spur midway through leads to a sandy lakeshore, along which you can find animal tracks and birds such as herons and egrets.

DESCRIPTION

Ray Roberts Lake, just north of Denton, is a 30,000-acre reservoir complete with boat ramps, camping, a swimming beach, trails, and a marina. The lake was originally called the Aubrey Reservoir but was renamed after a U.S. Congressman in 1980. It's a big attraction for anglers, who come to fish for crappie, white bass, catfish, and flathead, and is popular with nature lovers, who come to enjoy the various offerings of the state-park complex on its shores.

Part of the lake's state-park complex, Isle du Bois ("Island of the Trees") sits on its southern shore. The park opened in 1993, making it a few years older than the neighboring Johnson Branch Unit, which opened in 1996. Within the park, you'll find miles of hiking, biking, and equestrian trails, all of which see good use. The majority of these trails run

KEY AT-A-GLANCE INFORMATION

LENGTH: 1 mile

CONFIGURATION: Loop with spur

DIFFICULTY: Easy

SCENERY: Lake shoreline, hardwoods, pines

EXPOSURE: Shady–sunny

TRAIL TRAFFIC: Light

TRAIL SURFACE: Packed dirt trail, sand

HIKING TIME: 30 minutes

ACCESS: $5 per person for adults and children age 13 and up, kids age 12 and under free; open daily, 8 a.m.–10 p.m.

FACILITIES: Restrooms, picnic area, playground

WHEELCHAIR TRAVERSABLE: No

SPECIAL COMMENTS: This hike can be extended by walking along the lake shoreline. Bring along binoculars for bird-watching.

SUPPLEMENTAL MAPS: tpwd.state .tx.us/publications/pwdpubs/ media/park_maps/pwd_mp _p4503_137n.pdf

DRIVING DISTANCE FROM MAJOR INTERSECTION: 6 miles from FM 455 and US 377

Directions

When reading directional signs on the highway, keep in mind that there are two different state-park units: one on the north side of the lake and one on the south side. To get to the Isle du Bois State Park Unit, take I-35 North to Sanger, exit at FM 455, and go east about 10 miles toward Pilot Point to the park entrance. Park in the first parking area, just inside the park entrance.

GPS TRAILHEAD COORDINATES

Latitude: N 33° 21' 58"
Longitude: W 97° 0' 41"

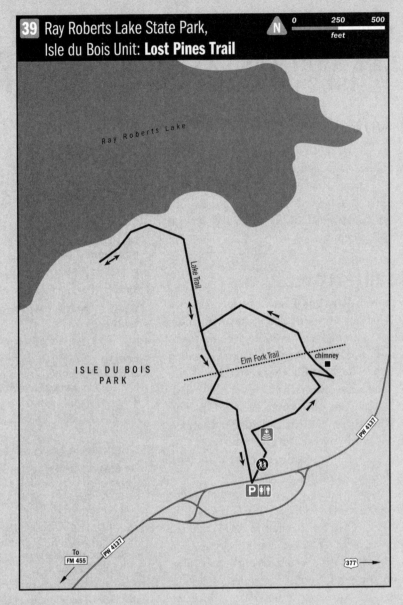

Ray Roberts Lake

Lake Trail

Elm Fork Trail   chimney

ISLE DU BOIS
PARK

PW 4137

P

To
FM 455   PW 4137

377 →

0   250   500
feet

N

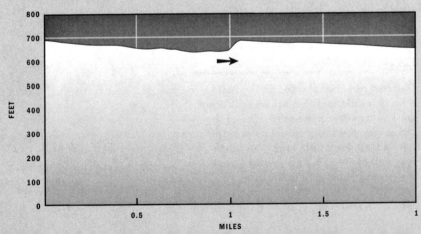

800
700
600
500
400
300
200
100
0

FEET

0.5   1   1.5   1

MILES

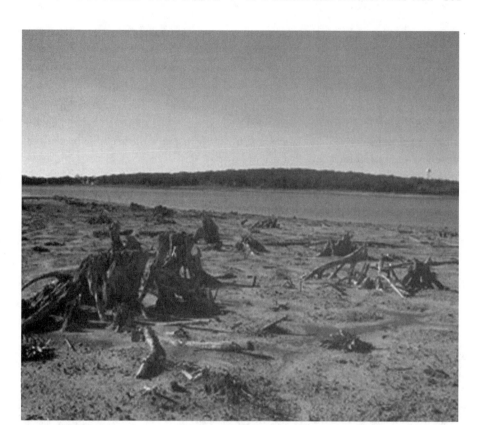

The trail offers a detour to the lake with great opportunities for beachcombing.

slightly inland from the shore, traveling for miles before looping back, making them ideal for long day treks. For shorter hikes, the park offers a paved loop trail through its center and a pretty interpretive nature trail near the park entrance, highlighted following.

The trailhead is just to the north of the parking area; you can see it from the lot. Pick up one of the brochures from the box at the trailhead to help you identify the flora along the trail; each plant has a numbered signpost. Heading down the trail, you'll immediately pass the first marker for Hercules' club—or toothache tree—a small tree whose bark, when chewed, can cause numbness in the mouth.

In about 400 feet, reach a small clearing and the amphitheater. Bear right, following the trail northeast through the woods. Here the trail is wide rather than singletrack, making it seem as if you've stepped into another world. At some points, I half-expected to see Little Red Riding Hood skipping through the woods on her way to a remote cottage.

Interpretive signs along the way will help you identify plants commonly found in this ecological woodland zone, known as the Eastern Cross Timbers region. Blackjack oaks and post oaks dominate the woods; bluejack oaks and live oaks are fewer in number. Watch for colorful birds such as the eastern bluebird and American robin.

At 0.25 mile, reach a clearing amid which you'll see the remains of a chimney fenced off on the right. Elm Fork Trail, a wide path of loose dirt ideal for equestrians, intersects the nature trail here, heading west–east. Cross Elm Fork Trail and continue onto the path marked PEDESTRIAN TRAFFIC ONLY. In the shade of a dense woodland canopy, sun filters through the trees only in small patches, keeping things cool even on a hot day. Pass trees such as the Chickasaw plum, gum bumelia, and eastern red cedar as you make your way northwest. As you walk along, read the interpretive brochure, which provides interesting information regarding the historical and common uses of many of these trees.

At 0.5 mile, reach a split in the trail. Bear right onto Lake Trail and toward the water. The trail breaks from the woods and winds through tall grasses growing in the sand near the lake. When the water is low, a huge expanse of beach is exposed to stroll along. If you feel like prolonging the hike, head right or left, following the shoreline as it curves out of sight. Binoculars are helpful—this is a great spot for bird-watching. Even novices will be able to identify egrets and gulls along the water's edge. You'll see animal tracks in the soft sand at the shoreline, including the prints of white-tailed deer, which live in the area.

When you're done exploring the shore, head away from the lake, retracing your steps to the start of Lake Trail. Once you reach the trail sign, continue straight to finish the loop. Markers along the path help you identify the American elm and cedar elm. Finally, at 0.89 mile, reach the trail's namesake, a grouping of slash pines dubbed "Lost Pines." The tall trees, with their needles and limbs hanging in gentle arches, present a captivating display that is completely unexpected amid the hardwood forest and greenbrier thicket.

Continuing along the trail, reach the soft dirt of Elm Fork Trail another 150 feet ahead. (Yield to horses and riders plodding along the trail.) Pass a few other native plants, such as the Texas prickly pear cactus, before reaching the amphitheater, where you'll retrace your steps the final few hundred feet to the trailhead.

NEARBY ACTIVITIES

Stop by Lake Ray Roberts Marina in the Sanger Unit along the lake for snacks or a fishing license and bait. For a small charge, you can fish from the marina's covered and lighted pier. Or try the fried catfish at Huck's Catfish Restaurant, adjacent to the marina. To get there, turn right onto FM 455 and drive 7 miles. At FM 2164, turn right, go 0.5 mile, then turn right again onto FM 1190. The marina is off Marina Circle, to the right.

RAY ROBERTS LAKE STATE PARK, JOHNSON BRANCH UNIT: Johnson Branch Trail

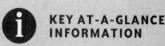

IN BRIEF

This flat, paved trail winds through the park, passing through terrain characteristic of the Eastern Cross Timbers region. Start with expansive views of the lake, then trek through the park toward campsites at its northern end.

DESCRIPTION

Ray Roberts Lake, just north of Denton, is a 30,000-acre reservoir with boat ramps, camping, a swimming beach, miles of trails, and a marina. The lake was originally called the Aubrey Reservoir but was renamed after a U.S. congressman in 1980. Popular with anglers, thanks to the crappie, white bass, catfish, and flathead in its waters, it also draws nature lovers who come to enjoy the various offerings of the state-park complex on its shores.

The Johnson Branch Unit is part of the state-park complex at Ray Roberts Lake and is on its northern shore in Valley View. Outdoorsy types will find both biking and hiking trails. The bike trail, which is also open to hikers, is a long trail in the western section of the park, offering loops through Dogwood Canyon and maintained by DORBA (the Dallas Off-Road Bicycle Association). For this hike, I've selected a long, paved trail that loops through the lake, woods, and camp areas on the eastern side of the park.

Directions

Follow I-35 North through Sanger, take Exit 483 onto Lone Oak Road/FM 3002, and head east 7 miles to the park, entering at the Johnson Branch Unit. There are signs, but keep in mind that there are two different state-park units, one on the north side of the lake and one on the south side.

GPS TRAILHEAD COORDINATES

Latitude: N 33° 24' 34"

Longitude: W 97° 3' 0"

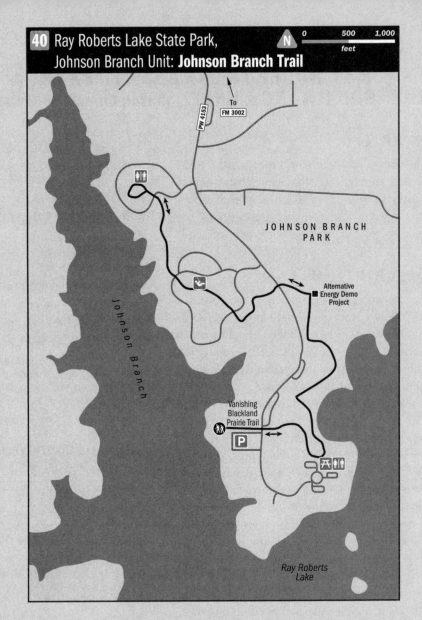

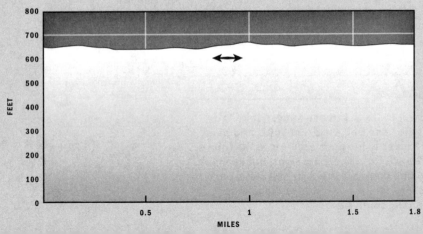

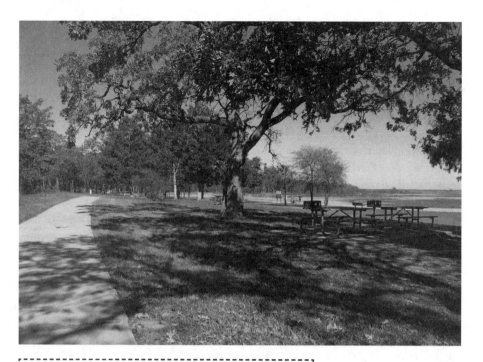

Picnic tables with lake views offer a nice spot for lunch or a snack.

When you arrive, stop by the park headquarters for a map and information on free events. Although some of the events, such as campfire programs and star-gazing parties (led by volunteer astronomers), occur during the evening, others, such as guided nature hikes, typically occur during the day.

Park in the large lot by the boat launch; the trailhead is just behind the fish-cleaning station, adjacent to the parking lot. Within a few steps, turn right, follow-ing the paved trail east through the trees. At 0.13 mile, reach a dirt trail turnoff on the left, with a sign identifying it as Vanishing Blackland Prairie Trail. Unfor-tunately, during my visit, the loop was closed. If it's open, it's worth a detour down the short trail with the interpretive guide that can be picked up at the visitor center. The small brochure describes the flora found along the trail—including trees such as honey locust, hackberry, pecan, cedar elm, and post oak, in addition to prairie grasses and wildflowers.

From the Vanishing Prairie Nature Trail turnoff, continue straight (east) along the paved trail, which crosses the park road and passes another parking area and a picnic area before reaching a split at 0.23 mile. Head right at the split, fol-lowing the trail toward the lake. The wide expanse of beach along the lakeshore is often busy with families playing ball, kids running through the sand in circles, and couples playing Frisbee. The trail makes a short loop around the peninsula, letting you take in lake views the whole way. Picnic tables along the trail tempt hikers to stay and enjoy the breeze.

At 0.28 mile, the trail splits—keep right. You'll come up behind some bathrooms, pass a playground, and then go left at 0.43 mile, looping back toward the beach. Turkey vultures can often be seen circling overhead as they search for leftover scraps of fish and other food. Also keep an eye out for water birds such as pelicans, herons, egrets, geese, and double-crested cormorants.

Turn away from the shoreline (left) at 0.55 mile, just before you reach the end. A few steps farther, bear right, then right again, following the trail north into some woods that quickly obscure the lake from view. The surrounding trees are characteristic of the Eastern Cross Timbers region and include honey mesquite, blackjack oak, winged elm, and pecan.

At 0.65 mile, turn right at the path split. The trail winds past some camping areas tucked into the woods, then emerges again at 0.88 mile, where you'll again bear right. The trail keeps straight here for 0.33 mile, following the park road, which is hidden off to your left. Birds you may spot in the woods include the Carolina chickadee and the tufted titmouse. Also look out for flycatchers, swallows, woodpeckers, and bluebirds.

Turn left at 0.98 mile, next to a booth marked ALTERNATIVE ENERGY DEMO PROJECT. Continuing west, cross the road at 1.08 miles. Off to your right, glimpse some campsites, folks pitching tents and walking dogs, and kids playing games.

At 1.28 miles, cross another park road. The path heads northwest past a playground to the left and crosses another road. Then enter a section of dense woods and heavy shade. After you cross a short footbridge spanning a small stream, you'll reach another park road. The restrooms are just opposite. Retrace your steps to the trailhead.

NEARBY ACTIVITIES

Stop by Lake Ray Roberts Marina in the Sanger Unit along the lake for snacks and a fishing license and bait. For a small charge, you can fish from the marina's covered and lighted pier. Or try the fried catfish at Huck's Catfish Restaurant, adjacent to the marina. To get there, head 6.6 miles west on East Lone Oak Road/FM 3002 toward Morrow Road. Turn onto I-35 South/US 77 South and go 4 miles, then take Exit 478 toward FM 455/Pilot Point/Bolivar. Turn left onto FM 455/West Chapman Drive, go 3 miles, then turn left onto FM 1190 and travel 0.9 mile. The marina is off Marina Circle, to the right.

SISTER GROVE LOOP 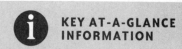 41

IN BRIEF

This excellent all-around hike loops through a pretty, green woodland interspersed with open fields and inhabited by coyotes, rabbits, and armadillos.

DESCRIPTION

This remote Collin County park, on the northeastern side of the expansive Lake Lavon, takes an unusual drive down two interconnected bridges to reach. It's a fun trail that will suit hikers whose tastes conflict—offering both open, sunny grassland and shady, lush green woodland. Expect to find some off-road bikers here—the trail is maintained by the Dallas Off-Road Bicycle Association (DORBA). It's not as popular as many of the DORBA trails closer to the city, so some days you might not find any bikers here at all. If you hike quietly, you might see some small wildlife along the trail—within a few minutes of starting the hike, I spotted a huge jackrabbit hopping alongside the path. Farther down the trail, I found what looked like coyote tracks.

The 21,400-acre Lavon Lake is operated by the U.S. Army Corps of Engineers and was impounded in 1953. More than a dozen lakeside parks dot its 83-mile shoreline. Sister Grove Park is not operated by the Corps but is part of Collin County Open Space. Its trails,

KEY AT-A-GLANCE INFORMATION

LENGTH: 2.96 miles

CONFIGURATION: Loop

DIFFICULTY: Easy

SCENERY: Open fields, thick woodlands, wildflowers

EXPOSURE: Sunny–shady

TRAIL TRAFFIC: Moderate

TRAIL SURFACE: Dirt

HIKING TIME: 1.25 hours

ACCESS: Free; open daily, sunrise–sunset (gate is locked at sunset, and hikers can get locked in)

FACILITIES: Toilet, picnic tables

WHEELCHAIR TRAVERSABLE: No

SPECIAL COMMENTS: Only the parking area, restrooms, and picnic area are wheelchair traversable.

DRIVING DISTANCE FROM MAJOR INTERSECTION: 8.3 miles from US 380 and CR 407

Directions ⟶

Follow US 75 North toward Sherman. Take Exit 41 toward US 380 and turn right onto West University Drive/US 380 East. Travel about 12.5 miles. In the middle of the bridge over Lavon Lake, turn left onto a smaller bridge, CR 559. After about 1 mile, turn left onto CR 561 to reach Sister Grove Park.

GPS TRAILHEAD COORDINATES

Latitude: N 33° 10' 58"

Longitude: W 96° 26' 48"

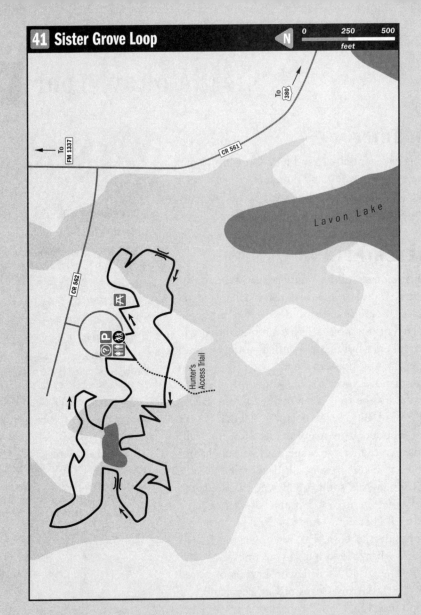

N

0   250   500
feet

To 380

To FM 1337

CR 561

CR 562

Lavon Lake

Hunter's Access Trail

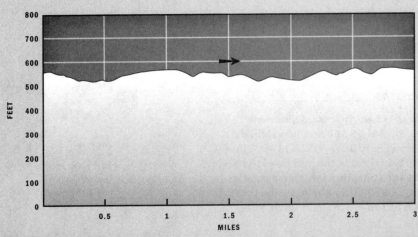

800
700
600
500
400
300
200
100
0

FEET

0.5   1   1.5   2   2.5   3

MILES

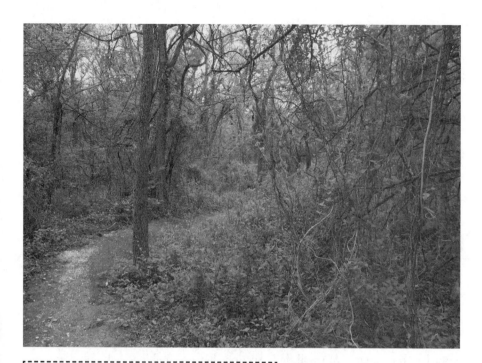

Thick vines dangle from tree limbs alongside the trail.

started in the early to mid-1990s, have been restored and extended by DORBA volunteers continually since then. The entire trail system is about 6 miles long and comprises two loops—the Sister Grove Loop, which forms the northern half (and is the route for this hike), and the Lake Loop, which forms the southern half. A third trail, Hunter's Access Trail, heads south to cut directly through the two loops, directing duck hunters down to the lake. Mountain bike tires have worn a narrow groove down the middle of a couple of the softer sections of the loop trails, making it sometimes awkward to hike; wear comfortable, sturdy shoes to avoid twisting an ankle.

From the trailhead, start the loop by taking the leftmost trail, next to Hunter's Access Trail. The path heads east past a picnic area and through a sunny, open field dotted with eastern red cedar. In the spring, small clumps of purple wildflowers grow in the grass, making for a cheerful scene.

As the trail rounds a curve, you'll trade open sky for a canopy of trees as you enter a woodland full of huge, gnarled trees with vines growing up their trunks and hanging from their branches. At 0.53 mile, cross a wooden bridge, then emerge from the trees and into a small pocket of wildflower-studded grassland. The trail weaves in and out of the open and wooded areas several times; it won't be long before you find yourself heading through shrubs and back into the cool green woodlands for a more prolonged hike through the shade.

At 0.88 mile, bear right at the junction, following the Sister Grove Loop west. Stay to the right at the next junction. At 1.2 miles, bear right for a short detour past a small pond hidden in the woods. After checking out its still, murky, green-brown waters, which are popular with birds, loop back up and rejoin the main trail. A few hundred feet farther, pass a wide dirt path, staying on the narrow singletrack instead. Then exit yet another small pocket of grassland and find yourself entering another thick section of woodland. Tiny holes in the tree trunks provide evidence of sapsuckers and woodpeckers. Birds are plentiful: watch for the colorful plumage of the easily recognizable cardinal, and keep an ear open for the melodies of warblers and thrashers. A thick understory of saplings and small trees colors everything a vibrant green. The thick foliage engulfs the trail, making this a haven on a hot day.

Keep left at the junction at 1.65 miles and go another 0.2 mile to cross a wooden bridge and pass another small pond. Traverse a few more sections of alternating grassland and woodland pockets before you finally emerge into the main grassland near the trailhead. Look out for springtime bluebonnets in the latter couple of grassland pockets.

Although the trailhead is just to your left, there's one last woodland section to hike before you complete the trail. Heading back into the trees, you'll work your legs on a couple of small, hilly sections before climbing back uphill and out of the woods for good. At 2.9 miles, reach Hunter Access Trail, where you'll turn left to head back north to the trailhead.

NEARBY ACTIVITIES

In nearby Greenville, visit the Audie Murphy/American Cotton Museum, which comprises exhibits and displays related to the cotton industry; the Ende-Gaillard House, Greenville's oldest residence; a collection of historic military memorabilia; and various special collections. The museum is open Tuesday–Saturday, 10 a.m.– 5 p.m.; admission is $6 for adults, $4 for seniors (60+), military veterans, and college students, and $2 for children age 18 and under. To get there, take US 380/ Audie Murphy Parkway east toward Greenville about 16 miles. Bear right onto US 69, then turn right onto I-30 East. The museum is at 600 I-30; for more information, call (903) 450-4502 or visit **cottonmuseum.com.**

WALNUT GROVE TRAIL

IN BRIEF

This trail appeals to hikers looking for a quiet, peaceful walk with plenty of solitude. Although frequented by local horse owners, trail traffic is very light. Several loops to the water's edge offer opportunities to explore the wild shoreline.

DESCRIPTION

Certified as a National Recreation Trail in 1991, this pleasant trail follows the southern shoreline of Grapevine Lake, offering almost a continuous view of the water. Unlike the northern side of the lake, where waters are a little rougher and trails more crowded, this side is calm and serene, with plenty of opportunities for being alone. The gentle waters on this side of the lake do little more than lap at the shoreline, and even the view is relaxing—only the occasional fishing boat can be seen sitting out in the tranquil waters. The trail is considered a hiking and equestrian trail, and you're likely to run across a few horseback riders clopping down the path. The horses add to the bucolic mood, though you'll want to keep an eye peeled for the occasional horse dropping.

The best feature of this trail is the constant beach access. The main path traverses the shoreline slightly inland, but if you're in the mood for beachcombing, you'll find a

KEY AT-A-GLANCE INFORMATION

LENGTH: 4.76 miles

CONFIGURATION: Balloon

DIFFICULTY: Easy

SCENERY: Lake, wild beach

EXPOSURE: Sunny–shady

TRAIL TRAFFIC: Light

TRAIL SURFACE: Dirt path

HIKING TIME: 2 hours

ACCESS: Free

FACILITIES: None

WHEELCHAIR TRAVERSABLE: No

SPECIAL COMMENTS: The closest restrooms are at nearby Bob Jones Park.

DRIVING DISTANCE FROM MAJOR INTERSECTION: 9.3 miles from I-35W and TX 114

GPS TRAILHEAD COORDINATES

Latitude: N 33° 00' 16"

Longitude: W 97° 09' 25"

Directions

Take TX 114 west into Southlake, then head north (right) onto White Chapel Boulevard. Follow the road about 3 miles past Bob Jones Park to the very end, where you'll dead-end in a small parking lot. The trailhead is on your right.

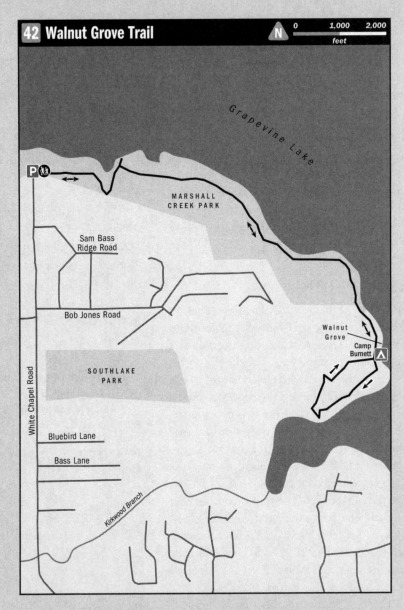

N

0   1,000   2,000

feet

Grapevine Lake

MARSHALL
CREEK PARK

P 🚶

Sam Bass
Ridge Road

Bob Jones Road

Walnut
Grove

Camp
Burnett

SOUTHLAKE
PARK

White Chapel Road

Bluebird Lane

Bass Lane

Kirkwood Branch

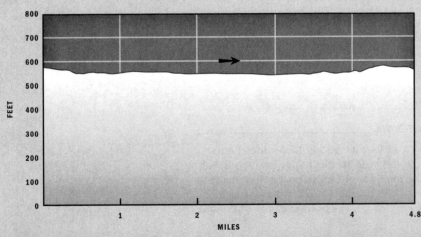

800
700
600
500
400
300
200
100
0

FEET

1   2   3   4   4.8

MILES

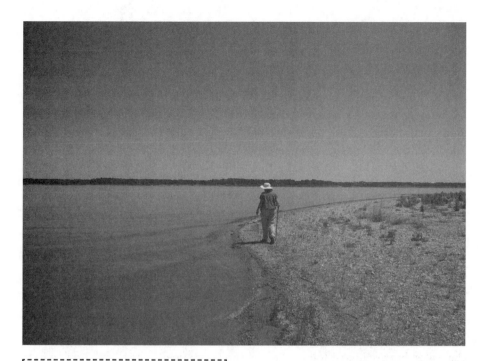

A hiker beachcombing along the lakeshore

number of paths branching off the main trail toward the lake that loop back to rejoin the main trail. At 0.25 mile into the hike, reach the first of these, branching off to the left. Bear right to stay on the main trail.

The dirt trail winds past glimpses of the lake on your left and woods and shrubs on the right. At 0.3 mile, encounter the next junction, where you'll stay to the right as the trail winds through some dense shade, then reemerges into the sun. At 0.5 mile, look for another loop heading out to the shoreline. If you decide to make a brief detour down the side trail on the left, as I did, you'll find a narrow, sandy beach with tall beach grass here and there—a completely wild and unmanicured shoreline. On my hike, I saw what is probably most typical—a couple of shorebirds standing along the water's edge and a lone woman and her dog picking their way down the shoreline. I didn't see anyone else on the shore the entire hike, until my way back, when a couple of horseback riders clopped slowly toward me, then disappeared down a lake loop, presumably for a slow ride along the beach.

When you're done beachcombing, rejoin the loop, heading up and to the left through the tall grass back toward the main path. The next four junctions are more loops down to the water; keep on the main path, going straight to bypass them.

As you hike, keep your eyes open for wildlife, including fox, deer, coyote, opossum, armadillo, and rabbit. While I was hiking, an instructor leading a group of horseback riders passed me. She stopped to chat, commenting that on a couple of recent visits here she had spotted what she believed to be a large cougar just off the trail. She notified the U.S. Army Corps of Engineers, who told her they had already received reports of a large cat on the trail. Chances of an encounter are probably rare, but be aware of the possibility. Although I saw few animals on my hike, I found plenty of scat and tracks on the trail. If you're interested in identifying animals that have recently traipsed through, bring along an animal-scat and print-identification book. Prints are best sighted after rain (though if it's rained too hard, the trail may be too muddy to hike).

At 1.2 miles in, turn left at a fork and soon reach a clearing overlooking a sandy beach strewn with driftwood. Adjacent to the trail, about a half a dozen structures resembling bat houses have been installed. At the next fork, stay to the left; at the next two forks, keep straight, following the main trail as it winds over grassy knolls with nice lake views.

At 2 miles in, reach a fork with a sign marked BOB JONES PARK/WALNUT GROVE/CAMP BURNETT. Continue straight, following the trail as it twists uphill away from the lake. At 2.4 miles, the path forks again; a sign directs hikers to Bob Jones or White Chapel. Continue straight toward Bob Jones. A couple hundred feet farther, you'll reach the next trail sign. From here, the return loop begins, so follow the trail to the right in the direction of White Chapel. At the next fork, at 2.5 miles, bear right and follow the trail through a field spotted with prickly pear cactus. At 2.65 miles, turn right at the split and follow the fence as the trail winds back and rejoins the main trail. You'll find yourself back at the BOB JONES PARK/WALNUT GROVE/CAMP BURNETT sign, where you'll turn left to head back toward the trailhead.

NEARBY ACTIVITIES

The huge Grapevine Mills Mall— with more than 190 shops and a 30-screen AMC movie theater—is only a short drive away. You'll also find a selection of restaurants both within and around the mall. To get there, take TX 114 South 2 miles and exit at Northwest Highway/East Southlake Boulevard. Turn left onto Northwest Highway and go about 5 miles; you'll see the signs for Grapevine Mills on your left.

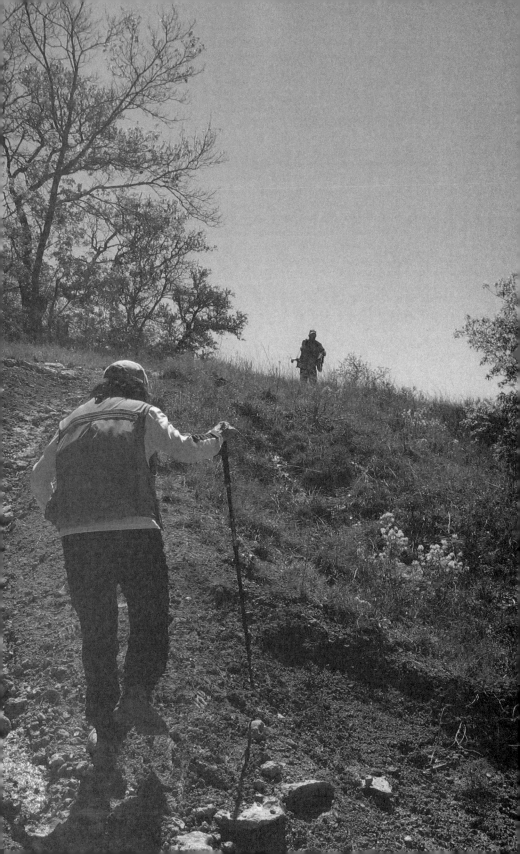

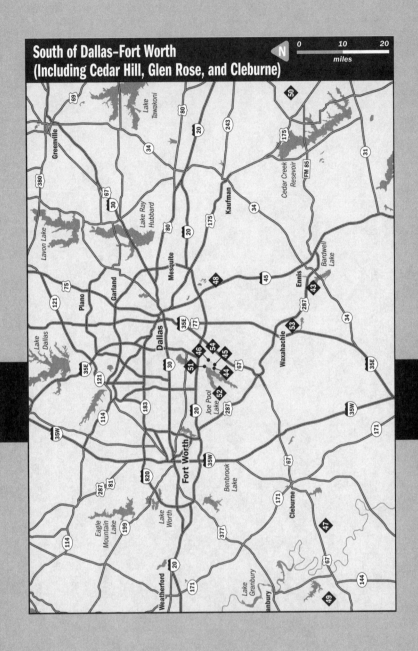

South of Dallas–Fort Worth
(Including Cedar Hill, Glen Rose, and Cleburne)

N

0   10   20
miles

43 Bardwell Lake Multiuse Trail **198**

44 Cedar Hill State Park:
Talala–Duck Pond Loop **202**

45 Cedar Mountain Trail **206**

46 Cedar Ridge Preserve Trail **210**

47 Cleburne State Park Loop Trail **215**

48 Cottonwood Creek Trail **220**

49 Dinosaur Valley Trail **224**

50 Purtis Creek Trail **229**

51 Visitor's Overlook:
Joe Pool Lake Dam Trail **233**

52 Walnut Creek Trail **237**

53 Waxahachie Creek Hike & Bike Trail **241**

54 Windmill Hill Preserve Trail **245**

SOUTH OF DALLAS-FORT WORTH
(INCLUDING CEDAR HILL, GLEN ROSE, AND CLEBURNE)

43 BARDWELL LAKE MULTIUSE TRAIL

KEY AT-A-GLANCE INFORMATION

LENGTH: 2.34 miles

CONFIGURATION: Loop

DIFFICULTY: Moderate

SCENERY: Grassland, wooded thickets

EXPOSURE: Sunny

TRAIL TRAFFIC: Moderate

TRAIL SURFACE: Dirt

HIKING TIME: 45 minutes

ACCESS: Free; open daily, 6 a.m.–10 p.m.

FACILITIES: Toilets, picnic tables

WHEELCHAIR TRAVERSABLE: No

SPECIAL COMMENTS: Trail etiquette gives equestrians the right-of-way.

SUPPLEMENTAL MAPS: www.swf -wc.usace.army.mil/bardwell/ Bardwell Multi Use Trail Map.pdf

DRIVING DISTANCE FROM MAJOR INTERSECTION: 9.6 miles from US 287 and I-45

GPS TRAILHEAD COORDINATES

Latitude: N 32° 17' 46"

Longitude: W 96° 41' 49"

IN BRIEF

Grassy meadows and sunny fields take center stage on this flat hike along Bardwell Lake. The second half of the trail loops back through wooded thickets. More than 13 miles of trails offer unlimited options for those seeking a longer hike.

DESCRIPTION

On Waxahachie Creek in Ellis County, the 3,570-acre Bardwell Lake is about 40 miles south of Dallas and 60 miles southeast of Fort Worth. It was impounded in 1965 to facilitate flood control and supply water, and today it also serves as a recreational spot. A half-dozen parks lie along its perimeter, including Waxahachie Creek Park, on the southwestern shoreline—the starting point for this hike. In addition to the hiking trails, the park also offers boating, picnicking, and camping.

Many folks familiar with Bardwell Lake have heard of it while visiting nearby Ennis—the "Bluebonnet City of Texas." The city's driving routes, known as the Bluebonnet Trails, lead visitors through the best of the springtime display. If you intend to tour the driving trails after you've done some hiking, you'll want to plan your visit around the end of April, when the bluebonnets should be in full bloom.

Directions

Take I-45 South toward Corsicana. In Ennis, take Exit 251A and turn left onto Creechville Road/FM 1181. Creechville Road becomes TX 34. Continue about 4.5 miles and turn right onto Bozek Road to reach Waxahachie Creek Park. The entrance to the park is about 1.5 miles down Bozek. Park in the westernmost parking lot, adjacent to the boat launch.

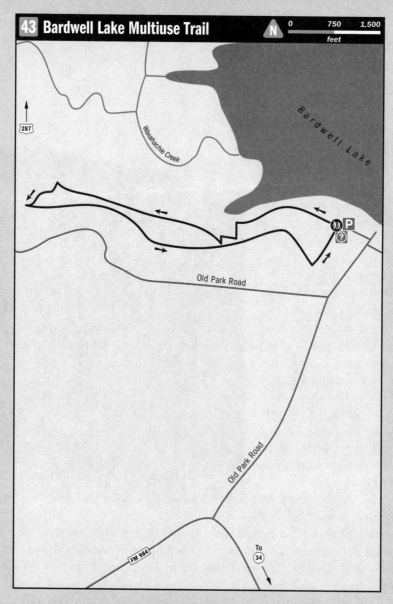

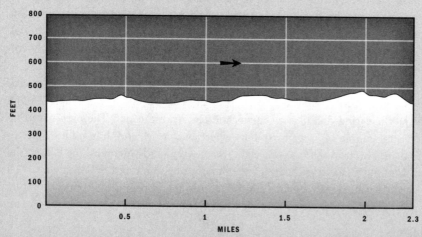

> Bring plenty of sunscreen, as
> much of the trail is exposed.

At the park entrance, pass through a gate; let the park worker there know you'll be hiking, and you should receive a general map of the trails. Admission is free for hikers, but if you plan to camp, you'll need to pay. Once you pass through the gate, turn left and park in the lot on the western-most side of the park, near the boat launch. Although the huge parking lot can easily accommodate a large number of cars, on my visit it was completely empty because most hikers were primarily campers who just walked over.

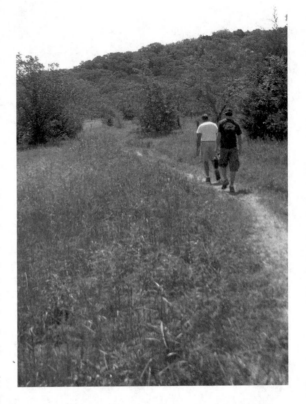

The Army Corps of Engineers website advises that this trail is within a hunting area, and hikers should be wary during hunting season. I did speak with a park ranger regarding safety issues, and he advised me that the trail receives a fair amount of traffic from campers, hikers, equestrians, and bikers year-round and that they have never encountered any type of a problem, even during hunting season. I felt very safe and would readily visit again at any time of year. Those still concerned, however, can check the dates of hunting season for Ellis County available in the Texas Parks and Wildlife *Outdoor Annual*. Some general tips for hiking close to or within a hunting area: wear brightly colored clothing in shades not found in nature, and stay on designated trails.

At the trailhead, take the path that heads straight out from the gate toward the west. A couple hundred feet down, bear right at the junction and hike through a grassland clearing dotted with cactus and eastern red cedar. The path winds up and down a couple of low, grassy hills where butterflies and dragonflies come to greet you as you pass. Off to your right, thick woodlands surround the lake to the north, forming a shield preventing any glimpse of the water.

At 0.48 mile, reach a wide, grassy lane running through the center of a long stretch of grassland meadow. Bear right onto the flat, sunny route, heading west.

This is an excellent trail to hike with the family, because the comfortable width of the trail allows you to walk three or four abreast. With the woodlands still to the far right, tree-dotted hillsides to the far left, and nothing but a grassy corridor before you, you'll be able to take in the peaceful scenery while still maintaining a conversation. Equestrian riders love the trail for just this reason, and you're likely to pass a few along this portion of the hike.

Bear left at 1.1 miles, leaving the grassland and heading south onto the narrow path through the short trees and berry-laden shrubs. The path winds slightly uphill and curves back east through the gently rolling, shrubby woodlands. You'll eventually emerge from the woods and back into the grassland, hiking parallel to the trail you came in on, which is hidden by the tall, dry grasses on your left.

Merge back onto the wide path at 1.9 miles, where you'll turn right, following the trail uphill. It's a pleasant walk through more open grassland until you reach 2.2 miles, where an alternate trailhead intended for equestrians appears. Bear left at the junction and follow the trail back to the final right turn at 2.3 miles, where you'll find the trailhead.

For hikers wanting a longer trail, instead of turning off the wide, grassy path at 1.1 miles, continue straight. The trail heads northwest past the Ennis Rotary Club, then turns east, leading all the way out to Mustang Point on the edge of the lake; in total there are more than 13 miles of trail.

NEARBY ACTIVITIES

For lunch, don't miss Bubba's Bar-B-Q & Steakhouse in Ennis, spotlighted in USA Today as an excellent roadside eatery ([972] 875-0036). Bubba's is right off I-45 at Exit 251.

If you're here in spring, don't miss Ennis's Bluebonnet Trails driving routes, which take you past fields of wildflowers. Springtime also brings the Bluebonnet Trails Festival, where you'll find arts, crafts, food, and music. Visit the city's convention and visitor bureau for the exact dates, or check online at **visitennis.org**.

44 CEDAR HILL STATE PARK:
Talala–Duck Pond Loop

KEY AT-A-GLANCE INFORMATION

LENGTH: 4.23 miles

CONFIGURATION: Loop with spurs

DIFFICULTY: Easy

SCENERY: Native plants, wildflowers, pond

EXPOSURE: Partially shady

TRAIL TRAFFIC: Light

TRAIL SURFACE: Packed dirt

HIKING TIME: 2 hours

ACCESS: $5 per person; open daily, 8 a.m.–10 p.m.

FACILITIES: Restrooms, water fountain, picnic area

WHEELCHAIR TRAVERSABLE: No

SPECIAL COMMENTS: Bring insect repellent in spring and summer. Pack a picnic to enjoy at a lakeside table.

SUPPLEMENTAL MAPS: tpwd.state .tx.us/publications/pwdpubs/ media/park_maps/pwd_mp _p4503_131l_1.pdf

DRIVING DISTANCE FROM MAJOR INTERSECTION: 9 miles from I-20 and US 67

GPS TRAILHEAD COORDINATES

Latitude: N 32° 36' 59"
Longitude: W 96° 58' 53"

IN BRIEF

This pleasant hike winds along an interpretive trail where markers help you identify native plants and grasses then loops around a small pond. A couple of overlooks along the trail provide peaceful spots to enjoy the scenery.

DESCRIPTION

Since Cedar Hill State Park's opening in 1991, it has become one of the most visited state parks in the state of Texas, in large part because it's so close to both Dallas and Fort Worth (about 20 miles from the former, and about 25 miles from the latter). Adjacent to Joe Pool Lake, the park's expansive 1,826 acres attract millions of outdoor enthusiasts each year. Although Joe Pool is not the most scenic of lakes, it's justifiably popular as a catalyst for getting outside and enjoying the park's array of activities, which include hiking, camping, biking, fishing, picnicking, and boating.

The park's several miles of trails include some open to both mountain bikers and hikers, and a couple open only to hikers. Before the hike, stop by the visitor center at the park's entrance and ask for the interpretive brochure for the Talala Trail. The small booklet is not usually out with the other park maps and information, but the park rangers do have brochures

----

Directions

Take I-20 to exit FM 1382 toward Cedar Hill. Cedar Hill State Park is about 4 miles south on the right. The trailhead is on the south side of the park. From the park entrance, turn left at the first intersection, onto South Spine Road. Continue straight, past some campsite turnoffs on the right, before you reach the trailhead parking lot, also on the right.

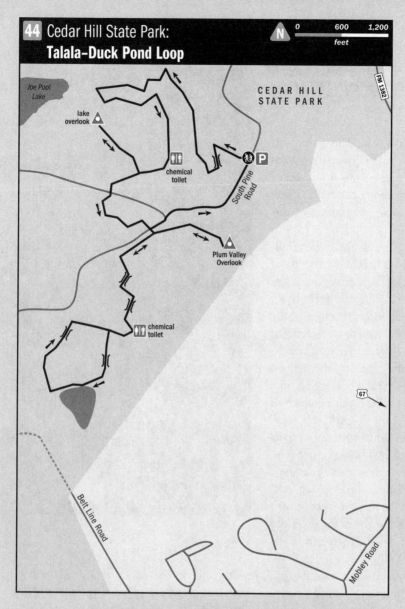

N

0   600   1,200
feet

Joe Pool Lake

CEDAR HILL
STATE PARK

FM 1382

lake overlook

chemical toilet

South Pine Road

P

Plum Valley Overlook

chemical toilet

67

Belt Line Road

Mobley Road

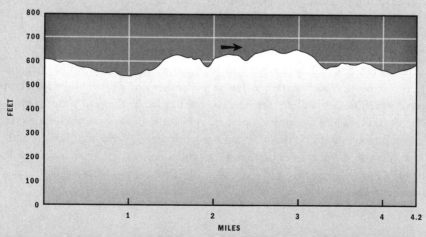

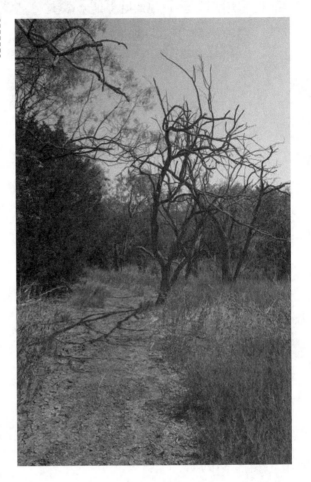

Animals such as the bobcat call the wild terrain home.

if you ask. The pamphlet, which describes native wildlife and plants at numbered posts along the trail, is useful at the beginning of this hike.

You'll find the trailhead adjacent to the parking lot. The first part of the hike is along the Talala Trail, which loops through a hilly terrain where you can use the interpretive brochure to identify points of interests. This trail is best hiked on a cooler day because much of the trail is exposed; small trees and brush cast partial shade on only some portions. I strongly suggest bringing a GPS or compass along, as it can be easy to get disoriented at the many junctions and secondary paths along the trail.

Starting down the trail, reach a split in the path at 0.13 mile and turn left, following the trail as it curves south through a grassy meadow with a few trees. At 0.18 mile, come to a wooden bridge (which, on my hike, spanned a dried-up creek), across which you'll find another trail junction, where you'll bear left. The next junction is at 0.21 mile and has the first marker, identifying the clasping coneflower, a yellow annual with a long, cone-shaped head.

The trail slopes slightly downhill, crosses another small, wooden bridge, and passes through some hackberries. A few steps farther on is the marker for giant ragweed, which flowers in late summer. For the next mile, the trail winds slightly uphill past trees such as the honey locust and grasses such as Texas wintergrass. In the spring, markers indicate that you can see wildflowers, including Indian paintbrush. You'll also see posts identifying the wildlife that lives in the area, including the painted bunting, red-tailed hawk, and cattle egret, along with larger animals such as the bobcat.

At about 1.1 miles, reach a clearing and see a small red outhouse intended for primitive campers, as well as a trail split, where you'll bear right. Watch for a marker identifying the mesquite tree, recognizable by its spiny branches. About 150 feet farther is the next junction, where you'll go right. Continue straight until you reach 1.18 miles, where the path splits. Head right to reach Lake Overlook, which offers a view of the glistening waters of Joe Pool Lake in the distance. This is a nice places to rest for a minute on the bench and take in the scenery. Retrace your steps to the overlook turnoff, this time taking the left split, to resume the trail. The path widens, still winding through the trees. You'll see a campground over to the left, and then you'll cross over a small road that heads past the campsites. Cross the street and pick up Duck Pond Trail at the yellow gate just to the left of some restrooms. The path winds downhill through the trees, crosses a bridge, and then starts to wind back uphill through grassy terrain.

At 1.88 miles, cross South Spine Road and resume the trail on the other side. A couple hundred feet farther, reach the next junction. To the left, the trail dead-ends at Plum Valley Overlook, where a bench is tucked away beneath some vine-covered trees and you can relax and enjoy the views of the surrounding hillsides.

When you're ready, head back to the overlook turnoff, then follow the trail to the right, which curls downhill through trees and native grasses and over a couple of long, wooden bridges spanning ravines. The path slowly winds uphill and then, at 2.63 miles, reaches a junction marked by another red outhouse, indicating another area for primitive camping. When I was here, however, I saw no evidence of any such adventurers.

Turn right, onto a wide gravel trail peppered with cacti. At 2.7 miles, reach the loop junction. Turn left onto the loop. The trail crosses a wooden bridge and then heads through some tall trees before passing two more bridges and finally reaching Duck Pond. The small pond is like an oasis amid the woods. There's only one small vantage point between the trees, however, discouraging anything more than a short rest.

Continuing past the pond, cross a bridge and turn right at the split at 3.18 miles. At 3.25 miles, you'll have completed the pond loop. From here, retrace your steps to South Spine Road. Turn right onto the road and walk along the grassy shoulder. The trailhead and parking lot are about 0.29 mile ahead on the left.

NEARBY ACTIVITIES

Within the park, you can explore Penn Farm Agricultural History Center, a restored farm exhibit. Ask at the visitor center for a self-guided interpretive booklet.

About 8.5 miles northwest of the park, you can visit Trader's Village—the largest weekend flea market in the state—open weekends from 8 a.m. to sundown. Thousands of booths sell all manner of products. To get there, take I-20 West to Exit 454, and turn right onto South Great Southwest Parkway. After 1 mile, turn left onto Mayfield Road. Trader's Village is about 0.3 mile down on the right.

45 CEDAR MOUNTAIN TRAIL

KEY AT-A-GLANCE INFORMATION

LENGTH: 1.2 miles

CONFIGURATION: Balloon

DIFFICULTY: Easy

SCENERY: Woodlands, cedar trees

EXPOSURE: Mostly shady

TRAIL TRAFFIC: Light

TRAIL SURFACE: Packed dirt

HIKING TIME: 45 minutes

ACCESS: Free; open daily, 6 a.m.–sundown

FACILITIES: None

WHEELCHAIR TRAVERSABLE: No

SPECIAL COMMENTS: Caution younger hikers on what they should do if they see a snake. Bring insect repellent. Bikes are prohibited on this trail.

DRIVING DISTANCE FROM MAJOR INTERSECTION: 8.4 miles from I-20 and US 67

GPS TRAILHEAD COORDINATES

Latitude: N 32° 36' 55"

Longitude: W 96° 58' 19"

IN BRIEF

This pleasant trail winds slowly uphill through a dense woodland. It's a nice hike for kids just getting interested in hiking, because the size and terrain are easy to manage, but it's still wild and secluded enough to feel like an accomplishment.

DESCRIPTION

The Cedar Mountain Preserve, a 110-acre section of hilly woodland next to Joe Pool Lake, draws a fair number of visitors, despite its proximity to larger trail systems, such as the Cedar Ridge Preserve (aka the Dallas Nature Center) and Cedar Hill State Park. This is in part due to Cedar Mountain's convenient, appealing location. The small parking lot is adjacent to the main road and is easy to stumble upon. If you happen to be driving by on a sunny day and see a couple of parked cars and a few folks disappearing down one of the trails, you'll undoubtedly want to pull over and investigate. Many of the hikers lured in to the preserve are on their way to or from the lake, a reservoir named after a 1960s congressman instrumental in its establishment. The lake lies just to the west of the preserve. Organized events are always happening somewhere along the lake and include bike rallies, fishing tournaments, outdoor-club meet-ups, and activities such as camping, picnicking, and bird-watching.

Directions ⟶

Take I-20 and exit onto FM 1382 toward Cedar Hill. The trail is in Cedar Mountain Preserve, about 5 miles south on the right, just past Cedar Hill State Park.

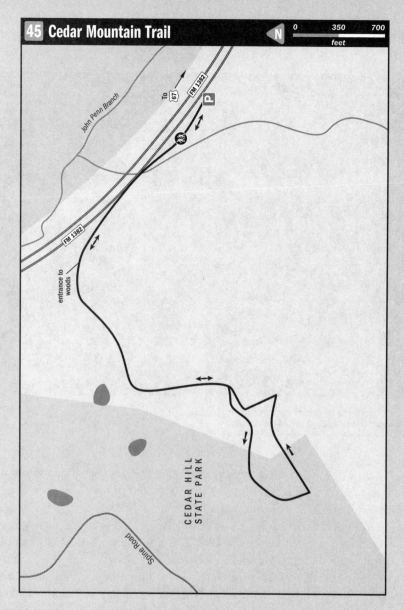

N

0   350   700
feet

To 67

FM 1382

FM 1382

P

John Penn Branch

entrance to woods

CEDAR HILL STATE PARK

Spine Road

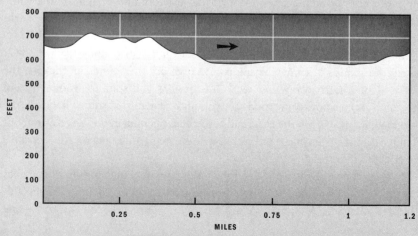

800
700
600
500
400
FEET
300
200
100
0

0.25   0.5   0.75   1   1.2
MILES

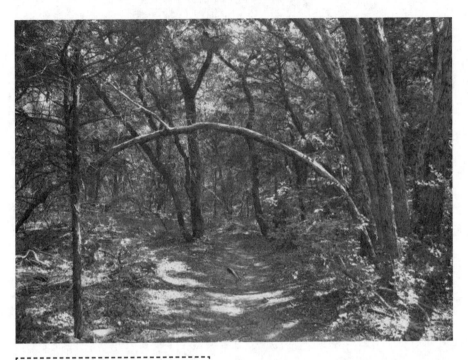

The trail winds through thick woodlands.

Because the trails in the preserve are not incredibly lengthy, visitors don't stay long, and parking is plentiful. It's popular with folks walking their dogs and families with children, who appreciate its manageable size.

In front of the parking lot, a kiosk displaying a map of the preserve gives you a chance to get oriented before the hike. To get to the trailhead from here, head right, following the sidewalk north. The trail curves away from the parking lot and, at about 0.1 mile, reaches the trailhead—a dirt path branching north off the paved trail. A sign here advises that bicyclists are prohibited and cautions hikers of the presence of poisonous snakes. (Many folks just continue straight on the wide, paved trail, which makes a small loop over level terrain back around to the parking lot.)

The dirt trail heads northwest onto the wide, grassy strip alongside FM 1382. Although the sounds of cars whizzing past drown out the sounds of crickets, the trail is well off the roadway and feels safe. Just as you start to wonder where you're going and become concerned that you may have missed some vital turn, the trail veers west, away from the road and toward an opening in the woods, at about 0.27 mile. A rustic sign mounted between two tree trunks marks the entrance where the trail disappears into the trees.

The trail climbs slightly and then descends, twisting and turning as it makes its way through the woods. The closely packed trees do an excellent job of shrouding the trail in shade. Although we did pass a couple of folks on the trail—one group with children and one couple—the trail still had a feeling of solitude and remoteness to it.

You'll soon reach a grove of trees where an intoxicating scent hangs thick in the air. A few deep breaths will help you identify it as the rich smell of cedar. In the summer, flying insects buzz regularly around the path. Apply plenty of insect repellent for your walk through this wooded hillside. I also found it impossible to ignore the thick spiderwebs that stretched across the ground and between trees, bridging gaps between logs, across branches, amid leaves, and in every trunk's knothole. Fortunately, most of the spiders stay in the woods, and unless you're one of the first hikers on the trail, their webs don't obstruct the path. The woodlands are also home to raccoons, coyotes, and armadillos.

At about 0.55 mile, head right onto the beginning of the trail loop, which makes a slow, mild uphill climb. The path passes an interesting section where a number of old, dead trees litter the ground, then bypasses a dried-out ravine. After you duck under a low-hanging branch that spans the trail, reach the top of a hill. Although you haven't climbed high enough to get above the trees for any kind of a view, the surrounding wilderness rewards you with a sense of being deep in the woods.

The trail then loops east, heading back downhill before rejoining the trail. At about 0.88 mile, you'll be back at the loop junction. From here, retrace your steps to the trailhead. To extend the hike, detour onto the paved pathway loop through the woods and back to the parking lot.

NEARBY ACTIVITIES

Just up FM 1382, Cedar Hill State Park, which lies along Joe Pool Lake, is popular with fishermen, boaters, picnickers, campers, and birders (see Hike 44, page 202). Inside the state park you'll also find the Penn Farm Agricultural History Center, a restored farm exhibit.

46 CEDAR RIDGE PRESERVE TRAIL

KEY AT-A-GLANCE INFORMATION

LENGTH: 3.25 miles

CONFIGURATION: Double loop

DIFFICULTY: Moderate

SCENERY: Pond, creek, abundant birdlife

EXPOSURE: Open–shady

TRAIL TRAFFIC: Light

TRAIL SURFACE: Dirt, rock

HIKING TIME: 2 hours

ACCESS: November 1–March 31: 6:30 a.m.–6 p.m.; April 1–October 1: 6:30 a.m.–8:30 p.m.; donations accepted

FACILITIES: Restrooms, benches, and water fountains

WHEELCHAIR TRAVERSABLE: Yes

SPECIAL COMMENTS: Bring sunscreen.

SUPPLEMENTAL MAPS: audubon Dallas.org/crp_trail_map.pdf

DRIVING DISTANCE FROM MAJOR INTERSECTION: 5.3 miles from I-20 and US 67

GPS TRAILHEAD COORDINATES

Latitude: N 32° 38' 12"

Longitude: W 96° 57' 32"

IN BRIEF

This rigorous hike takes you through varied terrain on some of the most enjoyable trails in the area. Hike up a modest hill, trek down a fossil trail, traverse a pond enclosed by hundreds of cattails, and meander down excellent bird-watching footpaths.

DESCRIPTION

A 10-mile network of paths of varying difficulty keeps the Cedar Ridge Preserve—a park that can be fairly busy on weekends—uncrowded and even desolate in parts. In spring the preserve is a great place to see butterflies, migrating and breeding birds, and beds of bluebonnets. In addition to hawks circling overhead, you may see a snake or two, as I did on another recent hike here. Signs clearly posted at several points along the trail warn of copperheads, rattlesnakes, water moccasins, and coral snakes; obviously, sticking to designated trails is a must.

Formerly known as the Dallas Nature Center, Cedar Ridge Preserve is managed by the Dallas Audubon Society, which has done an excellent job of maintaining the park. The amenities in particular are excellent and include picnic tables, restrooms, well-marked

Directions

From I-20 West, take Exit 458, then turn left onto Mountain Creek Parkway and follow it 2.8 miles to the Cedar Ridge Preserve. Access the reserve via a turnoff on the right where there is a small sign—keep an eye out for it. Follow the road into the preserve and turn right at the fork to enter the main parking lot; the left fork terminates at a smaller lot reserved for persons with disabilities.

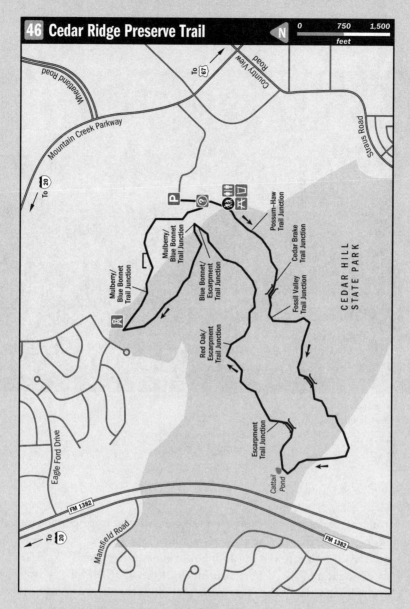

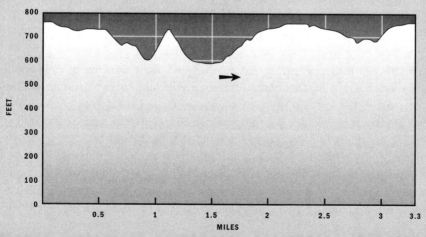

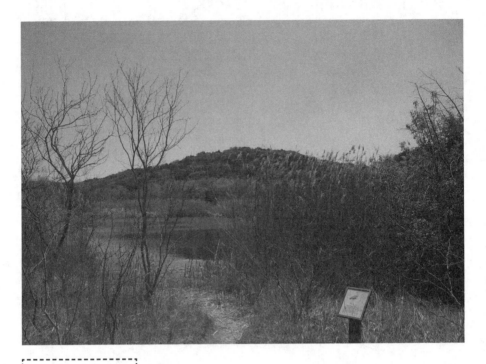

A view of Cattail Pond

trails, and water fountains . . . even one at ground level for hikes of the four-legged kind!

From the parking area, enter the preserve and stop to orient yourself at the visitor kiosk. The trailhead starts just behind the kiosk, so once you're ready to go, follow the main trail a few steps until you see a sign for Cattail Pond Trail. The trail is well kept, and you'll note that much of the first half mile is strewn with mulch, which makes walking fairly easy. You will, however, want to be watchful of low branches and exposed roots, especially as you venture farther down the trail and deeper into the preserve. Most of this section is enclosed by trees and shrubbery, keeping hot sun to a minimum. But you should expect it to be warm, even on an otherwise cool day, because trees tend to block the wind.

Follow the trail past prickly pear cactus and signs warning of poison ivy, until you reach a trail split at about 300 feet into the hike, where Possumhaw Trail branches off to the left. Continuing straight on Cattail Pond Trail, a short hike quickly leads you to another junction, where you can access Cedar Brake Trail (a 1.7-mile loop). For this hike, stay to the right on Cattail Pond Trail, which briefly descends a rocky path, then climbs gently. The path meanders through low trees and brush, past the spot where Cedar Brake Trail rejoins Cattail Pond Trail, and then over a small wooden bridge that spans a dry ravine. The preserve is particularly well known among birders; many birds visit and live here, particularly in the spring, including warblers, flycatchers, buntings, vireos, bluebirds, and hawks. The bridge is a good vantage point to catch sight of one of these residents, the Carolina wren—a small, rust-colored bird distinguished by a thin white stripe over its eye, further described on a plaque adjacent to the bridge.

A little more than 0.5 mile into the hike, turn left onto the path marked FOS-SIL VALLEY TRAIL. The trail curls downhill before starting a steep ascent. As you begin the uphill trek, scan the ground for fossils, which you may find embedded in rocks along the trail if you have a keen eye. The next 0.25 mile is the most challenging part of the hike—the trail climbs steeply to the summit of a small hill, passing a couple of benches, some grassy patches with dragonflies buzzing past and butterflies darting about, a wide shallow creek, and another wooden bridge. When you reach an unmarked trail split, with both paths continuing steeply uphill, take the path to the right for a more moderate climb. A short climb later, reach a small clearing that marks the hill's summit. Although trees obstruct the view of the surrounding terrain, there are several viewpoints on the descent that make the climb worthwhile. This is an excellent spot (with a conveniently placed bench) for taking a breather before you begin the downhill trek.

Your route downhill winds past a couple more benches before emerging into a small meadow teeming with purple wildflowers and offering excellent views of the surrounding hills and the surprisingly close highway. When you reach the bottom of the hill, you'll find yourself on the other side of Cattail Pond, which is hidden by hundreds of 6-foot-tall cattails. As you wind your way around the pond, take time to enjoy the scenery. You may discover animal tracks or spy the elegant great blue heron. This portion of the trail is much more exposed to the sun, so be prepared.

At the next trail split, look for signs for Escarpment Road Trail to the left and Cattail Pond Trail to the right. Head left down Escarpment Road Trail, which quickly widens and follows the remnants of an old wagon trail. This portion of the trail has a few scenic overlooks on its way slowly up another hill.

At about 1.85 miles into the hike, you'll reach the intersection of Red Oak Trail and Escarpment Road Trail. Continue right, up Escarpment Road Trail, then bear left onto Bluebonnet Trail. The past couple of summers have seen few bluebonnets, but if you're hiking in spring, you should see at least some bordering the trail. At the next trail split, take a hard left, continuing along Bluebonnet Trail. At the next unsigned junction, bear right. A few steps up this trail, at 2.75 miles into the hike, you'll find an observation tower that affords excellent views of the surrounding hills and woodlands. A few steps up the trail from the tower, turn left onto Mulberry Trail, where you'll find yourself at the top of a set of steep stairs built into the trail, overlooking what is one of the most striking parts of the hike. Tall trees threaded with vines rise out of a small valley and tower overhead, casting deep shadows on the trail and the surrounding dense, green vegetation. This little section of trail makes you feel as if you're deep inside a forest. The most curious feature—an old tree that has somehow curled in upon itself to form a C

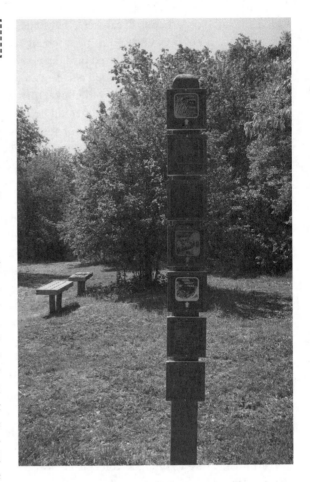

Signposts help direct visitors onto the preserve's many trails.

before reaching for the sun—is definitely worth a closer look. A few benches tucked next to the trail offer a spot from which to enjoy the special beauty of this portion of trail. At this point, you're close to 3 miles into the hike.

The final portion of the hike follows the trail until it reaches an unmarked split, where you turn left. The trail then emerges into an open meadow, where the trail splits, strategically circling the meadow—ideal for bird-watching. Turn left at the split to reach the trail's end, behind the restrooms; head toward and around them, and you're back at the trailhead.

NEARBY ACTIVITIES

Just 3 miles away, Cedar Hill State Park, which lies along Joe Pool Lake, is popular with fishermen, boaters, picnickers, campers, and birders (see Hike 44, page 202). Inside the state park you'll also find the Penn Farm Agricultural History Center, a restored farm exhibit. To get there, head north on Mountain Creek Parkway for 1 mile, then turn left onto Eagle Ford Drive. About 0.8 mile ahead, turn left onto South Beltline Road; the park entrance is about 1.7 miles ahead on the right.

CLEBURNE STATE PARK LOOP TRAIL

47

IN BRIEF

This rocky trail loops through the woods of the park's outer perimeter, offering a few steep sections that will raise your heart rate. Its highlight is an overlook with a view of an elaborate masonry spillway adjacent to the park's small Cedar Lake.

DESCRIPTION

The 528-acre Cleburne State Park was opened in 1938, thanks in part to the hard work done by the Civilian Conservation Corps, whose efforts are apparent in the elaborate masonry spillway they constructed adjacent to the park's spring-fed Cedar Lake. The park's amenities include camping and fishing (though at only 116 acres, the lake is quite small) and more than 5 miles of hiking trails. These trails, with names such as Whispering Meadow, Fossil Ridge, and Spillway, can be combined to form an exhilarating loop circumnavigating the park.

To get to the trailhead for the loop, enter the park, pass the bathrooms on the left, and pull off into the first small parking area on the right, just off the park road. The trail curls downhill through trees and brush and crosses a creek. Across the creek bed, continue straight, heading east. The trail starts to ascend a rough, rutted path strewn with small rocks.

Directions

Take US 67 South toward Cleburne. About 6 miles past Cleburne, follow the brown state-park signs left onto Park Road 21. Cleburne State Park is about 6 miles down on the right. Once inside, park in the first lot on the right, just after the restrooms.

KEY AT-A-GLANCE INFORMATION

LENGTH: 5.86 miles

CONFIGURATION: Loop

DIFFICULTY: Hard

SCENERY: Spillway, lake, woods, meadow, fossils

EXPOSURE: Partially shady

TRAIL TRAFFIC: Light

TRAIL SURFACE: Packed dirt

HIKING TIME: 2.75 hours

ACCESS: $3 per person; open daily, 7 a.m.–10 p.m.

FACILITIES: Restrooms, benches, and picnic tables in nearby day-use area

WHEELCHAIR TRAVERSABLE: No

SPECIAL COMMENTS: Bring a walking stick and wear good hiking shoes.

SUPPLEMENTAL MAPS: tpwd.state .tx.us/publications/pwdpubs/ media/park_maps/pwd_mp _p4503_013a.pdf

DRIVING DISTANCE FROM MAJOR INTERSECTION: 25 miles from I-35W and US 67

GPS TRAILHEAD COORDINATES

Latitude: N 32° 15' 33"

Longitude: W 97° 33' 11"

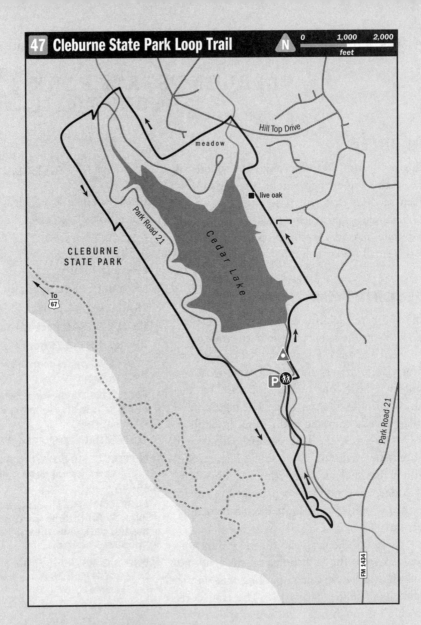

N

0   1,000   2,000
feet

Hill Top Drive

meadow

live oak

Cedar Lake

Park Road 21

CLEBURNE
STATE PARK

To
67

P

Park Road 21

FM 1434

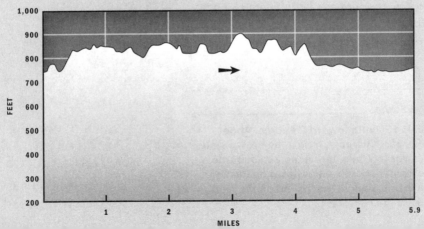

1,000
900
800
700
600
500
400
300
200

FEET

1   2   3   4   5   5.9

MILES

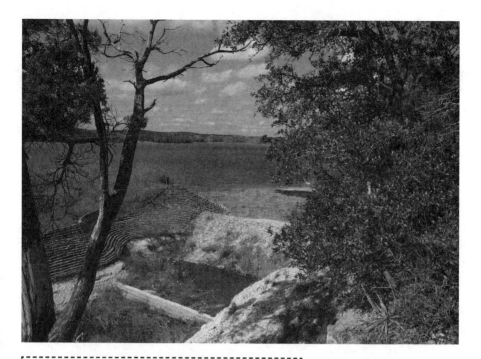

A short climb offers outstanding views of the spillway below.

At about 0.1 mile, bear left at the trail split. The path proceeds parallel to the creek you crossed and climbs toward an overlook. Be prepared for uneven footing; this ragged section of trail resembles a gully more than a path. Small bushes adjacent to the path cling to the hillside, offering little by way of scenery.

After a short climb, at 0.3 mile you'll come to the overlook, from which you'll have an exceptional view into the ravine and spillway below. When I first reached this overlook, I was unprepared for the spillway's massive size and beauty. Masonry built onto the sides of the bluff on the far side of the ravine accentuates a matching spillway that rises gradually in three massive tiers, appearing almost to resemble an ancient pyramid rather than a common spillway. Pick your way along the bluffs for a couple of great lookout spots.

When you're ready, continue down the trail, following the sign reading TO OVERLOOK AND LAKE LOOP, and bear right at the 0.35-mile junction. The path makes another short, strenuous climb up a rock-strewn stretch before reaching an old, gnarled tree clinging precariously to the edge of the bluff, beyond which is another fantastic view of the lake and spillway.

The trail continues through elm, mesquite, oak, and juniper; here you should keep an eye out for exposed tree roots. Bear to the right at the next couple of trail splits. You'll then begin a downhill trek through woods of mesquite, ash, oak, and elm. From here, the trail traces the state park's outer perimeter, marked by a barbed-wire fence. Note that, when in doubt at a trail split, keeping the fence to your right

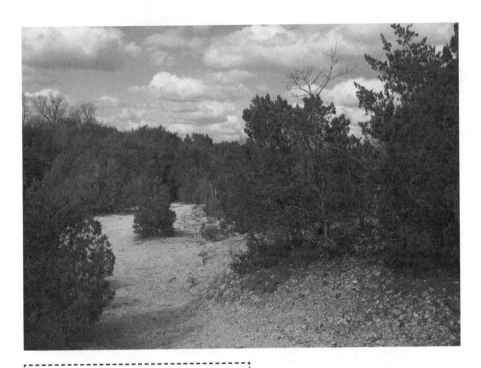

The hard-packed trail can be rough on the feet.

will keep you on the correct trail. The fence is almost invisible at most points, thanks to an overgrowth of vines and trees, and does not detract from the scenery.

Stay to the right at the next two junctions, continuing through terrain characterized by short, steep, rocky hills. The trail eventually flattens somewhat; however, it remains rocky and uneven for almost the entire hike. The path winds through the shade of the woods, keeping the sun from overheating you on sunny days.

Pass a sign marking a huge, beautiful old live oak tree before reaching a junction at 1.25 miles; bear right here. Continue across a babbling brook, then turn right at the next junction, where you'll trek through a small, cheery meadow. Briefly glimpse some private houses to the right before the next split at 2 miles, where you continue straight. When you get 0.35 mile farther down the path, reach a paved road in Shady Spring's camping area; if you've brought your lunch, you might stop at one of the shaded picnic tables for a rest and a quick bite to eat.

To resume the trail, head southwest along the road and look for a narrow dirt trail disappearing into the woods off to the right. It will be the first trail you see, only a few hundred feet from where you emerged. It is unmarked, so watch for it: it's easy to miss. You'll know you're on the correct trail by the familiar barbed-wire fence, which reappears a few feet down the trail on the right.

The trail continues straight, adjacent to the park's southwestern boundary and along a rocky slope appropriately named Fossil Ridge Trail. I spotted a couple of excellent imprints of ammonites (extinct mollusks with spiral shells) embedded in the trail's rock bed. Stay to the right at the next few junctions.

The property to the southwest of the park is being developed for its natural resources, and at various points along this section of the park's boundary you'll see signs advising you not to cross out of the state park and into the adjacent property. A barbed-wire fence continues along this section, clearly demarcating the boundary; be sure, however, youngsters don't get too curious and try to explore—the adjacent property is a lime quarry and can be dangerous. As you hike farther south, you'll also start to hear the rumble of heavy machinery, the source of which is a huge natural-gas rig on the next property off to the right.

Continue past the rig, bearing right at the next junction, at 4.3 miles, where the path reaches the park road. The sound of machinery will fade. The trail continues straight, stretching toward the southern park boundary before looping back through the woods and along a narrow creek. At 5.53 miles, it again intersects the park road, which you'll cross to resume the trail on the far side. Continue another 0.33 mile alongside the densely wooded creek before finally emerging at the trailhead from which you started.

NEARBY ACTIVITIES

Dinosaur Valley State Park, where you can explore dinosaur footprints fossilized in the park's riverbed, is in nearby Glen Rose. The Fossil Rim Wildlife Center, an 1,800-acre drive-through park where animals such as antelopes, rhinos, giraffes, ostriches, and zebras roam the fields and hillsides, is also close by. You can drive through the 10 miles of road in your own vehicle. Guided tours are available with advance booking. To get there from Cleburne State Park, return to US 67 and head west about 15 miles. You'll see a brown state-park sign for Dinosaur Valley on your right. The wildlife center is about 3 miles beyond it, down CR 2008, on the left. Hours vary by season. For more information, call (254) 897-2960.

48 COTTONWOOD CREEK TRAIL

KEY AT-A-GLANCE INFORMATION

LENGTH: 2.17 miles

CONFIGURATION: Loop

DIFFICULTY: Easy

SCENERY: Pecan grove, creek

EXPOSURE: Shady–sunny

TRAIL TRAFFIC: Light

TRAIL SURFACE: Grass

HIKING TIME: 40 minutes

ACCESS: Free; open daily, year-round

FACILITIES: Picnic tables

WHEELCHAIR TRAVERSABLE: No

SPECIAL COMMENTS: Watch your step if you leave the trail; there are patches of poison ivy along the creek.

DRIVING DISTANCE FROM MAJOR INTERSECTION: 7 miles from I-20 and I-45

GPS TRAILHEAD COORDINATES

Latitude: N 32° 36' 10"
Longitude: W 96° 40' 23"

IN BRIEF

This peaceful trail winds alongside a creek toward a tall pecan grove. Interpretive signs along the way identify the flora, and a pretty bridge at the far end crosses the creek to take you back to the beginning.

DESCRIPTION

Hidden down a small, bumpy road behind an old neighborhood in Wilmer, the 220-acre Cottonwood Creek Preserve was private land before it was given to the city. Its original owner planted the land with pecan trees. The pecan grove, which remains, comes as a pleasant surprise halfway through the hike.

During your visit, you'll probably see only one or two other hikers, more because of the hidden location than anything else. We arrived to an empty parking lot and empty trails and took our time enjoying the scenery before having a leisurely lunch at the picnic table. It wasn't until we were about to leave that others arrived—one local who quietly let his dog out for some romping, then left shortly thereafter, and another local couple who arrived with pecan pie in mind; they headed down the trail to quietly collect a few nuts from the thousands strewn through the grove.

From the parking lot, take the road past the entrance gate toward the creek. Initially it

Directions

Follow I-45 South toward I-30 and take Exit 270 onto Beltline Road. Turn left onto East Beltline Road and go 0.4 mile, then make a left onto North Goode Road and travel 0.3 mile. Turn right onto Cottonwood Valley Road to reach Cottonwood Creek Preserve.

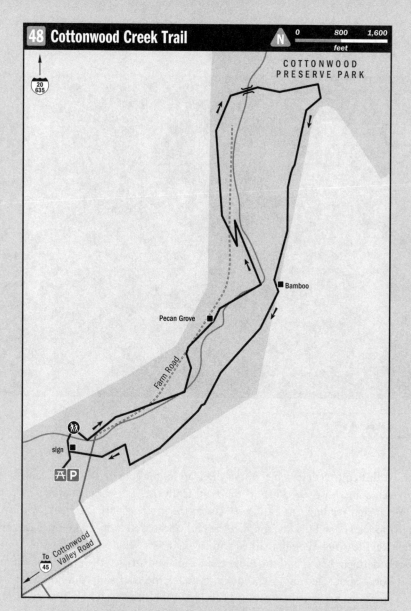

N

0   800   1,600

feet

20
635

COTTONWOOD
PRESERVE PARK

Bamboo

Pecan Grove

Farm Road

sign

To Cottonwood
Valley Road

45

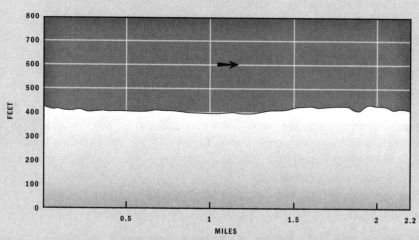

800
700
600
500
400
300
200
100
0

FEET

0.5   1   1.5   2   2.2

MILES

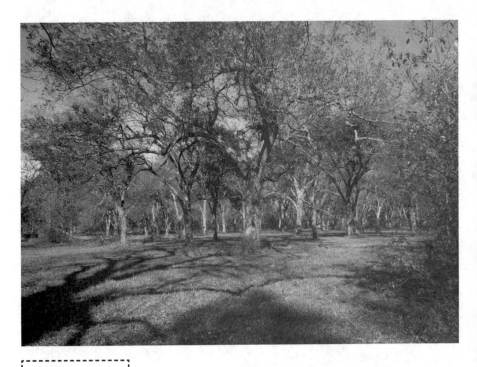

A quiet pecan grove

can be difficult to determine where the trail is: on your right, a low cable strung between some posts cordons off the road from the rest of the landscape. A small wooden sign reading CREEK TRAIL sits in the grass against the creek, with seemingly no trail in sight. This is in fact the end of the trail loop. In many places along the hike, the trail—though marked with regular wooden signs pointing the way—is poorly defined, being nothing more than a mowed strip in the tall grass. You need not worry about getting lost, though, because the trail simply follows the creek out, crosses a bridge, then comes back along the other side. Helpful signs along the way identify trees and point to the trail.

The trailhead is down the road and over the creek a few hundred feet past the CREEK TRAIL sign. Turn right onto the mowed, grassy strip, and you'll see a sign identifying the path as the Green Trail, which is where the hike starts. A sign next to it advises that archaeological remains, which you may see in the preserve, are not to be disturbed.

The trail heads northeast. To your right, between the trees, catch sight of the wide creek running along the bottom of a deep gully. Trees loom on either side, forming a shady canopy over the water. To your left, a small treeless meadow soaks in the sun, stretching alongside the path. Lime-green, softball-sized fruits known as horse apples (sometimes referred to as "green brains" because of their mottled appearance) litter the trail. An old farm road, now mostly grass, runs a couple dozen feet off to the left along the length of the trail. It stays mostly hidden from view, except at 0.2 mile, where the trail curves to join the road temporarily before veering east back toward the creek.

Along the trail, you'll spot a number of wooden signs in front of various plants and trees. The signs identify the honey locust, a thorny tree identifiable by its long brown seedpods; the grapevine, a climbing vine; the saw greenbrier, a vine that can form thick thickets; and poison ivy. Other signs along the trail advise that the area is a poisonous-snake habitat.

The trail continues along the creek, offering a couple of nice overlooks with views of the water on the right. Pass more signs identifying native plants, including coralberry, chittamwood, and privet. The meadow ends as you enter a large grove of pecan trees where the creek curves. In the fall, leaves litter the ground, hiding the trail.

Continue alongside the creek, traversing the outskirts of the grove. On the banks you'll spot trees such as chinaberry, dogwood, cedar elm, and hackberry. At various points, the trees open a little, and you can peer into the creek and see the intricate patterns of exposed tree roots clinging to the sides of the steep bank.

The preserve narrows into a lane with the creek on the left and a fence on the right. The trail then merges onto the park road, overgrown and barely discernible, before it curves toward a wooden bridge. The bridge, built atop two huge logs that bounce with each step, marks the hike's halfway point. Cross the bridge and follow the trail signs on the opposite side of the creek for Creek Trail. The path winds through another grove, then curves back south along the creek. In the fall, the grove's small leaves turn a brilliant yellow. When they fall in the breeze, the sun glints off them, in an entrancing snowlike effect.

At 1.5 miles, traverse a patch of bamboo. At 1.6 miles, the trees recede and the trail is exposed to sun as it passes through a small meadow of tall grass. Droves of crickets and grasshoppers, including some up to two inches long, live along this section. With your every step, they spring up and fly out of the way in a wide spray. Stay in the mowed area alongside the creek. Before long, you'll pass another CREEK TRAIL sign and find yourself back at the trailhead.

NEARBY ACTIVITIES

The Rogers Wildlife Rehab and Farm Sanctuary is in Hutchins, only 6 miles away. The facility is a nonprofit organization that rehabilitates injured birds and farm animals. Visitors are welcome to roam the property free of charge; donations are accepted. On the grounds, you'll find dozens of outdoor cages serving as temporary homes for rehabilitating hawks, owls, blue jays, vultures, and herons, among others. Geese and pheasants wander around unfettered. To get there, follow I-45 North 2 miles and take Exit 274 (Dowdy Ferry Road). Stay on the service road about 0.5 mile, then turn right onto East Cleveland Street.

49 DINOSAUR VALLEY TRAIL

KEY AT-A-GLANCE INFORMATION

LENGTH: 4.31 miles

CONFIGURATION: Loop

DIFFICULTY: Moderate–hard

SCENERY: Hills, valley, river, dinosaur tracks

EXPOSURE: Partially sunny

TRAIL TRAFFIC: Light

TRAIL SURFACE: Packed dirt

HIKING TIME: 2 hours

ACCESS: $5 per person; open daily, 8 a.m.–10 p.m.

FACILITIES: Restrooms, picnic area, store

WHEELCHAIR TRAVERSABLE: No

SPECIAL COMMENTS: If the water level is high, be prepared to ford a couple shallow rivers. Bring your swimsuit for a dip in the swimming hole after the hike.

SUPPLEMENTAL MAPS: tpwd.state .tx.us/publications/pwdpubs/ media/park_maps/pwd_mp _p4503_094r.pdf

DRIVING DISTANCE FROM MAJOR INTERSECTION: 7 miles from TX 144 and US 67

GPS TRAILHEAD COORDINATES

Latitude: N 32° 14' 59"

Longitude: W 97° 48' 45"

IN BRIEF

This hike gains a little altitude to offer excellent overlooks of the park, then winds down to the riverbed, where you trek along million-year-old fossilized dinosaur tracks.

DESCRIPTION

Dinosaur Valley State Park is known internationally for the well-preserved dinosaur tracks in the riverbed that runs through the park. The tracks date back about 110 million years to the Cretaceous period. It is believed that at that time this area was an ancient shoreline, along which the dinosaurs may have been migrating or feeding. The mud tracks of these huge creatures eventually fossilized and were buried by limestone and sandstone in what is now the Paluxy riverbed. Today, the river cuts through these sheets of rock, exposing the tracks buried within. In summer, the river dries out and many of the tracks are exposed on the dry, stony riverbed. The park allows you to roam freely among these sites, and in summer you'll find hoards of visitors closely examining the imprints left by these prehistoric reptiles.

Although the park is heavily visited, you'll find that the hiking trails are fairly empty, because most folks head straight for

Directions

Take US 67 south to Glen Rose and Dinosaur Valley State Park. Just before you leave Glen Rose, turn right onto FM 205 (Barnard Street); the DINOSAUR VALLEY sign is small, so watch for it. At about 3 miles, bear right at the fork onto Park Road 59. The park entrance is about 1 mile farther. When inside the park, take the first two right turns, following the signs toward the camping area. The parking lot is on the right, just before the campsites.

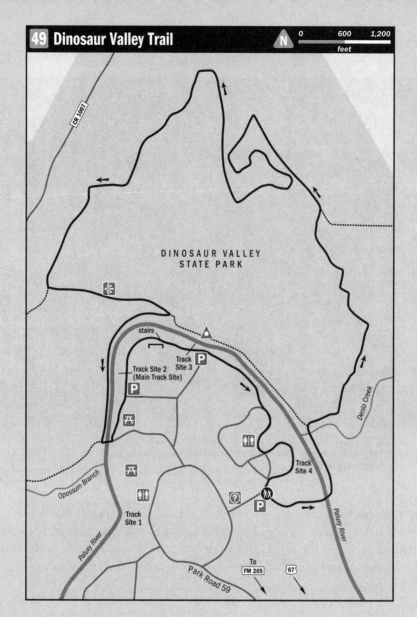

0   600   1,200
feet

N

DINOSAUR VALLEY
STATE PARK

CR 1007

stairs

Track
Site 3

P

Track Site 2
(Main Track Site)

P

Track
Site 4

Track
Site 1

Opossum Branch

Paluxy River

Paluxy River

Denio Creek

P

To
FM 205

67

Park Road 59

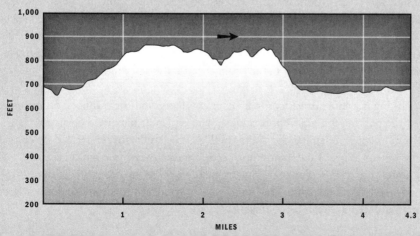

1,000
900
800
700
600
500
400
300
200

FEET

1   2   3   4   4.3

MILES

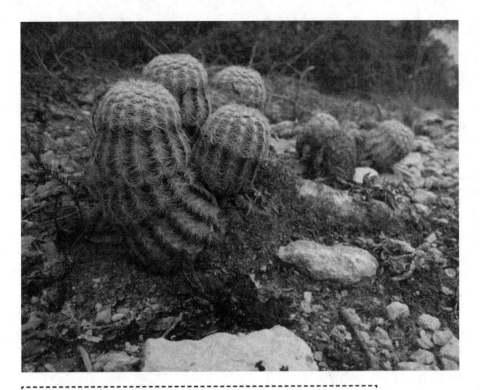

Only a couple of inches tall, these small cacti can be seen growing along some parts of the trail's edge.

the main track sites or for a dip in the nearby swimming hole. In fact, the day we set out on this hike, we passed no other hikers on the trail, although footprints and bike marks in the dirt indicate that the trails do see some use. Those who don't venture onto the hillside trails are missing out on one of the more fun hikes in the area.

The route I've selected starts with a decent workout as it climbs into the hills alongside the river, offers inspiring views of the surrounding hillsides midway through, and finally rewards you with the excitement of discovery as you reach the ancient dinosaur tracks at its end. When you arrive, stop by the park's headquarters at the main entrance to pick up a trail map, check out the interpretive display, and find information on any ranger-led talks or events happening during your visit.

Parking is a short drive from the main entrance; find the trailhead on the east side of the parking lot, adjacent to a kiosk with a map displaying the various trails. Take a moment to examine the map; you'll see the trails are referenced by color. On the hike, the trail's corresponding color appears every few hundred feet on a tree. Watch for these color markings to ensure you're on the correct route—it's easy to get lost. The park's trail maps are a good reference, though they are slightly outdated and can be confusing.

Follow the trail past the kiosk through a grassy field dotted with trees. When the path splits at 0.18 mile, keep left to follow the main trail. Descend a brief switchback and a few steep stairs before reaching the riverbed. Hop across the rocks or wade through the shallow river to resume the trail on the opposite bank. If you've come late in summer, as I did, chances are that the river will be dry, allowing you to stop and investigate Track Site 4, which is in the riverbed about 500 feet to the left. Look for the three-toed tracks, which are about a foot long, on the left bank of the river. Many of them are so well defined that it's hard to believe that they're not fresh and that one of the huge beasts isn't waiting around the bend for you.

After you cross the river, you'll be on White Trail, which leads steadily up through a wooded hill, paralleling the river. Keep straight, following this trail and ignoring any secondary paths branching into the woods, until you reach a pole marking Junction A, at about 0.36 mile. The trail to the right heads southeast into the primitive-camping area; take the left branch, following the trail downhill into the Denio Creek riverbed. Cross the shallow river and pick up the trail across the river, slightly to the right. Head back uphill until you reach another junction at about 0.43 mile, where you bear left. Stay on this path, following it as it slowly climbs into the hills, through woodlands peppered with grassy clearings and cacti; you should see paint on the trees marking this as the Green Trail. During the summer months, dragonflies, crickets, and, curiously enough, flies buzz across the trail often, so you'd be well advised to bring insect repellent along. As for animals, in the early morning, you can hear movement in the brush adjacent to the trail as they clear out of your way. The area is home to deer, armadillos, coyotes, and skunks. Though we spotted nothing more than lizards (of which there are many), we came very close to seeing a raccoon, as indicated by the fresh scat on the trail.

The trail passes a barbed-wire fence marking the boundary of the park, then switchbacks downhill. Pass a small pool on the right, followed by some excellent unobstructed views of the surrounding valley, before reaching the next junction at 2.41 miles. To the right, catch glimpses between the trees of the park's entrance down below. A better overlook is not far off; stay to the left and, at 2.61 miles, reach another junction, with a path heading steeply downhill to the right. Again, stay to the left, and at 2.81 miles come to an overlook where you'll have a bird's-eye view of the Main Track Site below and the scores of visitors bending over to examine the ground.

Continuing on the trail, you'll see yellow markings on the trees, indicating that you've reached the Yellow Trail. The trail descends and then, at 2.96 miles, reaches a pole (which, during my visit, had a huge vulture perched atop it), marking yet another junction. Head right, onto the Blue Trail. The trail descends steadily toward the river peeking through on the left. At 3.29 miles, just past a field on the right, you'll see the turnoff on the left to get to the river; a small sign marks it as the continuation of the Blue Trail. Turn left here and, at 3.36 miles, reach the edge of the

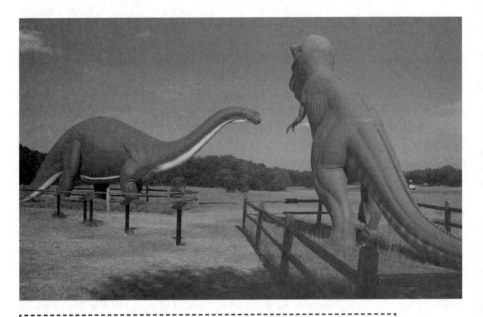

A 45-foot tall *T. rex* and a 70-foot tall *Apatosaurus* guard the entrance to the park.

river and the Main Track Site, where you can see the tracks of theropods (three-toed prints from large carnivorous dinosaurs) and sauropods (elephant-like prints from gigantic herbivorous dinosaurs, resembling brontosaurs).

The trail resumes on the left, adjacent to the entrance steps, on the other side of the river. In summer you probably won't have to ford the river to get there but can simply walk across the dried-out riverbed, examining the tracks as you go. You might even catch one of the park rangers giving an impromptu presentation there. When you're done exploring, continue on the trail. At about 3.69 miles, reach some benches and stairs climbing up out of the riverbed, and at about 3.71 miles, pass a parking lot and an overlook to the theropod tracks at Track Site 3. The trail continues along the sidewalk through the woods and to the camping area. At about 3.96 miles, arrive at the camping area, where you'll turn left onto the road, following it 0.35 mile past the restrooms and back to the trailhead.

NEARBY ACTIVITIES

The nearby Fossil Rim Wildlife Center is an 1,800-acre drive through a park where animals such as antelopes, rhinos, giraffes, ostriches, and zebras roam the fields and hillsides. You can drive the 10 miles of road in your own vehicle. Guided tours are also available but require advance booking. To get there from Dinosaur Valley, take US 67 southwest 3 miles and turn left onto CR 2008; from here it's about 1 more mile to the park. Hours vary by season. For more information, call (254) 897-2960.

PURTIS CREEK TRAIL

IN BRIEF

This shady trail loops through the woods in an area used for primitive camping. Several access points to the water and a photo blind make it a good morning hike for bird-watchers.

DESCRIPTION

Almost exactly 60 miles from Dallas, Purtis Creek State Park is known specifically for its excellent fishing. The waters, stocked with largemouth bass (catch-and-release), catfish, and crappie, attract anglers from throughout the Metroplex. The lake has speed limits and permits only 50 boats on the water at a time, resulting in a quiet, mellow atmosphere. The park was acquired in 1977 and opened to the public in 1988. It includes a 355-acre lake with a swimming area, fishing pier, boat ramp, and bait shop. If you're interested in getting out on the water after the hike, you can rent a canoe or a kayak.

According to the Texas Parks and Wildlife Department, the Caddo and Wichita tribes originally inhabited the area, and some petroglyphs have been found nearby. The petroglyphs cannot be viewed from the park, however, because they are on private land. Pick up a map, an interpretive brochure, and a pamphlet on the park's history from the rangers in the park headquarters. The brochure, in

KEY AT-A-GLANCE INFORMATION

LENGTH: 1.73 miles

CONFIGURATION: Balloon

DIFFICULTY: Easy

SCENERY: Woods, lake

EXPOSURE: Shady

TRAIL TRAFFIC: Light

TRAIL SURFACE: Packed dirt

HIKING TIME: 40 minutes

ACCESS: 7 a.m.–10 p.m.; $3 per day for adults and for children age 13 and older

FACILITIES: Restrooms, playground, water fountain

WHEELCHAIR TRAVERSABLE: No

SPECIAL COMMENTS: Pets are allowed but must be leashed. A couple of days a year, in the winter, are for hunting only. Before your visit, check tpwd.state.tx.us/spdest/findadest/parks/purtis _creek for trail closures. Canoes and kayaks are available for rent.

SUPPLEMENTAL MAPS: tpwd.state .tx.us/publications/pwdpubs/ media/park_maps/pwd_mp _p4508_105d.pdf

DRIVING DISTANCE FROM MAJOR INTERSECTION: 20 miles from I-20 and FM 47

Directions

From Dallas, take US 175 to Eustace. Follow the signs to Purtis Creek State Park, exiting left (north) onto FM 316 to travel 3.5 miles. From the park entrance, take the first left, pass the fish ponds, and head into the camping area. Take the left fork and park in the small parking lot on the left.

GPS TRAILHEAD COORDINATES

Latitude: N 32° 21' 50"

Longitude: W 96° 0' 10"

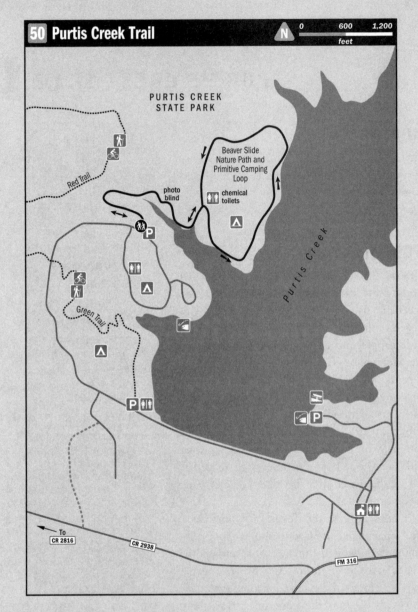

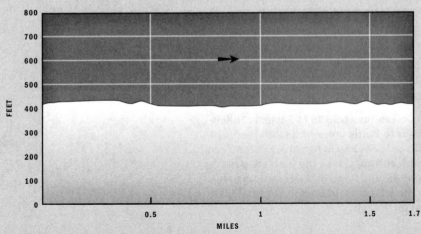

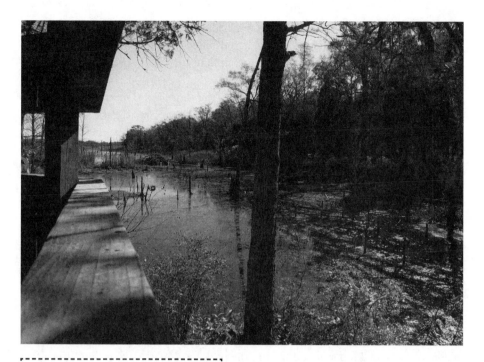

Looking through the photo blind for birds

conjunction with numbered signposts along the trail, will help you identify the local flora.

The trailhead is adjacent to the parking area. Head southeast down a narrow dirt path bordered by dense thickets. Plants you'll spot along the trail include the American beautyberry, which bursts with purple berries in the fall. Also look for the flowering dogwood. In the fall, this short tree produces small red fruits that look like berries; in the spring, they sport hundreds of pretty, small, white flowers.

The trail continues, winding its way through the woods before reaching a lookout over a swampy inlet of the lake. Across the water, you can sometimes spot hikers peering out of the narrow slats of a wooden photo blind on the opposite bank.

Back on the trail, cross a couple of bridges spanning small streams before reaching the first trail junction. Bear right at the path split, then right again at the next split. This portion of the trail loops through the woods and around a primitive-camping area. As you venture onto the loop trail, you'll first reach the photo blind you glimpsed earlier on the hike. When waters are low, the narrow inlet in front of the blind is very shallow, exposing numerous tree stumps. The main portion of the lake is farther to the left. This is a nice spot for spying some of the park's birds. More than 200 species inhabit the area, including the downy and hairy woodpeckers, the warbling and red-eyed vireos, the belted kingfisher, and the yellow-billed cuckoo. I lingered in the photo blind a while and spotted a turkey vulture, an egret, and some mallards. Farther down the trail, a fellow hiker spied what he believed to be a red-tailed hawk before it disappeared behind the trees. Birders can pick up a complete list of all bird species found in the area at park headquarters.

Continue along the loop, which follows the shoreline. The trail stays inland, offering only brief glimpses of the water through the trees. Pass a number of shorter side trails shooting off to the right from the main trail. These trails lead to primitive-camping spots at the water's edge and provide nice overlooks and access to the water. Investigate as many of these trails as you'd like; each gives a different view of the lake. Just be sure no campers are settled into the sites you explore. Each of these sites is designed for boat (and pedestrian) access. Trails lead from the campsite itself to small beaches along the adjacent shoreline. Small numbered signposts on the water's edge allow boaters to float up to their site from the lake.

The trail continues through dense woods that close in on both sides. If you've failed to spot any birds, you won't fail to hear the cawing of crows as you walk along. Old, gnarled trees in a couple of spots along the trail add interest to the mass of woodlands.

If you enjoy geocaching—using a GPS unit to locate items hidden in various public places—pick up a handout from the park headquarters that describes a few caches hidden here.

Pass some chemical toilets, then find yourself back at the beginning of the loop. From here, retrace your steps to the trailhead.

NEARBY ACTIVITIES

If you're interested in getting on the lake after the hike, rent a canoe, kayak, or paddleboat. Outside the park, stop by the Texas Freshwater Fisheries Center, which has a hatchery, an aquarium, a wetlands trail, and a 1.2-acre lake, where rods and bait are provided (closed Mondays; [800] 792-1112; **tpwd.state.tx.us/ spdest/visitorcenters/tffc**). To get there, turn left onto US 175 heading south, then take Loop 7 East to FM 2495, where you'll turn left and go about 3 miles.

VISITOR'S OVERLOOK:
Joe Pool Lake Dam Trail

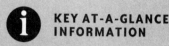

IN BRIEF

This flat trail runs across the top of Joe Pool Dam, rewarding you with unobstructed views of the lake. The trail is kid-friendly, dog-friendly, and bike-friendly.

DESCRIPTION

Though not the prettiest lake in the Metroplex, Joe Pool Lake has, since its recent completion in 1989, been surprisingly popular—and for good reason. The lake is ideally located, about 20 miles southwest of Dallas and about 25 miles southeast of Fort Worth. A state park and several city parks border the lake, making it a natural choice for summer outings. Large and sprawling amid nondescript tree-filled terrain, the lake is unlikely to inspire awe. But what it lacks in beauty, it makes up for in activities: the parks offer everything from camping and hiking to boating, fishing, and swimming. Organized events are always happening somewhere along the lake and include bike rallies, fishing tournaments, and outdoor-club activities.

Named after a 1960s congressman instrumental in its establishment, the lake is a huge reservoir created by impounding creek waters with a long embankment dam. The dam is made of earth fill, composed of compacted soils that form a raised wall on the northern side of the lake. An old road that runs along the top of the dam and over the lake is popular with cyclists and joggers—this is the route for the following hike.

- -

Directions ⟶

From I-20, head west toward Fort Worth. Exit onto FM 1382 and turn left (south). The entrance is 3 miles down on the right and has a small sign identifying it as Visitor's Overlook.

KEY AT-A-GLANCE INFORMATION

LENGTH: 3 miles

CONFIGURATION: Out-and-back

DIFFICULTY: Easy

SCENERY: Lake, spillway

EXPOSURE: Sunny

TRAIL TRAFFIC: Moderate

TRAIL SURFACE: Paved

HIKING TIME: 1.5 hours

ACCESS: Free; open sunrise–sunset, year-round facilities: Restrooms

WHEELCHAIR TRAVERSABLE: No

SPECIAL COMMENTS: Bring plenty of water, a hat, and sunscreen—there's no shade on this trail. Restrooms are at the trailhead.

DRIVING DISTANCE FROM MAJOR INTERSECTION: 9 miles from I-20 and US 67

GPS TRAILHEAD COORDINATES

Latitude: N 32° 38' 28"

Longitude: W 96° 58' 34"

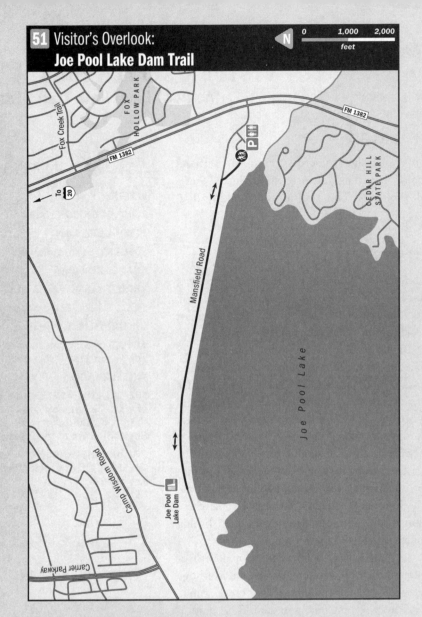

51 Visitor's Overlook: **Joe Pool Lake Dam Trail**

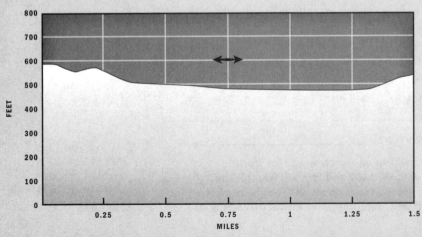

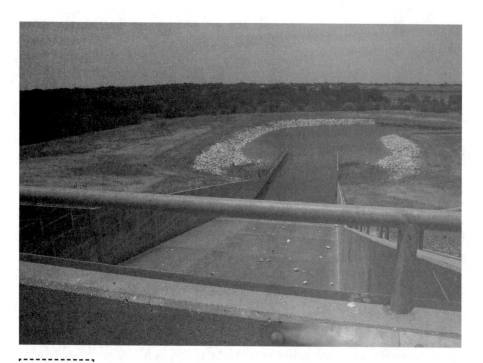

The spillway

The trail is flat and there is little nature along the route, but that's why it's an excellent spot for those who want to hike with their dogs and those looking for an easy walk. From any point along the trail, you have unparalleled views of all lake activity, and thanks to nearby Cedar Hill State Park, which is just 1 mile south on FM 1382, there's always something to see on the waters, be it kayakers, sailors, fishermen, or seabirds. Wear plenty of sunscreen—the trail is completely sun-drenched, though a strong breeze helps keep the trail cool on even the hottest days.

Adjacent to the parking area, a long walkway twists back and forth, leading to the restrooms and ending at an overlook, which curiously enough looks out onto nothing but grass and shrubs. Several trails disappear into the brush from this area, heading toward the lake. This hike starts at the trailhead just to the right of the restrooms and is marked by a sign advising that all pets must be leashed. The trail heads into the trees and within 100 feet ends at a service road, where you'll turn left toward the lake. This road serves as the trail for the duration of the hike and is open only to pedestrian and bicycle traffic. At 0.25 mile, the trail meets the lake's edge and continues straight along the top of the dam toward the far side of the lake.

On a clear, sunny day the opposite bank looks close, making you think you can reach the other side of the lake fairly quickly. The distance, however, is greater than it appears, and as much as you walk, the far side of the lake is likely to stay just out of reach. In fact, the trail continues along the dam for 1.5 miles before reaching the far side of the lake, where it continues another couple miles inland.

As you hike along the dam, enjoy unobstructed views of the lake on the left and a vacant, low-lying floodplain on the right. A pair of binoculars comes in handy—the vastness of the lake makes it hard to see much detail along the shoreline. Without binoculars you'll be able to make out little more than some of the closer tents pitched by state-park visitors.

Wildlife along the route consists of only a few butterflies and birds, although nearby Cedar Hill State Park's website (**tpwd.state.tx.us/spdest/findadest/parks/cedar_hill**) identifies more than 200 types of birds that have been found here, including several varieties of hawks, herons, and pelicans, and more than a dozen types of sparrows. The bald eagle even makes the list, although on my hike I saw only a few gulls swooping over the water.

At 2 miles, reach the far side of the lake and the end of the dam, marked by a tower and a concrete spillway. This is a good place to turn around—from here the trail quickly heats up as you leave the water and loses the breeze coming off it.

NEARBY ACTIVITIES

Visitor's Overlook is adjacent to Cedar Hill State Park, which is only 1 mile south down FM 1382 (see Hike 44, page 202). The state-park visitor center is a good place to get maps and brochures. Check with the staff for event information; the park also regularly schedules nature walks and talks.

WALNUT CREEK TRAIL

IN BRIEF

A shady trail with multiple overlooks for bank fishing follows the creek through the woods. After the hike, enjoy a picnic overlooking Joe Pool Lake; the picnic area is just down the road in the northern section of the park.

DESCRIPTION

Loyd Park, on the northwest banks of Joe Pool Lake in Grand Prairie, is operated by the city's parks and recreation department. The lake is a reservoir named after a 1960s congressman instrumental in its establishment. Cedar Hill State Park sits on the shores on the opposite side of the lake.

At this scenic park, aside from hiking and equestrian trails, you'll find more than 200 campsites, eight cabins, a beach, a designated swimming area, a boat ramp, fishing piers, and an assortment of picnic areas along the lakeshore. The park sometimes appears empty, but a quick drive from end to end reveals considerable activity; the amenities are fairly spread out, and so too are the visitors. From the hiking trailhead on the west side of the park, you'd never know how many boaters are coming and going at the easternmost side or how many kids are romping on the beach just to

KEY AT-A-GLANCE INFORMATION

LENGTH: 2.16 miles

CONFIGURATION: Out-and-back

DIFFICULTY: Easy

SCENERY: Woods, lake

EXPOSURE: Shady–sunny

TRAIL TRAFFIC: Light

TRAIL SURFACE: Sections of loose- and packed-dirt trail

HIKING TIME: 45 minutes

ACCESS: Open 24 hours, quiet time after 10 p.m.; $10 per vehicle, per day

FACILITIES: Restrooms, picnic area, fishing pier, swimming beach

WHEELCHAIR TRAVERSABLE: No

SPECIAL COMMENTS: Up to 6 people per car for the 1 entrance rate. There is a special senior citizens' rate of only $2 per person.

DRIVING DISTANCE FROM MAJOR INTERSECTION: 6.4 miles from I-20 and TX 360

Directions

Follow I-20 West toward Fort Worth and take Exit 453B onto TX 360 South toward Frontage Road/Watson Road. Go about 3 miles and turn left onto Arlington Webb Road/CR 2017, which becomes Ragland Road. The entrance to Loyd Park is on your right at 3401 Ragland Road. The trailhead is on the western side of the park; to reach it, turn right after you enter the park.

GPS TRAILHEAD COORDINATES

Latitude: N 32° 35' 52"
Longitude: W 97° 4' 6"

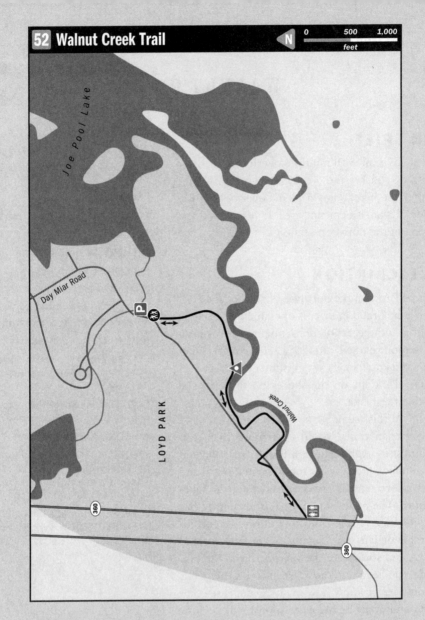

0   500   1,000
feet

N

Joe Pool Lake

Day Miar Road

P

LOYD PARK

Walnut Creek

360

360

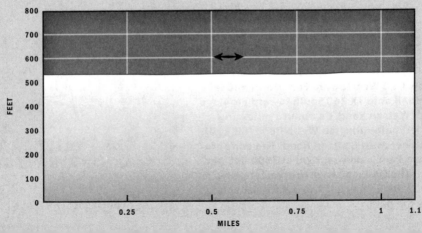

800
700
600
500
400
300
200
100
0

FEET

0.25   0.5   0.75   1   1.1

MILES

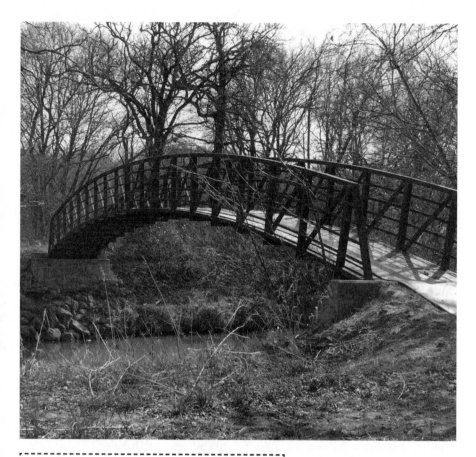

A bridge provides easy access to additional sections of trail.

the west. Leashed pets are allowed in the park, except at the swimming beach and playgrounds.

There is an admission fee, which may seem a bit high for just a day hike, considering the other options. However, you'll find this park spotlessly clean and the trail well maintained. And after the hike you can enjoy the roped-off swimming beach and other amenities. Another tip: come with a couple of friends—the charge per car is the same whether you have two people in the car or six.

The trail starts on the park's west side. A small wooden WALNUT CREEK TRAIL sign welcomes you onto a wide path that disappears into the trees. Tall grasses beneath the towering trees provide good cover for snakes. I didn't spot any, and you're unlikely to have a problem, but it's always a good idea to watch where you step. The trail is easily wide enough to walk two abreast and allow you to step around anything you might see. Because the trail also welcomes equestrians, you'll want to keep an eye out for horse manure, although I found little evidence of horses. At the first trail junction, bear right.

The trail winds through the woods; bear left at the next junction to follow it alongside a creek connected to the lake. There are a couple of pretty water overlooks at the beginning of the hike; after that, the water is hidden from view behind the trees to your left. Plenty of paths lead over to the water, though, and you'll pass a number of spurs from the main trail heading left toward the bank. The spurs, which are marked with BANK FISHING signs, attest to the trail's popularity with fishermen. I ventured down some of these trails and found a father fishing with his son at one, a young teen fishing alone at another, and only the soft rustling of leaves at the third. It comes as no surprise that fishermen like the area—most of the trail has a quiet, mellow feel, the only sounds being the wind rustling in the leaves and the occasional bird chirp.

Because most of the trail winds through the woods, the fall is an excellent time to hike here. The reds, yellows, and greens of the changing leaves add to the trail's beauty. This is also a good hike for a bright, sunny day, because the trees cast most of the trail in deep shade. Pick a different trail if it rained the day before your hike; some sections of the trail are loosely packed soil, making for a muddy walk if the trail gets even slightly wet.

At 0.63 mile, the trail emerges from the woods onto a grassy maintenance road. Head left and pick up the trail that disappears back into the woods on the left. Wind through more woods before you finally reemerge onto the maintenance road at 0.9 mile. Go left down the service road. You'll hear the sounds of cars coming from US 360, which you'll see ahead, beyond the park's boundary.

At 1.08 miles, within view of the highway, reach a small building—the Walnut Creek Restroom. Continue past it to the next trail junction, where signs indicate that left will take you down the Guide's Trail and right will take you on the Creek Trail. Turn left onto the Guide's Trail, following it through the woods. You'll eventually rejoin the main trail and spot a pretty bridge to your left. This is a good place to turn around; just go right, following the path straight. It will take you back to the restroom, where you can retrace your steps to the trailhead.

Note: Crossing the bridge at the last trail intersection will take you to the Blackland Federation Trail. This section is very confusing, with many junctions that can easily get you lost. I highly suggest bringing a compass or GPS if you choose to explore the section across the bridge.

NEARBY ACTIVITIES

Lone Star Park, site of the 2004 Breeders' Cup, is a huge racetrack that offers horse racing in the spring, early summer, and fall ([800] 795-7223; **lonestarpark .com**). The park also hosts special events such as live music throughout the spring and fall. To get there, follow TX 360 North 6 miles and exit at I-30/Six Flags Drive toward Dallas. Go 3 miles and take Exit 34. Turn left onto Belt Line Road. Lone Star Park will be on your right.

WAXAHACHIE CREEK HIKE & BIKE TRAIL

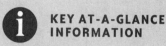

53

IN BRIEF

A surprisingly charming hike down a rural path running alongside Waxahachie Creek and ending at the remnants of the historic Interurban Railway. The lush, green setting and abundance of bird boxes make this trail a must-visit for birders.

DESCRIPTION

Dubbed "Gingerbread City," thanks to the ornate carpentry on some of its Victorian-style homes, Waxahachie is the seat of Ellis County. It also has the distinct honor of being associated with the Texas state shrub, having been designated the Crape Myrtle Capital of Texas. A third nickname refers to the city as the Movie Capital of Texas, thanks to a number of feature films having done location shooting here. About 30 miles south of Dallas and 40 miles southeast of Fort Worth, the city is easy to reach from anywhere in the Metroplex.

The Texas Parks and Wildlife Department helped fund the trail, which currently offers about 6 miles of paved path. The trailhead is hidden just outside downtown Waxahachie in Lion's Park, a small city park that's dominated by soccer and softball fields. As you enter the park, you'll see a huge field with a pavilion at the northeastern end. Park in the small lot adjacent to the pavilion, where you'll find the trailhead.

KEY AT-A-GLANCE INFORMATION

LENGTH: 5.54 miles

CONFIGURATION: Out-and-back

DIFFICULTY: Easy

SCENERY: Historic bridges, rail tracks, creek, birds

EXPOSURE: Partially sunny

TRAIL TRAFFIC: Moderate

TRAIL SURFACE: Paved

HIKING TIME: 1.75 hours

ACCESS: Free; open daily, sunrise–10 p.m.

FACILITIES: Restrooms, picnic tables, benches

WHEELCHAIR TRAVERSABLE: Yes

SPECIAL COMMENTS: A good option if it's recently rained.

DRIVING DISTANCE FROM MAJOR INTERSECTION: 3 miles from I-35E and US 77

Directions

Follow I-35E south toward Waxahachie and take Exit 408 onto US 77 South. Go about 9 miles, then turn left onto Howard Street. Lion's Park is about 1.3 miles ahead on the left. Park in the lot next to the pavilion, at the northeast end of the road.

GPS TRAILHEAD COORDINATES

Latitude: N 32° 22' 5"

Longitude: W 96° 50' 1"

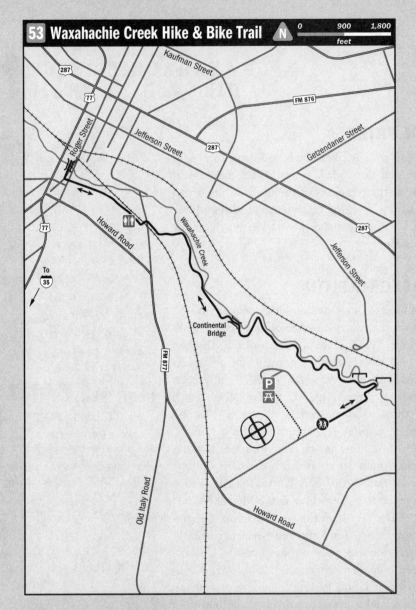

N

0   900   1,800
feet

Kaufman Street

287

77

FM 876

Roger Street

Jefferson Street

287

Getzendaner Street

77

Howard Road

Waxahachie Creek

287

Jefferson Street

To
35

FM 877

Continental
Bridge

P

Old Italy Road

Howard Road

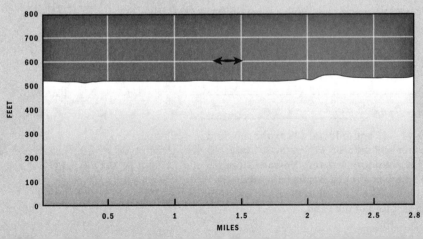

800
700
600
500
400
300
200
100
0

FEET

0.5   1   1.5   2   2.5   2.8

MILES

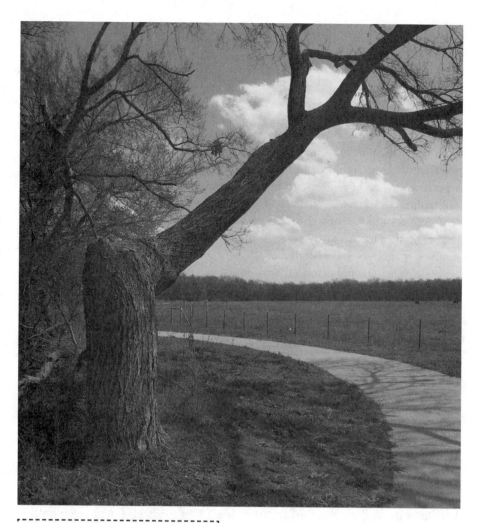

Horse-filled pastures line this pretty trail.

The trail heads a few hundred feet northeast until it meets Waxahachie Creek, then turns left, following the curves and bends of the creek as it heads northwest. For the duration of the hike, the creek gurgles and babbles just beyond the hardwoods to your right. Lion's Park soon disappears from view and is replaced by fenced-in pastures where horses graze and trot lazily through sunny fields. The trail is very well maintained, and in addition to trash bins placed discreetly at various points along the trail, you'll find large, handsome stone mile markers at quarter-mile intervals, helping you keep track of where you are on the trail.

As you hike, you'll hear the near-constant chirping and whistling of birds, many attracted by the wooden bird boxes that have been set up at various points along the trail. Benches at key spots overlooking the creek offer opportunities for you to rest and pull out your binoculars. Especially in spring, this trail is so full of life that even if you don't have any binoculars, you won't leave disappointed—the birds swoop and flit across the trail, disregarding hikers. Watch for colorful cardinals, bluebirds, robins, and warblers. If you're lucky, you'll even spot a few hummingbirds—as I stood taking a swig from my water bottle, a couple of them buzzed boldly past me, seeming to ignore my very existence.

At 0.38 mile, a small clearing offers a scenic overlook where you can view the creek. Trees loom on either side, partially shading its clear waters. If you look carefully, you're likely to spot turtles warming themselves in the small patches of sun that filter through the tree branches. Just ahead, environmentalists have built a bat house. Just beyond it and behind the trees across the river, glimpse some railroad tracks paralleling the creek.

At 1.53 miles, reach the short, wooden Continental Bridge. Beyond it, the trail continues to curl lazily through the lovely rural setting, framed by pastures on the left and a dense clustering of hardwood trees growing up against the creek on your right—a combination that is utterly peaceful and entirely relaxing without being boring.

The trail crosses Matthews Street at 2.15 miles; if you glance to the right as you cross the street, you'll see the top of the Ellis County Courthouse towering in the distance. Continuing along the trail, cross the railroad tracks and hike another 0.3 mile to Interurban Park, named for the Interurban Railway (aka Texas Electric Railway), which ran from Dallas through Waxahachie to Waco until December 31, 1948. Signposts show old photographs of the 1,442-foot trestle bridge that spanned Waxahachie Creek here. Though the bridge is long gone, the supports are still intact. The scenery hasn't changed much since the photographs were taken, and with a little imagination you can almost see the bridge disappearing north toward downtown.

Continue northwest down the trail until you reach Rogers Street, at 2.58 miles. Cross the street and turn right toward the old red metal truss bridge, known as the Rogers Street Bridge. This Texas Historic Bridge, now open only to pedestrians, was built in 1889 when the area was first settled; vehicles used it until 1990, when a newer bridge replaced it. Cross back over Rogers Street and explore the old depot, sitting just in front of the railroad tracks. Adjacent to the depot, an old feed store reminds you of the city's agricultural roots. This is an ideal spot to turn and retrace your steps to the trailhead. If you want to extend the hike, the trail continues northwest to Getzendaner Park.

NEARBY ACTIVITIES

Stop by Waxahachie's Downtown Historic District, where you can browse antiques shops and boutiques, visit the Ellis County Museum, and admire the Ellis County Courthouse, which dates to 1895. To get downtown, turn right onto Howard Street, then right onto South Elm Street (US 77).

WINDMILL HILL PRESERVE TRAIL 54

IN BRIEF

This shady trail loops through a small, heavily wooded preserve, making it an excellent spot for hiking on a hot, sunny day. Though not especially scenic, the trail is appealing to those who enjoy exploring because the myriad junctions allow you to digress with little risk of becoming too lost.

DESCRIPTION

The local community lobbied to get this plot of land set aside, and now, thanks to their efforts, it is part of the Dallas County Trail and Preserve Program. The 72-acre nature preserve has a large network of trails crisscrossing the woods and is well used by those in the area.

Be prepared for a network of paths branching left and right as you hike along the trail. Though these unmarked trails split off in different directions every few hundred feet, it's almost impossible to get lost for long because almost all trails eventually lead back to the center of the preserve, where a trail runs west–east through its center. All trails funnel into this central trail and go across the Stevie Ray Vaughan Memorial Bridge, which divides the western side of the preserve from the eastern side. The bridge honors the famous 1980s blues-rock guitarist Stevie Ray Vaughan. Vaughan played lead guitar on David Bowie's *Let's Dance* album and became very popular

KEY AT-A-GLANCE INFORMATION

LENGTH: 1.8 miles

CONFIGURATION: Double loop

DIFFICULTY: Moderate

SCENERY: Woodlands, bridge

EXPOSURE: Mostly shady

TRAIL TRAFFIC: Light

TRAIL SURFACE: Packed dirt

HIKING TIME: 50 minutes

ACCESS: Free; open daily, 6 a.m.–10 p.m. year-round

FACILITIES: None

WHEELCHAIR TRAVERSABLE: No

SPECIAL COMMENTS: Leashed dogs and mountain bikers are welcome on this trail.

DRIVING DISTANCE FROM MAJOR INTERSECTION: 3 miles from US 67 and I-20

Directions ➤

Take US 67 south toward Cleburne, and exit at Duncanville Road/Main Street, turning left. Head south on Main about 0.75 mile; the parking lot is at Windmill Hill Preserve on the left, at the corner of Wintergreen Road.

GPS TRAILHEAD COORDINATES

Latitude: N 32° 37' 1"

Longitude: W 96° 54' 29"

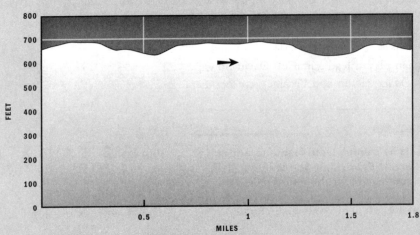
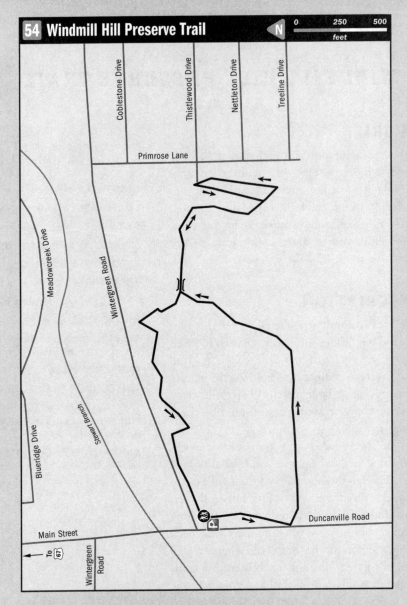

N

0   250   500
feet

Coblestone Drive

Thistlewood Drive

Nettleton Drive

Treeline Drive

Primrose Lane

Meadowcreek Drive

Wintergreen Road

Blueridge Drive

Stewart Branch

Duncanville Road

Main Street

To 67

Wintergreen Road

FEET

800
700
600
500
400
300
200
100
0

0.5   1   1.5   1.8

MILES

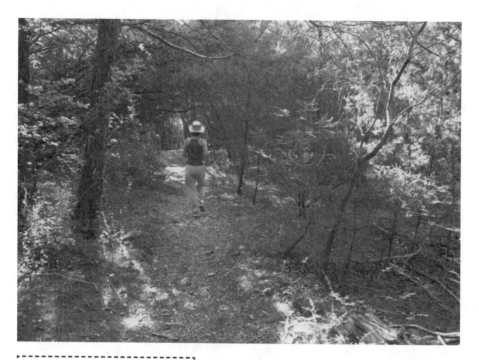

A hiker enjoys the trail's shady path.

with his own band, Double Trouble. The guitarist died in a helicopter crash following a concert on August 26, 1990. Vaughan is memorialized here because he was born and raised in Dallas.

The trail I've mapped out is a rough loop around the preserve and has lots of small ups and downs through hilly terrain, providing a nice workout. If you miss a turn—highly possible with so many trails branching out—don't become overly concerned. Explore as you wish, and you'll eventually find yourself back at the bridge, which is a good reference point.

There are two main entrances from the parking lot. Take the trailhead on the right (the one on the left is where you'll come out at the trail's end). Immediately, you'll be on a somewhat rocky trail. The scenery for most of this hike is what you see here: dense woods that shade much of the trail. About 250 feet into your trek, the trail splits; bear right. At the next trail split, at 0.13 mile, bear left. At this point, the trail has some small steep uphill and downhill climbs. The ruggedness here appeals to mountain bikers, who maintain the trail. On my hike, however, I didn't see a single biker, just a couple of hikers whose dogs were thoroughly enjoying their workout.

At the next junction, 0.28 mile into the hike, continue straight and downhill. The preserve abuts some backyards, and through the trees you'll catch sight of houses before the trail returns to the woods. Finally, at 0.55 mile into the hike, come to the Stevie Ray Vaughan Memorial Bridge, a very pretty brick-red truss bridge spanning a dry creek bed.

Cross the bridge and a small gully, then turn right at the next split, at about 0.65 mile. This will take you on an 0.5-mile loop through the eastern half of the preserve. Hang a right at the junction at 0.8 mile, and the trail will loop through a piney grove and emerge into a small field with a few pine trees. Bear right at the next turnoff to climb up and down some small hills before yet another turnoff, where you continue straight. The trail then curls around a small field and meets up with a creek before putting you back at the Stevie Ray Vaughn Bridge.

Cross back over the bridge and turn right, heading down a concrete trail. A picnic table sits to the left; a little farther down, at 1.45 miles, is a small clearing to the right, where you'll see some large dirt ramps for mountain bikers.

Turn left just before the dirt mounds onto the trail heading west; the path switchbacks down a small, steep hill. A couple hundred feet farther, reach the next turnoff, where you should go right.

To exit the preserve, follow the right split at the next three turnoffs. If you prefer a little more exercise, do as I did and head left and uphill, staying to the left at the next couple of turnoffs. The trail emerges into a small field on the eastern side of the parking lot.

NEARBY ACTIVITIES

Joe Pool Lake, along which lies Cedar Hill State Park, is nearby and is popular with fishermen, boaters, picnickers, campers, and birders (see Hike 44, page 202). Inside the state park, you'll also find Penn Farm Agricultural History Center, a restored farm exhibit. To get there, take US 67 South. After about 1.5 miles, exit to the right, onto Pleasant Run Road. Turn right onto South Belt Line Road (FM 1382). The park is about 2 miles down on the left.

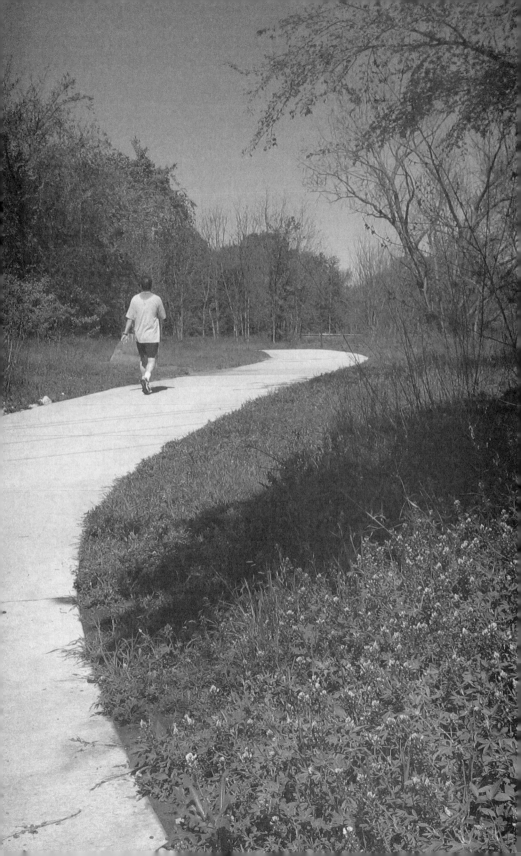

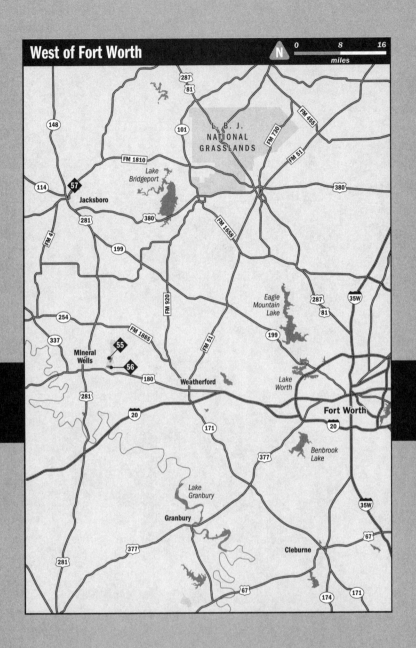

55 Lake Mineral Wells State Park: Cross Timbers Trail 252

56 Lake Mineral Wells State Trailway 257

57 Lost Creek Reservoir State Trailway 261

WEST OF FORT WORTH

55 LAKE MINERAL WELLS STATE PARK:
Cross Timbers Trail

KEY AT-A-GLANCE INFORMATION

LENGTH: 4 miles

CONFIGURATION: Balloon

DIFFICULTY: Easy

SCENERY: Rocks, cactus, grasslands

EXPOSURE: Sunny

TRAIL TRAFFIC: Light

TRAIL SURFACE: Packed dirt, rock

HIKING TIME: 1.5 hours

ACCESS: $5 per person entrance fee; open daily, 6 a.m.–10 p.m.

FACILITIES: Restrooms, picnic tables

WHEELCHAIR TRAVERSABLE: No

SPECIAL COMMENTS: Bring along an animal-tracking and scat-identification book.

SUPPLEMENTAL MAPS: tpwd.state .tx.us/publications/pwdpubs/ media/park_maps/pwd_mp _p4503_103f.pdf

DRIVING DISTANCE FROM MAJOR INTERSECTION: 5.5 miles from US 180 and US 281

GPS TRAILHEAD COORDINATES

Latitude: N32° 50' 4"

Longitude: W 98° 2' 10"

IN BRIEF

This wide trail is great for spotting animal tracks after a rainstorm—check with the park, though, to ensure the path has dried out enough to hike. The route starts in a wooded area, then loops through some sunny cactus-dotted grasslands.

DESCRIPTION

About 46 miles west of Fort Worth, Lake Mineral Wells State Park is popular among outdoor enthusiasts for good reason—not only does it have a generous trail system that welcomes bikers, hikers, and equestrians, it also has a fishing pier, which attracts anglers; beach access for lake swimming; and, most uniquely, a section of canyons and boulders open to rock climbers. The park, which opened in 1981, covers more than 3,200 acres, including the 646-acre Lake Mineral Wells. The lake was originally designed to supply water to the expanding city of Mineral Wells. It served its purpose for 40 years before an alternate water supply was found in 1963.

On the northwest side of the lake, find the park's camping areas and the backcountry trail this hike traverses. On the southeast side of the lake, locate the trailhead for the Lake

Directions

Follow I-20 West toward Abilene. Take Exit 414 onto Fort Worth Highway/US 180 West toward Mineral Wells. Continue about 21 miles (about 14 miles past Weatherford), then turn right onto Park Road 71, following the brown state-park signs. To get to the trailhead, enter the Lake Mineral Wells State Park and make a sharp left, crossing over the spillway. Bear left at the next juncture. The parking lot is at the end of the road.

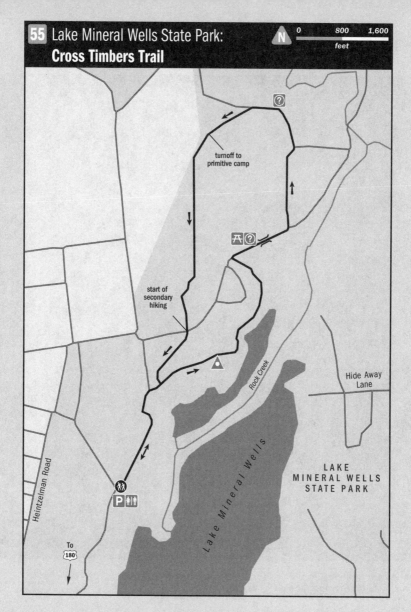

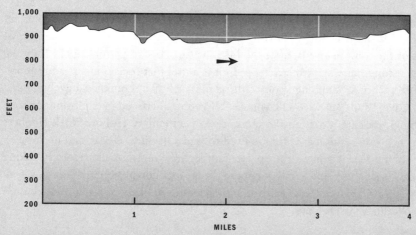

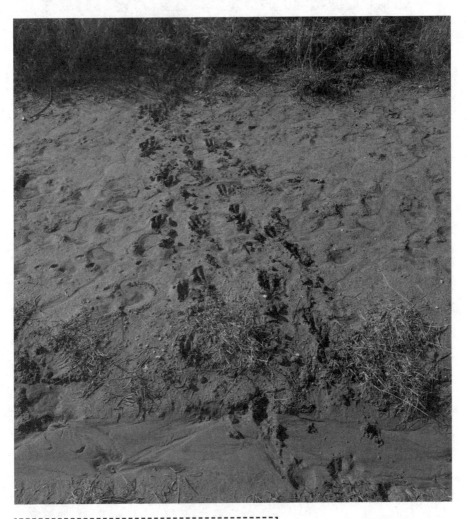

Animal tracks crisscross the path the day after a rainstorm.

Mineral Wells State Trailway and the rock-climbing area, known as "Penitentiary Hollow." Its narrow, rocky canyons are in stark contrast to the wide, open grasslands of the trail; before or after the hike, be sure to stop by for a look. Running down a stone stairway to the canyon floor is a trail that rock climbers and rappellers use to access climbing spots with names such as "Scrambled Egg Boulder," "The Cave," and "Pee Wee's Playhouse." If you're interested in exploring (or rock climbing), pick up a map at the entrance to Penitentiary Hollow. Rock climbers bring their own equipment, are required to sign a liability release, and must pay a $3 climbing fee. If you're not up for another hike and just interested in taking a look, a scenic overlook only a couple dozen feet down the rock-climbing trail offers fantastic views of the canyon and lake. You're likely to see a rock climber or two scaling the far walls.

To get to the trailhead from the park entrance, take a sharp left at the first road juncture, then follow the road across the spillway. At the next intersection, stay left. The road dead-ends at the parking area, and you'll find the trailhead on the northeast side of the lot.

The trail is very wide and stays this way for most of the hike, easily accommodating both hikers and equestrians. You'll also find that the combination of partially rocky surface and sunny exposure allows for the trail's quick drying after rains. I encountered few problems with mud or puddles, even though I visited at the end of a very rainy week. And because I hiked it just after it had rained, I was rewarded with some of the best animal tracks I've ever encountered on a trail—clear prints from raccoons, opossums, white-tailed deer, coyotes, and birds zigzagged all across the path throughout the entire length of the hike. Though I did not spot any of the animals themselves, I had a lot of fun reconstructing the scenes of skirmishes, crossings, and encounters that I imagined had occurred the night before my visit. A sign at the trailhead does indicate that the trail is closed when wet, so be sure to call ahead to check on trail conditions and possible closures.

The trail is bordered by cactus to your right, beyond which the woods shroud all but brief glimpses of Lake Mineral Wells in the distance. To your left, a chain-link fence marks the boundary of the state park.

The trail soon curls away past the fence, and at 0.5 mile, you'll find yourself at a split, where you should veer right. You'll soon pass the junction to a small singletrack hiking trail that heads off to the primitive camping area. Bypass this, staying on the wide trail as it heads slightly uphill through rocky terrain. Close examination of the ground reveals the rocks to be varying shades of pink, glittering with flecks of mica or some other mineral.

To the right you'll catch glimpses of the surrounding hillsides through breaks in the trees. You'll find a better vantage point at 0.83 mile, where a small path to the right leads to an overlook.

Continuing on, you'll bypass a turnoff heading back the way you came. A few dozen feet beyond, a trail forks; veer right to continue north. Rest areas have been placed at each of the major trail junctures, and at 1.68 miles you'll reach the first one, which has both a kiosk with a map of the entire backcountry trail and a shady picnic table just off the trail.

At 1.85 miles, veer left at the next trail fork. The trail passes through a sun-baked grassland dotted with the occasional tree. In the winter, the flatlands can be uninspiring, but in the spring, wildflowers peek from tall grasses, adding interest and beauty to the setting. At 2.28 miles, reach another junction and rest area with a kiosk. Turn left (south), to begin the trek back toward the trailhead. If you wanted to extend the hike another few miles, you could instead turn right (north) to follow the trail onto another loop.

The trail back continues through grassland another 0.8 mile, passing the turnoff to the primitive camping area and another split, where you'll continue straight. Finally, at 3 miles, reach a junction with a smaller singletrack hiking

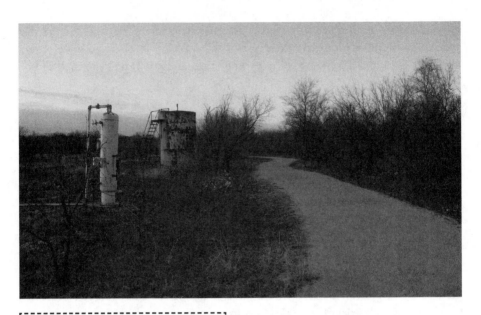

The wide trailway curls through grasslands.

trail. For a change of scenery, veer right into the trees and onto the narrow trail; it winds slightly uphill through dense woods. The path crosses the wide trail once, disappearing into the woods on the far side. At 3.5 miles, it crosses back onto another section of the main trail you just left. This time you should veer right, back onto the main trail, to retrace your steps to the trailhead. Alternatively, if you're enjoying the woods, you can cross the wide trail and pick the singletrack path where it runs through the woods back toward the trailhead parallel to the main trail.

NEARBY ACTIVITIES

You can buy bottled mineral water and souvenirs at Mineral Wells' Famous Mineral Water Company. The company was founded in 1904 by the pharmacist Edward Dismuke, who believed the town's mineral waters could cure ailments—including his own. At the age of 40, he was told he had only a short time left to live; he ended up dying at the age of 97, attributing his longevity to the mineral waters. The Texas Historical Commission has honored the building with a historical marker.

To get to Mineral Wells, follow US 180 West 4 miles. Turn right onto Northwest Sixth Street; the building is number 209. The Famous Mineral Water Company is open Tuesday–Friday, 8 a.m.–5:30 p.m., and Saturday, 9 a.m.–5 p.m. If you have more time, take US 180 West 15 miles to Palo Pinto, where you can visit the Palo Pinto Museum, in a jail from the mid-1800s just off US 180 in Palo Pinto.

LAKE MINERAL WELLS STATE TRAILWAY 56

IN BRIEF

This packed-gravel trail runs atop an old railway bed and connects the cities of Mineral Wells and Weatherford. It will appeal most to folks looking more for exercise than for scenery.

DESCRIPTION

With four access points along its 20-mile route, Lake Mineral Wells State Trailway stretches between Mineral Wells and Weatherford along a converted railway line. The multiuse trail, which opened in 1998, runs through countryside peppered with ranches. Because of its length, it is well suited to joggers and to walkers looking for a good section of uninterrupted trail upon which to stretch the legs. Access points for bicyclists, hikers, and equestrians are, from east to west, just outside Weatherford, in Garner, and at Lake Mineral Wells State Park. The fourth access point at the far western end of the trail is in the Mineral Wells; access here is restricted to hikers and bicyclists.

Besides the trailway, you'll find an excellent backcountry trail within the park, which I've also highlighted. The park's more unusual attraction, however, is a rock-climbing area

KEY AT-A-GLANCE INFORMATION

LENGTH: 3.16 miles

CONFIGURATION: Out-and-back

DIFFICULTY: Easy–moderate

SCENERY: Hills, grass, chaparral, old railway bed

EXPOSURE: Sunny

TRAIL TRAFFIC: Light–moderate

TRAIL SURFACE: Packed gravel

HIKING TIME: 1 hour

ACCESS: $2 adults, $1 senior citizens over age 65 and children under age 12, $5 state-park admittance fee; state park open 6 a.m.–10 p.m., trail open sunrise–sunset

FACILITIES: Restrooms, benches

WHEELCHAIR TRAVERSABLE: Yes

SPECIAL COMMENTS: You can extend this hike for just about as long as you like—there are about 20 miles of trail.

SUPPLEMENTAL MAPS: tpwd.state .tx.us/publications/pwdpubs/ media/park_maps/pwd_mp _p4503_103h.pdf

DRIVING DISTANCE FROM MAJOR INTERSECTION: 5.5 miles from US 180 and US-281

Directions

Follow I-20 West toward Abilene, then take Exit 414 onto Fort Worth Highway/US 180 West toward Mineral Wells. Follow the highway about 21 miles (about 14 miles past Weatherford), then turn right onto Park Road 71, following the brown state-park signs. To get to the trailhead parking, enter Lake Mineral Wells State Park and stay right at the junction. The parking lot is on the right.

GPS TRAILHEAD COORDINATES

Latitude: N 32° 48' 48"

Longitude: W 98° 1' 54"

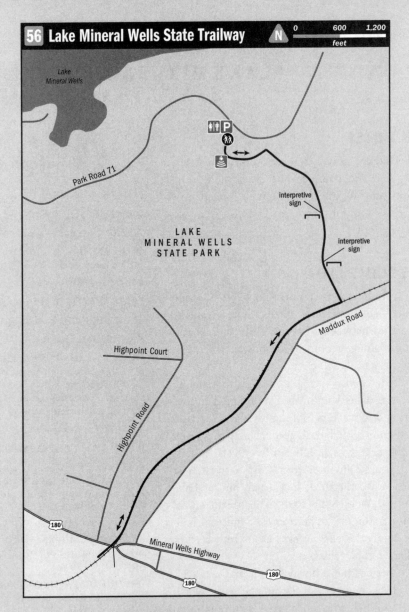

N

0   600   1,200
feet

Lake
Mineral Wells

Park Road 71

L A K E
M I N E R A L   W E L L S
S T A T E   P A R K

interpretive
sign

interpretive
sign

Maddux Road

Highpoint Court

Highpoint Road

180

Mineral Wells Highway

180

180

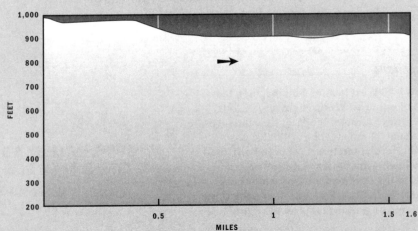

FEET

1,000
900
800
700
600
500
400
300
200

0.5   1   1.5   1.6

MILES

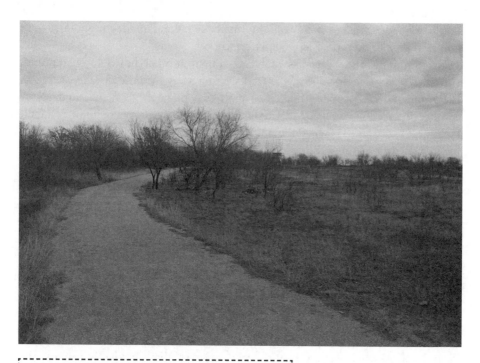

Cactus and isolated trees dot the grasslands along the trail.

known as "Penitentiary Hollow"—a section of narrow canyons on the eastern side of the lake near the trailhead for this hike. See the Description for Hike 55, Cross Timbers Trail (page 252), for more details about the area.

To get to the trailhead, stay to the right at the first fork after you enter the park. A short drive down on the right, you'll find the huge parking lot. There is a small trail fee, and a self-pay box has been set up adjacent to the trailhead for hikers' convenience.

As you head down the paved trail, the path immediately starts to switchback down a steep hill. Pass an open outdoor amphitheater off to the right; the trail then turns into packed gravel. This section of trail is actually a small spur that connects the state park with the trailway itself, which is 0.6 mile to the southeast. The spur curls toward the main trail, cutting through grassy fields peppered with cactus and the occasional isolated tree.

At 0.38 mile, pass a bench alongside an interpretive sign identifying native wildflowers of the area. The sign advises you to keep an eye out for the vivid hues of more than a dozen wildflowers, including the Texas bluebonnet, the standing cypress, and the Texas yellow star. Unfortunately, when I visited (in the middle of winter), the dry grasses were devoid of all color but brown. Although in winter it's not at its most picturesque, it is at its most pleasant, temperature-wise. Sections of this little-shaded trail—which would normally be baking midday in summer—are mild and gentle, even on a late-winter afternoon.

Continuing on, the trail switchbacks down another hill. As you descend, you'll have a charming view of the trail snaking away into the distance against a backdrop of small wooded hills. The path cuts through grasslands and passes another interpretive sign identifying the red-tailed hawk, a common resident. Finally, at 0.63 mile, reach the main juncture with the trailway. The trail splits here, extending 14 miles to the left (east) to Weatherford, and 6 miles to the right (west) into Mineral Wells.

I opted for a shorter hike, heading right toward Mineral Wells. Both directions are equally pleasant, offering wide, paved trails atop an old railway bed, suitable for comfortable walking shoes, strollers, or bikes. The trail runs parallel to a road, so expect the sound of cars occasionally passing as folks head to and from their ranches. Traffic is light, however, and not distracting. The section of trail between Garner and Weatherford on the far eastern portion of the trailway does not run near any roads, something to consider if you're looking for a more remote feel.

Turn right (west) onto the trailway. The scenery along the trail is mostly trees and shrubs, and, unlike the hilly spur from the state park, this section is fairly level. As you near US 180, the trail starts to climb gradually to cross the highway via an overpass. The other side of the bridge marks exactly 1.5 miles into the hike and is the point where I turned around. If you're interested in continuing on, the trail stretches another 4.5 miles west into downtown Mineral Wells.

NEARBY ACTIVITIES

You can buy bottled mineral water and souvenirs at Mineral Wells' Famous Mineral Water Company. See Nearby Activities for Hike 55, Cross Timbers Trail (page 252), for more information.

LOST CREEK RESERVOIR STATE TRAILWAY 57

IN BRIEF

In an area rich with the history of the North Texas frontier settlement, this sunny, peaceful hike winds through grasslands and over the dam of the Lost Creek Reservoir toward Fort Richardson State Park. Ranchlands abut the trailway, and you'll sometimes be greeted by the curious stares of bulls or livestock as you hike along.

DESCRIPTION

In Jacksboro, along the banks of Lost Creek, the Fort Richardson State Park, Historic Site, and Lost Creek Trailway's amenities include fishing, hiking, and camping. The trailway portion opened in 1998 and is about 10 miles long (one way), connecting the state park with the Lost Creek Reservoir. Trailheads are at both the park and the reservoir. The reservoir trailhead is a few miles away from the state park and historic site, a short drive northeast.

If you want to explore Fort Richardson itself, it will require a separate stop before or after the hike but is well worth it. Consider making a weekend of this trip—not only is there a lot to explore, but the state park has been named one of the top 100 family campgrounds among U.S. federal and state parks.

KEY AT-A-GLANCE INFORMATION

LENGTH: 5.35 miles

CONFIGURATION: Balloon

DIFFICULTY: Easy

SCENERY: Grassland, ranches, reservoir, dam

EXPOSURE: Sunny

TRAIL TRAFFIC: Light

TRAIL SURFACE: Pavement and crushed rock

HIKING TIME: 2 hours

ACCESS: $3 per person; daily

FACILITIES: Composting toilet and picnic tables near the swimming beach

WHEELCHAIR TRAVERSABLE: No

SPECIAL COMMENTS: This trail can be very hot in summer; bring a hat, sunscreen, and plenty of water—there are no drinking fountains along the route.

SUPPLEMENTAL MAPS: tpwd.state .tx.us/publications/pwdpubs/ media/park_maps/pwd_mp _p4506_025k.pdf

DRIVING DISTANCE FROM MAJOR INTERSECTION: 2.5 miles from TX 59 and South Main Street in Jacksboro

Directions

Take Jacksboro Highway/TX 199 west toward Jacksboro. Fort Richardson State Park is on the left, just off the highway, about 1 mile outside Jacksboro. To get to the trailhead itself, bypass the state park and continue straight into downtown Jacksboro. Turn right onto East Belknap Street; the road curves left and becomes Bowie Street/TX 59. The parking lot is about 2 miles ahead on the right.

GPS TRAILHEAD COORDINATES

Latitude: N 33° 14' 42"

Longitude: W 98° 8' 18"

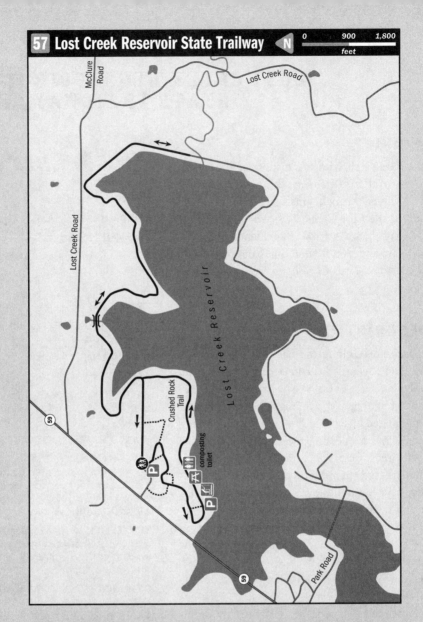

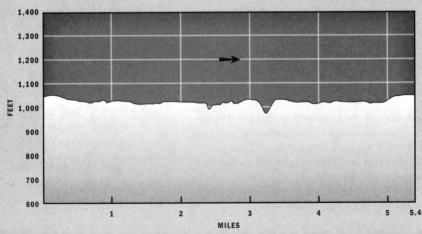

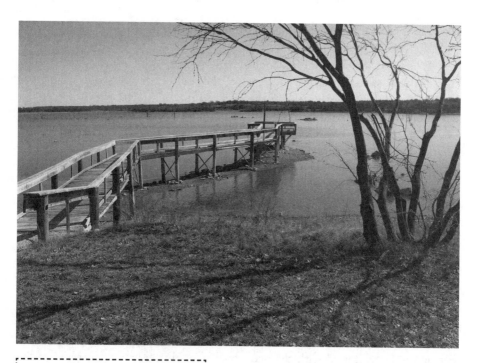

A wooden fishing pier attracts anglers.

The fort was established to protect frontier settlements against raids from Southern Plains Indian tribes after the Civil War. Named after Civil War general Israel Bush Richardson, it is associated with many battles, including the Salt Creek Massacre (aka the Warren Wagon Train Massacre). The massacre involved a bloody raid against a wagon train by a group of Kiowa and Comanche. The chiefs were eventually arrested and tried for murder—the first trial of its kind. In 1878, 11 years after its establishment, the unsettled frontier plains were secured and the fort was finally abandoned.

In 1963 the fort was named a National Historic Landmark. In 1968 the Texas Parks and Wildlife Department claimed it, opening it to the public as a state park and historic site a few years later. A few of the buildings from the fort's original complex have been restored or preserved, including the commanding officer's quarters, the post hospital, and the magazine. Pick up a walking-tour pamphlet at the visitor center to guide you around the site. The tour starts at the Interpretive Center, where you'll find displays and information about the fort's history.

This hike starts at the trailhead at the reservoir. If you want to pick up a map or other park information, be sure to stop by the state-park visitor center before heading to the trailhead; the trailway is unmanned. A self-pay booth allows you to pay the marginal trail fee; state-park pass holders should just hang their pass inside their car. Park rangers do patrol the area, so be sure you've paid your dues.

The trail is open to hikers, bikers, and equestrians, though on the gorgeous weekend day I visited, I encountered no one.

When you arrive, you'll find a huge parking area with trailheads on both the east and west sides of the lot. Head down the trail on the west side; facing the back of the lot, it'll be the trail at the back on the right. The path is actually a paved one-way park road bordered by woods and shrubs, which loops downhill toward the reservoir. Within a few hundred feet of starting down the path, you'll see the waters come into view and will pass a charming wooden fishing pier stretching into the still blue-green waters; anglers come here to fish for channel and blue catfish. Looking across the reservoir, the opposite shoreline is dotted with trees and shrubs and is pleasantly devoid of development or construction.

Just past the pier, you'll pass a huge day-use area replete with a long pavilion and picnic tables overlooking the water. Just before and below it, a swimming beach with a wide stretch of sand beckons visitors on hot days. The park road continues its loop then splits at 1.45 miles; follow the crushed-limestone multiuse trail. (Continuing to the left—on the road—would take you back to the parking lot and the opposite trailhead.) To the right, the reservoir's water is still visible, glinting in the sunlight just beyond the tall prairie grasses.

The trail winds around a small inlet of the reservoir and heads east through flat prairie lands dotted with the occasional tree. To the left, a fence marks the boundary of a local ranch. On the sunny day of my visit, I was greeted here by the steady gaze of a couple of huge bulls eyeing me through the fence.

At 2.1 miles, reach a large old metal bridge nestled among the prairie grasses, mysteriously spanning nothing more than flat grassland. Cross the bridge and continue following the trail east. The scenery is mostly trees and rocks to the right, blocking the nearby reservoir from view, and ranchland to the left. Eventually, the eastern edge of the reservoir comes into view between the trees to the right, and you have a glimpse of the dam. The trail winds toward them atop the dam. From the middle of the dam, you'll have a fabulous view of a lush green valley to the left. I spotted some type of livestock grazing there (though from the height of the dam, they looked like nothing more than white dots). To the right, the reservoir spreads out before you, shimmering in the sunlight. This is a great spot for taking a break and enjoying lunch before retracing your steps to the trailhead. If you want to extend the hike, you can follow the trail about 6 more miles across the dam, around the southern side of the reservoir, past the local airport, and to the state park.

NEARBY ACTIVITIES

If you're hiking the trailway, be sure to stop by Fort Richardson itself before or after the hike to explore the old buildings on the fort grounds. Within Jacksboro, you can visit the Jack County Museum, a historical house with period furnishings. It's near the town square, at 237 W. Belknap St.

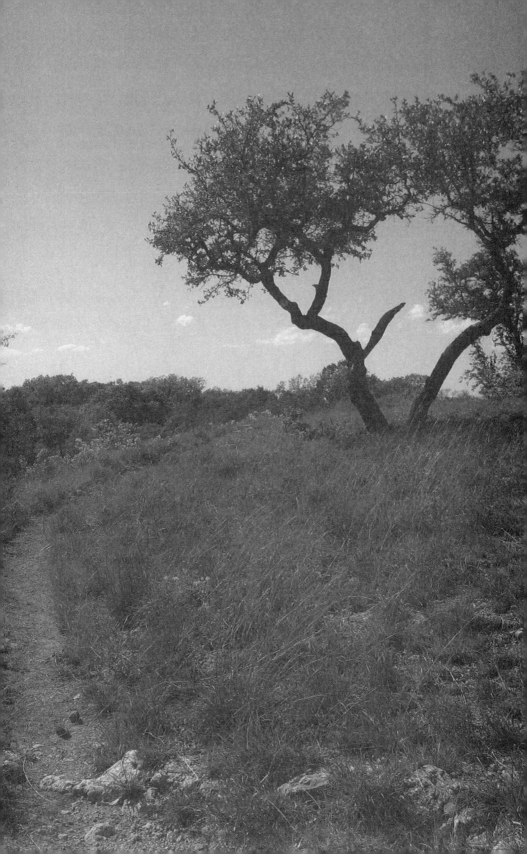

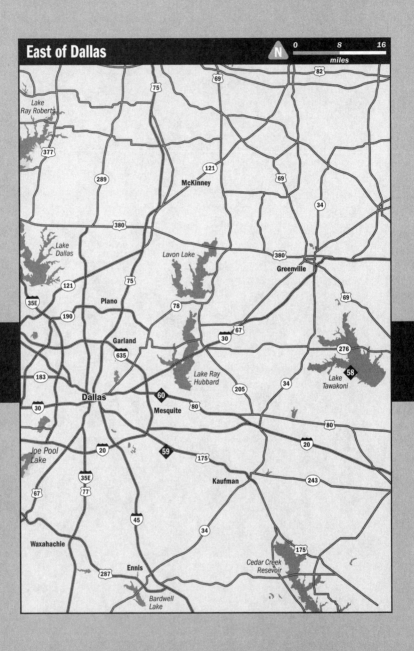

East of Dallas

N

0   8   16
miles

58 Lake Tawakoni Nature Trail 268

59 Post Oak Trail 272

60 Samuell Farm Trail 276

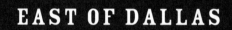

EAST OF DALLAS

58   LAKE TAWAKONI NATURE TRAIL

KEY AT-A-GLANCE INFORMATION

LENGTH: 1.72 miles

CONFIGURATION: Balloon

DIFFICULTY: Easy

SCENERY: Hardwood forest, birds

EXPOSURE: Partially shady

TRAIL TRAFFIC: Light

TRAIL SURFACE: Packed dirt

HIKING TIME: 45 minutes

ACCESS: $3 per person; open daily, 7 a.m.–10 p.m.

FACILITIES: Restrooms, picnic area, benches

WHEELCHAIR TRAVERSABLE: No

SPECIAL COMMENTS: Look for the unusually knobby bark of a couple of trees along the first half of the trail.

SUPPLEMENTAL MAPS: tpwd.state .tx.us/publications/pwdpubs/ media/park_maps/pwd_mp _p4508_142.pdf

DRIVING DISTANCE FROM MAJOR INTERSECTION: 4.5 miles from FM 2475 and FM 47

GPS TRAILHEAD COORDINATES

Latitude: N 32° 50' 44"
Longitude: W 95° 59' 39"

IN BRIEF

Near the "Bluebird Capital of Texas," this trail winds through the woods near Lake Tawakoni and is great for bird-watching.

DESCRIPTION

The 36,700-acre Lake Tawakoni (tuh-WOCK-o-nee) is a huge reservoir on the Sabine River occupying the corners of three counties—Hunt, Van Zandt, and Rains. Its dam (the Iron Bridge Dam) and spillway are 5.5 miles long. The reservoir serves as a municipal and industrial water supply and a recreational spot. Along its 200-plus-mile shoreline, boaters will find a half-dozen boat ramps, hunters will find three units of the Tawakoni Wildlife Management Area, and hikers and campers will find a state park. The lake is also known among anglers as an excellent spot for catfishing in particular; striped, largemouth, and white bass can also be found in good numbers.

At only 376 acres, Lake Tawakoni State Park sits like a tiny speck on the reservoir's southern shoreline. Opened in 2002, the state park is refreshingly remote, being just a 20-minute drive down a secondary road. Even the closest town—Wills Point—has a population of

----

Directions

Take US 80 east toward Terrell. When you reach Wills Point, turn left onto FM 47/North Fourth Street, then bear right and go about 5 miles. Turn left onto FM 2475, then travel about 4 miles, following the brown state-park sign to enter Lake Tawakoni State Park. You can pick up a map of the park at the headquarters as you drive in. As you head into the park, stay to the left at the first junction, and you'll reach the day-use area on your left, where you should park in the first parking lot.

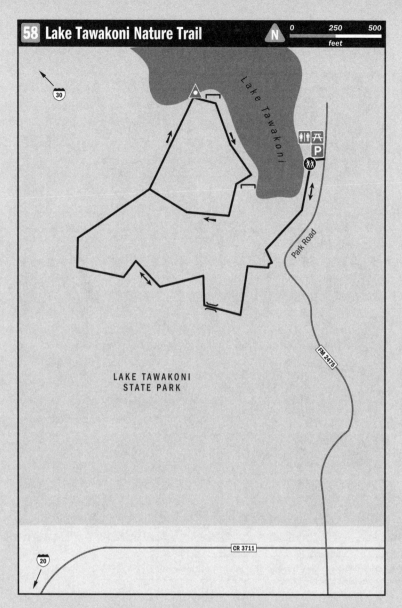

N

0   250   500
feet

Lake Tawakoni

30

Park Road

FM 2475

LAKE TAWAKONI
STATE PARK

CR 3711

20

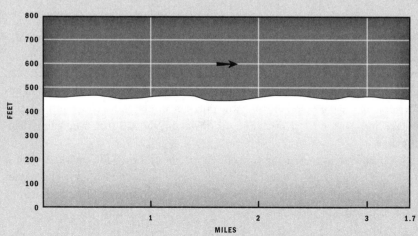

800
700
600
500
400
300
200
100
0

FEET

1   2   3   1.7

MILES

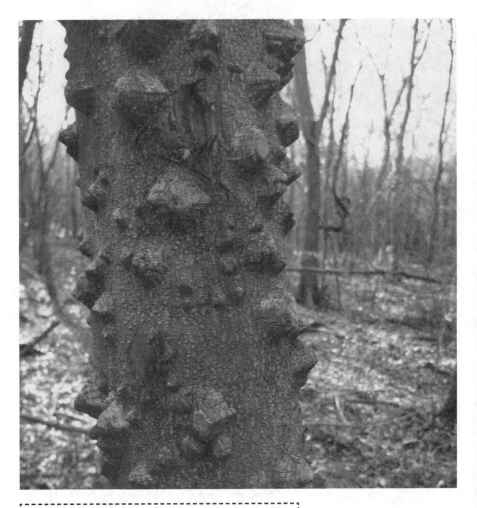

The curious bark of a tree trunk on the trail invites closer study.

fewer than 5,000 people. Although it's a drive to get there, the effort will reward you with a couple of charming trails, including a short loop along the lake's shoreline, and a longer trail through woodland adjacent to the lake. The park's atmosphere is laid-back and will appeal most to hikers looking for a mellow, quiet hike. If you come during the winter, it's not unusual to find yourself one of only a handful of visitors in the park, and certainly the only one on the trails. The unusual name of the lake and park are a reference to the Tawakoni Indians that originally inhabited the area.

The trailhead is in the far left corner of the parking lot, marked with a NATURE TRAIL sign and a notice that it is only open for use when dry. The single-track path winds southwest through the woods. A thick mixture of American elms and post oaks provide a pleasant canopy of shade as you hike.

At 0.3 mile, come to a split in the trail and turn right, heading west through more hardwood forest. Vines hang thick from the surrounding tree limbs, shrouding any wildlife in the vicinity from view. Occasionally, however, a rustling in the leaves indicates something is nearby—typically birds hopping through the underbrush. As you continue, keep an eye out for poison ivy.

The trail continues west, crosses a bridge spanning a small creek, heads slightly uphill, then reaches a junction at 0.57 mile. The entire trail is open to both bike and foot traffic, with one section exclusively for bikes. If you were to head left at this juncture, you'd reach the loop reserved for mountain bikes. You should therefore veer right at the juncture, following the path 1 mile farther, where you will reach a three-way junction. The first trail, to the right, loops to the south, from whence you just came. The second trail, straight ahead, loops north toward the lake, curls around, and comes back out onto the third trail to your right. Continue straight, following the second (middle) trail north, where you'll find the hardwood trees starting to mix with junipers such as eastern red cedar. The elevation is slightly higher than that of the lake, and as you reach the farthest point of the loop, you'll catch glimpses of the water to the left through the trees. If you've brought your binoculars, you'll find a couple of benches at 0.83 mile and 0.93 mile, just before you loop back. Just off the trail, beneath the trees, the benches provide ideal shade-covered spots for bird-watching. Keep an eye out for the eastern bluebird, which is commonly found in the park; the nearest town of Wills Point, is called the Bluebird Capital of Texas. State-park materials indicate more than 200 species of birds have been identified here.

At 0.93 mile, veer right, following the red arrow, and after about 500 feet, you'll be back at the start of the loop. From here, retrace your steps to the trailhead. If you're interested in extending the hike, drive to the northern end of the park and pick up the trailhead just to the right of the swimming beach to hike along the lake. The first half of the trail hugs the shoreline, providing inspiring views of the lake, before looping back through the woods, making it a little more than 1 mile round-trip. Keep an eye out for bird-attracting plants such as the American beautyberry, a shrub that produces clusters of vibrant purple fruit in the autumn, and yaupon holly, a berry-bearing evergreen shrub.

NEARBY ACTIVITIES

In 1995 Wills Point was recognized as having the most bluebirds in the State of Texas and was officially proclaimed the Bluebird Capital of Texas. In honor of this fact, the town hosts an annual bluebird festival each spring, with food, exhibits, and live entertainment. Check the official website (**willspointbluebird.com**) to see if your visit will coincide with the April festival. Year-round, you can explore the town's historic buildings, Depot Museum, and pioneer cabin. You can also take a wagon tour (starting and ending at the Depot Museum) that hits the historic spots around town.

59 POST OAK TRAIL

KEY AT-A-GLANCE INFORMATION

LENGTH: 1.69 miles

CONFIGURATION: Loop

DIFFICULTY: Easy

SCENERY: Pond, thickets, woods, meadows

EXPOSURE: Partially sunny

TRAIL TRAFFIC: Light

TRAIL SURFACE: Dirt

HIKING TIME: 45 minutes

ACCESS: Daily; free

FACILITIES: Picnic tables

WHEELCHAIR TRAVERSABLE: No

SPECIAL COMMENTS: Birding is excellent around the small lake.

DRIVING DISTANCE FROM MAJOR INTERSECTION: 6.5 miles from US 175 and I-20

GPS TRAILHEAD COORDINATES

Latitude: N 32° 38' 28"

Longitude: W 96° 34' 8"

IN BRIEF

A shady hike looping through a pretty preserve, the first half of the trail is through a predominately thickly wooded area, whereas the second half winds through smaller clearings of native grasses. A small lake midway through the hike attracts birds.

DESCRIPTION

As part of an effort to provide students with environmental learning programs, the Dallas Independent School District established the Environmental Education Center. In southeast Dallas County, in the small town of Seagoville (named for its founder, T. K. Seago), the center was established in the 1970s and offers students an outdoor education experience; in addition, there is a museum complete with ecosystem exhibits, learning labs, and interactive video stations. Although the center is mainly intended for students, it also manages the Post Oak Preserve, which is just across the street, where this hike begins. The preserve's namesake—the post oak—is a small, acorn-producing, drought-resistant tree, commonly used to make fence posts.

Open to the public, the preserve offers nature trails winding through a small remnant of post oak savannah. The 334-acre preserve is also regularly used by the center as an

----

Directions ⟶

Take US 175 east toward Kaufman. In Seagoville, take the exit for Simonds Road/Kimberly Drive. Turn right onto Simonds Road and travel 2 miles to Bowers Road, then turn left. The Post Oak Preserve is about 1.5 miles down on the right, across from the Environmental Education Center.

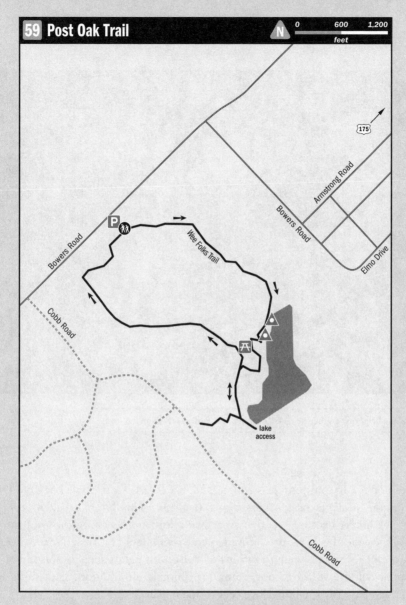

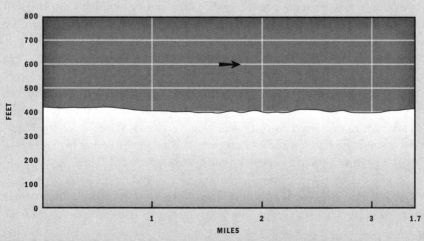

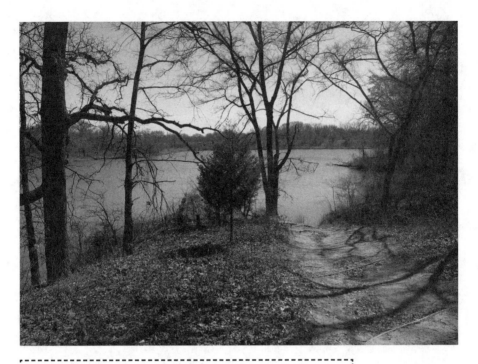

Take a brief rest on the shores of a small pond midway through the trail.

extension of its outdoor classroom, and if you visit on a weekday, you may encounter students or teachers along the trail. This is an excellent trail for younger hikers because wooden signs at various points along the trail instruct less experienced hikers, providing general reminders and tips, such as keeping an eye out for snakes, being cautious of poisonous plants such as poison ivy, and keeping wildlife wild by not feeding the animals. In addition, the trail is wide and flat—easy for small, curious feet to maneuver.

Start the hike by heading past the picnic area and bearing left onto the trail heading east (the path on the left is where you'll exit at the end of the hike). The trail winds through a thick woodland dotted with cedars and sporadic clumps of prairie grasses. Faced with all these trees, many of you may wonder, as I did, where the savannah is. Interestingly, natural fires and grazing bison are the two key forces in maintaining a savannah. The former keeps the woodlands at bay, allowing the prairie grasses to thrive, while the latter spreads the seed. Without these forces, the woodlands start to take over. As you hike along, you'll pass some educational signposts, which indicate that a woodland takeover is what you're seeing here.

As you continue, the trail becomes more densely wooded. Thick vines tangle themselves in the branches of the surrounding trees, hiding all signs of wildlife from view, though occasional rustling in the leaves and branches hints at their presence. At 0.3 mile, a small sign with bright-green lettering marks the split for the easy Wee Folks Trail. Stay to the left, bypassing the turnoff. As you continue along, the trees start to thin and you'll catch a few brief glimpses of water sparkling in the distance before you reach a signpost marking the "moderately easy" Lake Shore Trail. Another 0.27 mile down the trail, reach a quiet overlook of the preserve's 12-acre lake. A large old tree offers a shady spot for you to sit and observe the birds that frequent the small oasis. Most commonly, you'll spot teams of ducks paddling through the marshy waters or herons wading along the shoreline. If you glance up, you're likely to spot at least one slow-circling bird peering down at you—most likely a resident turkey vulture monitoring the ground for any food it can scavenge.

Back on the trail, you'll notice the scenery start to change as the woodlands thin dramatically and mix with patches of cactus and clumps of prairie grasses. At 0.92 mile, turn left onto a wide, paved road framed by short trees and shrubs. The road heads west and passes a picnic area before reaching another juncture a few hundred feet down. Bear left, following the paved path to its end, where it fades to join the soft, sandy banks of the lake. The gentle, sandy slopes offer you another chance to take a brief break and scope the pond-sized lake for waterfowl.

After exploring the short shoreline, head back up the trail and bear right at the next juncture to head northwest. The trail winds through patches of grassland dotted with small shrubs and cedar trees, markedly different from the dense woodlands characterizing the first half of the trail. You'll start to notice the shrubs and trees thin out, and then a sign advises that you've entered the Thickets and Meadow Trail. Throughout this section of trail, you'll find a couple of small, sunny meadows, framed by bright blue skies. Dragonflies and butterflies buzz and flutter as you round the final bend and turn back northeast toward the trailhead. From the final turn, it's a mere 0.2 mile before you emerge back at the trailhead, completing the loop.

NEARBY ACTIVITIES

The Rogers Wildlife Rehab and Farm Sanctuary is in nearby Hutchins, about 14 miles away. The facility is a nonprofit organization that rehabilitates injured birds and farm animals. Visitors are welcome to roam the property free of charge; donations are accepted. On the grounds, you'll find dozens of outdoor cages serving as temporary homes for rehabilitating hawks, owls, blue jays, vultures, and herons, among others. Geese and pheasants wander around unfettered. To get there, turn left, heading west on Simonds Road about 1.6 miles, then bear left onto Beltline Road and drive 4.6 miles. Turn right onto I-45 North, and go 3.6 miles to Exit 274, Dowdy Ferry Road/Palestine Street. Stay on the service road for about 0.5 mile, then turn right onto East Cleveland Street. The sanctuary is about 1 mile down on the left.

60 SAMUELL FARM TRAIL

KEY AT-A-GLANCE INFORMATION

LENGTH: 2.93 miles

CONFIGURATION: Triple loop

DIFFICULTY: Easy–moderate

SCENERY: Ponds, meadows, woods, birds, antique tractors

EXPOSURE: Sunny

TRAIL TRAFFIC: Light on weekdays, heavy on weekends

TRAIL SURFACE: Packed dirt

HIKING TIME: 1.5 hours

ACCESS: Free; open Tuesday–Sunday, 9 a.m.–5 p.m.

FACILITIES: Restrooms, picnic area

WHEELCHAIR TRAVERSABLE: No

SPECIAL COMMENTS: Hike in the morning to avoid the heat of the day on this sunny trail.

DRIVING DISTANCE FROM MAJOR INTERSECTION: 2.5 miles from US 80 and I-635

GPS TRAILHEAD COORDINATES

Latitude: N 32° 47' 12"

Longitude: W 96° 35' 2"

IN BRIEF

This cheerful hike through an old farm traverses a couple of pretty meadows and offers plenty to see, including a windmill, log cabins, and vintage tractors.

DESCRIPTION

Just off the service road of busy US 80 in Mesquite, Samuell Farm may seem like an unlikely spot for an enjoyable hiking experience, but don't let its location mislead you. The 340-acre farm is surprisingly beautiful, with miles of hiking trails and scores of birds. The farm is often used as an educational resource for school field trips and is also a regular monthly walk on the Dallas Trekkers Walking Club agenda. The atmosphere on the farm switches easily from festive and active to quiet and peaceful, so be prepared for either. I arrived one afternoon to find the huge gravel parking lot teeming with schoolkids and families. I set off expecting a lively hike; however, within 30 minutes of my arrival, the school buses had packed up and driven off, leaving me almost the only visitor on the entire farm. I enjoyed a couple of hours of quiet hiking and exploring and encountered only one other family, just as I was leaving.

The City of Dallas inherited the land in 1937 from the late Dr. W. W. Samuell. In 2001, budget constraints forced its closure,

Directions ————————————➤

Take I-30 East to US 80 East toward Terrell. Exit at Belt Line Road. Cross Belt Line Road and continue 0.3 mile on the service road. The entrance to Samuell Farm is just off the service road on the right and is marked by a huge tractor.

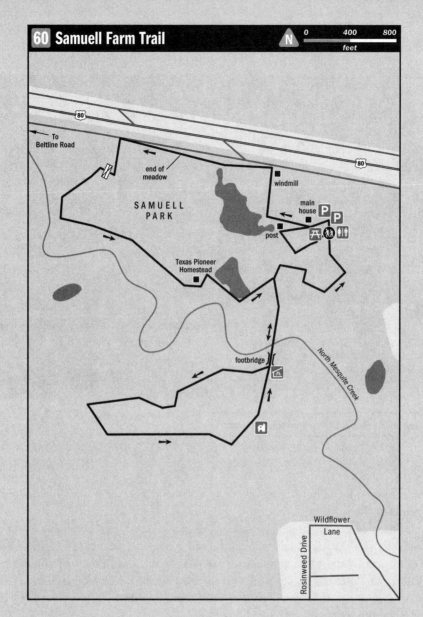

N

0   400   800
feet

To
Beltline Road

80

80

end of
meadow

windmill

SAMUELL
PARK

main
house

P P

post

Texas Pioneer
Homestead

North Mesquite Creek

footbridge

Wildflower
Lane

Rosinweed Drive

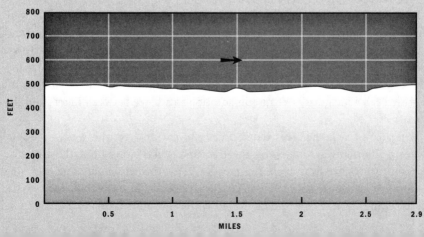

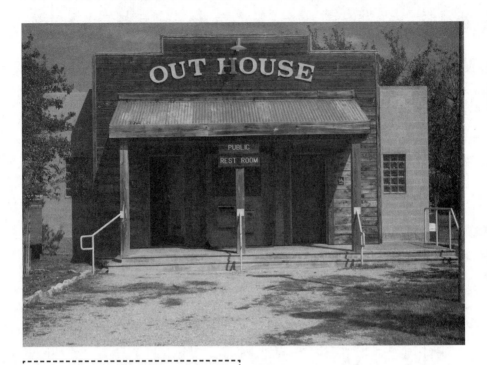

The cheery facade of a modern-day outhouse

and it has reopened in the past couple of years only with help from the nonprofit Friends of the Farm.

Enter the farm through the gate just to the left (east) of the main building. To your left, you'll see a small wooden building housing the restrooms. Begin the hike by turning right to take the dirt path passing in front of the main building. A picnic area dotted with colorful vintage tractors and a few tables fills a large expanse of grass off to your left. On your right, you'll pass a small working garden, then the trail splits in several directions.

Follow the wide dirt path to the right as it curves back toward the highway between a small pond and the parking lot. The trail heads toward the highway and at 0.57 mile reaches a windmill, where you'll turn left. The trail then narrows, following a faint grassy trail between the highway on the right, and a pretty meadow on the left. (Although the cars are distracting, the trail is safe for all ages—there is a wide grassy expanse in addition to a fence between hikers and the roadway.)

When you reach the trees that border the meadow on the west, turn left, away from the highway, following the tree line. Hike along until the tree line ends, then turn right, away from the meadow. Pass through a gate and continue 0.1 mile until the next split, where you'll turn left. The trail then loops back southeast alongside a wide meadow dotted with trees. Insects are abundant, so be sure you've applied repellent. On a sunny day, you may see small yellow butter-flies flitting across the trail. Crickets and grasshoppers are also abundant and are likely to smack you in the chest as they hop out of your way and back into the tall meadow grasses. The meadow also attracts birds and is a good spot to see the scissor-tailed flycatcher, easily identified by its forked tail.

Straight ahead, you'll see the Texas Pioneer Homestead, a picturesque old log cabin, whose cramped quarters and tiny rooms are open to exploration. Con-tinue along the path past a small pond, to the next split at 1.5 miles, where you'll turn right, following the gravel trail south. The trail heads slightly downhill into a dip where a shallow creek cuts the trail and prevents further progress. Instead of wading through the water, cross the grass to your right, following the creek a few dozen feet to a small red footbridge hidden behind the trees. Rejoin the trail, keeping the gazebo to your left. Another pond off to the right sets the bucolic mood as you pass rolls of hay and approach a large barn. At 2.15 miles, follow the trail to the right, passing the barn and a picnic area. The trail continues past a huge sunny meadow with tall grasses and brilliant yellow sunflowers.

You'll soon reach the next trail split, where you'll hang a right, following the shady remnants of a wide dirt road. Stay to the right at the next path split at 2.33 miles. After about another 0.2 mile, the gazebo will pop back into view. Before you reach it, bear left back onto the footbridge and cross the creek heading back toward the entrance.

At 2.7 miles, turn right on the path just before the picnic area. If you've brought lunch, grab a table and a bite; otherwise, continue along the trail, which passes between dozens of antique tractors. Take the next two lefts to do a small loop. Another picnic area and a small log cabin to the right invite closer inspec-tion. From here, it's just a few hundred feet back to the trailhead.

NEARBY ACTIVITIES

From spring through early fall, you can catch the Mesquite Championship Rodeo, which features bull riding, chuck-wagon races, clowns, cowboys, and cowgirls. Shows typically start in the early evenings. Check **mesquiterodeo.com** for the cur-rent season's hours and rates. The rodeo is 8 miles away. To get there, take US 80E west 3 miles. Merge onto I-635 South and travel 2 miles, then exit at Scyene Road/TX 352. Stay on the service road for about 0.5 mile, then turn right onto Rodeo Drive.

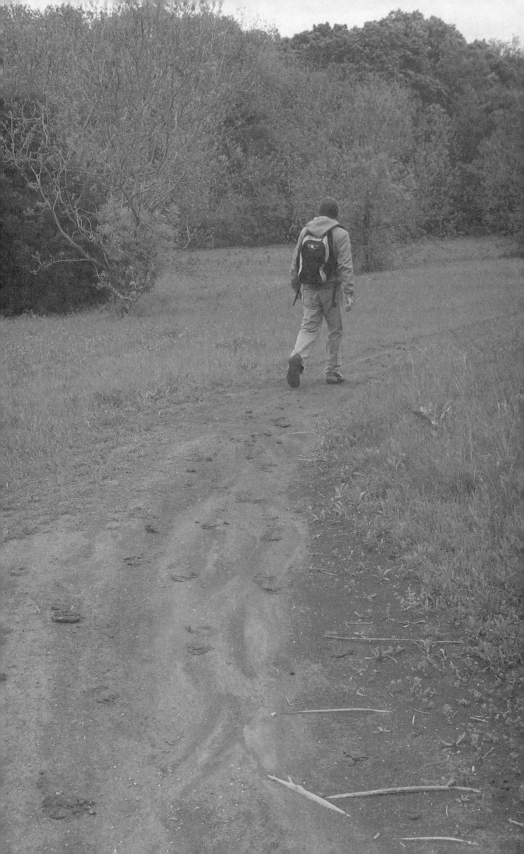

APPENDIXES AND INDEX

APPENDIX A:
OUTDOOR SHOPS

ACADEMY SPORTS + OUTDOORS
academy.com

6101 I-20 (at Bryant Irvin Road)
Fort Worth, TX 76132
(817) 361-1240

(See Academy website for more locations throughout the Metroplex.)

BASS PRO SHOPS
basspro.com

2501 Bass Pro Dr.
Grapevine, TX 76051
(972) 724-2018

5001 Bass Pro Dr.
Garland, TX 75043
(469) 221-2600

CABELA'S
cabelas.com

12901 Cabela Dr.
Fort Worth, TX 76177
(817) 337-2400

CAMPING WORLD
campingworld.com

10100 South Fwy.
Fort Worth, TX 76140
(866) 393-6441 or (817) 568-1991

5209 I-35 N.
Denton, TX 76207
(800) 527-4812 or (940) 898-8906

DICK'S SPORTING GOODS
dickssportinggoods.com

Parks at Arlington
3891 S. Cooper St.
Arlington, TX 76015
(817) 987-4800

13838 Dallas Pkwy.
Dallas, TX 75240
(972) 239-5455

8030 Park Ln.
Dallas, TX 75231
(214) 696-5800

(See Dick's website for more locations throughout the Metroplex.)

MOUNTAIN HIDEOUT
5643 Lovers Ln.
Dallas, TX 75209
(214) 350-8181

MOUNTAIN SPORTS
mountainsports.com

2025 W. Pioneer Pkwy.
Arlington, TX 76013
(800) 805-9139 or (817) 461-4503

REI
rei.com

4510 LBJ Freeway
Dallas, TX 75244
(972) 490-5989

2424 Preston Rd.
Plano, TX 75093
(972) 985-2241

SPORTS AUTHORITY
sportsauthority.com

9100 N. Central Expy., #123
Caruth Plaza
Dallas, TX 75231
(214) 363-8441

4830 SW Loop 820
Overton Plaza
Fort Worth, TX 76109
(817) 377-1515

(See Sports Authority website for more locations throughout the Metroplex.)

SUN & SKI SPORTS
sunandski.com

1100 W. Arbrook Blvd.
Arlington, TX 76015
(682) 433-0027

11170 N. Central Expy.
Dallas, TX 75243
(214) 442-7007

2943 Preston Rd., #1400
Frisco, TX 75034
(214) 494-4288

3000 Grapevine Mills Pkwy.
Grapevine, TX 76051
(972) 355-9424

WHOLE EARTH PROVISION CO.
wholeearthprovision.com

5400 E. Mockingbird Ln.
Dallas, TX 75206
(214) 824-7444

APPENDIX B:
PLACES TO BUY MAPS

DeLORME
delorme.com

KAPPA MAP GROUP
universalmap.com

MAPTECH, INC.
maptech.com

NATIONAL GEOGRAPHIC
nationalgeographic.com

ONE MAP PLACE, INC.
onemapplace.com

1620 Surveyor Blvd.
Carrollton, TX 75006
(972) 416-5071

REI
rei.com

TRAILS.COM
trails.com

USGS MAP STORE
store.usgs.gov

TEXAS PARKS & WILDLIFE
tpwd.state.tx.us

*(Free downloads of many
Texas State Park maps)*

USDA FOREST SERVICE
www.fs.fed.us/r8/texas

APPENDIX C:
HIKING CLUBS

AMERICAN HIKING SOCIETY
americanhiking.org

DALLAS SIERRA CLUB
texas.sierraclub.org/Dallas

DFW OUTDOORS
dfwoutdoors.com

FORT WORTH SIERRA CLUB
texas.sierraclub.org/fortworth

TEXINS OUTDOOR CLUB
outdoorclub.org

TEXAS OUTDOORS WOMAN NETWORK
towndallas.org

INDEX

A

Adolphus Hotel, 33
African American museums, 42, 178
Airports
    Love Field, 18–21
    Red Bird, 22–25
Allen Premium Outlet Mall, 150
Ameriquest Field, 83, 119
Animal hazards, 9–10
Aquariums, 21, 42
Arbor Hills Loop, 138–41
Arlington
    Linear Trail, 43–46
    River Legacy Trail, 116–19
Art Deco buildings, 39–42
Audie Murphy American Cotton Museum,
    190
Audubon Trail, Trinity River, 64–68

B

Bachman Lake Trail, 18–21
Backcountry camping, 13
Bardwell Lake Multiuse Trail, 198–201
Baseball, 83, 119
Bear Creek–Bob Eden Trail, 80–83
Benbrook Dam Trail, 84–87
Benbrook Lake Trail, 88–91
Bicycle trails
    Cedar Hill State Park, 202–5
    Erwin Park Loop, 159–62
    Horseshoe Trail, 104–7
    Knob Hill Trail, 108–11
    Lake Mineral Wells State Park, 252–56

    Lake Mineral Wells State Trailway,
        257–60
    Ray Roberts Lake State Park, 183–86
    River Legacy Trail, 116–19
    Sansom Park Trail, 124–27
    Sister Grove Loop, 187–90
    Trinity River Trail, 128–36
    Visitor's Overlook, 233–36
    White Rock Lake Trail, 73–77
Bird-watching, xx
Bison, 100–103, 151–54
Black Creek–Cottonwood Hiking Trail,
    142–46
Blackland Prairie, Arbor Hills Loop, 138–41
Blue Bird Capital of Texas, 271
Bluebonnet Trail, 213
Bluebonnet Trails Festival, 201
Boating
    Benbrook Lake, 88–91
    Cedar Hill State Park, 202–5
    Lake Mineral Wells State Park, 252–56
    Lake Tawakoni Nature Trail, 268–71
    Pilot Knoll Trail, 171–74
    Purtis Creek Trail, 229–32
    Ray Roberts Lake State Park,
        179–82, 183–86
    Trinity River, 99, 103
    Visitor's Overlook, 233–36
Bob Eden Trail, 80–83
Botanic gardens, 87
Boulder Park Trail, 22–25
Breckenridge Park Trail, 147–50
Bridges, Old Alton, 155–58
Bubba's Bar-B-Q & Steakhouse, 201
Buffalos, 100–103, 151–54

C

Caddo Park, 170
Caddo–Lyndon B. Johnson National
      Grasslands, 142–46
Camping
   advice for, 13
   Cedar Hill State Park, 202–5
   Cleburne State Park Loop Trail, 215–19
   Erwin Park Loop, 159–62
   guidelines for, 13
   Lake Mineral Wells State Park, 252–56
   Lake Tawakoni Nature Trail, 268–71
   Lavon Lake, Trinity Trail, 163–66
   Pilot Knoll Trail, 171–74
   Purtis Creek Trail, 229–32
   Ray Roberts Lake State Park,
      179–82, 183–86
   Visitor's Overlook, 233–36
   Walnut Creek Trail, 237–40
Campion Trail, 26–29
Canoeing, Trinity River, 99, 103
Canyon Ridge Trail, 96–99
Cattail Pond Trail, 212–13
Cattle drive, 127
Cedar Brake Trail, 212
Cedar Hill State Park
   Cedar Mountain Trail, 206–9
   Cedar Ridge Preserve Trail, 210–14
   Talala–Duck Pond Loop, 202–5
   Visitor's Overlook, 233–36
Cedar Lake, 215–19
Cedar Mountain Trail, 206–9
Cedar Ridge Preserve Trail, 210–14
Children, hiking with, xiv–xv, 7
Cicada–Cottonwood Loop, 151–54
Clear Fork River, 132–35
Cleburne State Park Loop Trail, 215–19
Clothing recommendations, 6
Coffee Mill, Lake, 142–46
Colleyville Nature Trail, 92–95
Continental DAR House, 41
Copper Canyon, Elm Fork Trail, 155–58
Cotton Bowl, 42
Cotton museums, 190
Cottonwood Creek Trail, 220–23

Cottonwood Lake, 142–46
Creeks, hikes along, xvi
Cross Timbers Trail, 252–56

D

Dallas Aquarium, 42
Dallas area, 17–77
Dallas Nature Center, 210–14
Dallas World Aquarium, 21
DAR House, 41
Davy Crockett, Lake, 142–46
Dealey Plaza, 34
Deep Ellum, 34
Denton
   Knob Hill Trail, 108–11
   Lewisville Lake, 158
   Ray Roberts Greenbelt, 175–78
Denton Creek, 108–11
Dinosaur Track, 115
Dinosaur Valley State Park, 219
Dinosaur Valley Trail, 224–28
Dogs, hiking with, xvii
Downtown Dallas Urban Trail, 30–34
Drinking water, 5–6
Duck Creek Greenbelt, 35–38
Dutch Branch Park, 85

E

East of Dallas, 266–79
Elevation, 2
Elm Fork Trail, 155–58
Elm tree, 26, 29
Ennis, 198–201
Equestrian trails
   Black Creek–Cottonwood Hiking Trail,
      142–46
   Lake Mineral Wells State Park, 252–56
   Lake Mineral Wells State Trailway,
      257–60
   Lavon Lake, 163–66
   Walnut Creek Trail, 237–40
   Walnut Grove Trail, 191–94
Erwin Park Loop, 159–62
Escarpment Road Trail, 213

Etiquette, trail, 13–14
Exercise stations, 82

F

Fair Park Loop, 39–42
Famous Mineral Water Company, 256
Farms
  exhibits of, 209
  Rogers Wildlife Rehab and Farm
    Sanctuary, 223, 275
  Samuell Farm Trail, 276–79
Ferris wheel, 39, 42
Firewheel Town Center, 38, 59, 63
First-aid kit, 7
Fish Creek Linear Trail, 43–46
Fishing, 182, 229–32
  Benbrook Dam Trail, 84–87
  Benbrook Lake, 88–91
  Cedar Hill State Park, 202–5
  Cicada–Cottonwood Loop, 151–54
  Cleburne State Park Loop Trail, 215–19
  Colleyville Nature Trail, 92–95
  Lake Mineral Wells State Park, 252–56
  Lake Tawakoni Nature Trail, 268–71
  North Shore Trail, 112–15
  Pilot Knoll Trail, 171–74
  Purtis Creek Trail, 229–32
  Ray Roberts Lake State Park,
    179–82, 186
  Sansom Park Trail, 124–27
  Visitor's Overlook, 233–36
  Walnut Creek Trail, 237–40
Forest Trail, 67
Forests, Great Trinity, 64–68
Fort Richardson State Park, 261–64
Fort Worth area, 78–135
Fort Worth Botanic Gardens, 87
Fort Worth Nature Center
  Canyon Ridge Trail, 96–99
  Prairie Trail, 100–103
Fossil(s)
  Dinosaur Valley State Park, 224–28
  Fossil Ridge Trail, 215, 218
  Fossil Rim Wildlife Center, 219, 228
  Fossil Valley Trail, 213

Sansom Park Trail, 124–27
Founders Square Park, 30

G

Gardens, 42, 87
Garland
  Duck Creek Greenbelt, 35–38
  Rowlett Creek Nature Trail, 56–59
Gaylord Texan, 115
Global positioning trailhead coordinates, 2
Golden Triangle Mall, 178
Grand Prairie
  Linear Trail, 43–46
  Walnut Creek Trail, 237–40
Grapevine Lake
  Horseshoe Trail, 104–7
  Rockledge Park, 112–15
  Rocky Point Trail, 120–23
  Walnut Grove Trail, 191–94
Grapevine Mills Mall, 194
Grapevine Vintage Railroad, 107
Grasslands, 142–46
Great Trinity Forest, 64–68
Greenbelt
  Bear Creek–Bob Eden Trail, 80–83
  Duck Creek, 35–38
  Ray Roberts, 175–78
Greenville, 190
Greer Island, 99, 103

H

Hall of State, 41
Hardwick Interpretative Center, 103
Heard Natural Science Museum, 162
Heritage Park Plaza, 128
Hikes
  best-maintained trails, xv
  birding, xx
  busiest trails, xv
  for children, xiv–xv
  along creeks, xvi
  difficult, xviii
  for dogs, xvii
  easiest, xv

H (*continued*)

Hikes (*continued*)
  flat, xvi
  for historical interest, xx
  lake, xvii
  over 5 miles, xiv
  along rivers, xvi
  for runners, xvi–xvii
  scenic, xviii
  for solitude, xv
  steepest, xviii
  under 3 miles, xiii
  3–5 miles, xiii–xiv
  urban, xviii–xix
  wheelchair-accessible, xix
  wildflower, xix
  wildlife, xix
Hiking clubs, 284
Historic trails, 26–29
Historical sites, xx, 87
  Cicaca–Cottonwood Loop, 151–54
  Elm Fork Trail, 155–58
  Lost Creek Reservoir State Trailway,
    261–64
  Samuell Farm Trail, 276–79
  Talala–Duck Pond Loop, 205
Horse racing, 240
Horse trails. *See* Equestrian trails
Horseshoe Trail, 104–7
Houston, L. B., Nature Trail, 52–55
Hutchins, 223, 275

I

Insects, 10–11
Interurban Park, 244
Iron Bridge Dam, 268–71
Isle du Bois, Ray Roberts Lake State Park,
  Lost Pines Trail, 179–82

J

Jacksboro, Lost Creek Reservoir State
  Trailway, 261–64
Joe Pool Lake, 206–9, 237–40, 248
Joe Pool Lake Dam Trail, 233–36

John Neely Bryan Cabin, 30
Johnson Branch Trail, Ray Roberts Lake
  State Park, 183–86

K

Katy Trail, 47–51
Kennedy Memorial Plaza, 30–34
Knob Hill Trail, 108–11

L

L. B. Houston Nature Trail, 52–55
Lake(s), hikes along, xvii
Lake Mineral Wells State Park, Cross
  Timbers Trail, 252–56
Lake Mineral Wells State Trailway, 257–60
Lake Tawakoni Nature Trail, 268–71
Lake Worth Monster, 98
Las Colinas, 55
Lavon Lake, 163–66, 187–90
LBJ National Grasslands, 142–46
Leonhardt Lagoon, 42
Lewisville Lake, 151–54, 155–58, 171–74
Little Bear Creek, 95
Log Cabin Village, 87
Lone Star Park, 240
Lost Creek Reservoir State Trailway,
  261–64
Lost Pines Trail, Ray Roberts Lake
  State Park, 179–82
Love Field Airport, 18–21
Loyd Park, 237–40

M

McCormick Park, 83
McKinney, Erwin Park Loop, 159–62
Magnolia Hotel, 33
Maps, 1, 12–13, 284.
  See also individual trails
Marathon, White Rock Lake, 73
Marion Sansom Park, 124–27
Marshall Creek Park, 192
Memorial Oak, 135
Mesquite, Samuell Farm Trail, 276–79
Mineral Wells, Lake, 252–56, 257–60

Mosquitoes, 10–11
Mulberry Trail, 213
Murrell Park, 113, 115
Museums, 41–42
    African American, 42, 178
    art, 83
    baseball, 83, 119
    cotton, 190
    Denton County, 178
    Ellis County, 244
    Jack County, 264
    natural history, 41, 162
    Wills Point, 271
    women's, 41–42

N

Nancy Dillon National Recreation Trail, 43
NASCAR racing, 111
Nature centers
    Fort Worth, 96–103
    Trinity River, 64–68
North East Mall, 95
North Garland, Spring Creek Park
    Nature Trail, 60–63
North Irving, sculptures in, 55
North of Dallas, 137–94
North Shore Trail, 112–15

O

Oak Grove Park, 104–7
Oakmont Park, 132–35
Old Alton Bridge Park, 155–58
Old Mill Inn, 41
Old Red Courthouse, 30

P

Parkhill Prairie Trail, 167–70
Parks
    Bob Eden, 80–83
    Boulder, 22–25
    Breckenridge, 147–50
    Caddo, 170
    Cedar Hill State Park, 202–5, 206–9,
        210–14, 233–36

Cleburne State Park, 215–19
Dinosaur Valley State Park, 219
Dutch Branch, 85
Erwin, 159–62
Fair Park, 39–42
Fish Creek, 43–46
Fort Richardson State Park, 261–64
Founders Square, 30
Interurban, 244
Isle du Bois, 179–82
Johnson Branch, 183–86
Katy Trail State Park, 47–51
Lake Mineral Wells State Park,
    252–56, 257–60
Lone Star, 240
Loyd, 237–40
McCormick, 83
Marion Sansom, 124–27
Marshall Creek, 192
Murrell, 113, 115
Oak Grove, 104–7
Oakmont, 132–35
Old Alton Bridge, 155–58
Pecan Valley, 132–35
Pike, 48
Pilot Knoll, 171–74
Purtis Creek State Park, 229–32
Ray Roberts Lake, 179–82, 183–86
Reverchon, 48, 51, 69–72
River Legacy, 116–19
Rivercrest, 56–59
Robert E. Lee, 48, 69–72
Rockledge, 112–15
Rocky Creek, 88–91
Samuell, 276–79
Sister Grove, 187–90
Southlake, 192
Spring Creek, 60–63
Twin Coves, 113
Victory, 50–51
Waxahachie Creek, 198–201
Pecan Valley Park, 87, 132–35
Penitentiary Hollow, 259
Penn Farm Agricultural History Center,
    205, 209, 248

P (*continued*)

Pike Park, 48, 51
Pilot Knoll Trail, 171–74
Pioneer Plaza Cattle Drive, 32
Planetarium, 46
Plano, Arbor Hills Loop, 138–41
Plant hazards, 10
Poisonous plants, 10
Possumhaw Trail, 212
Post Oak Trail, 272–75
Prairie Dog Town, 100–103
Prairies
    Arbor Hills Loop, 138–41
    Parkhill Prairie Trail, 167–70
    Prairie Trail, 100–103
Primitive camping, 13
Purtis Creek Trail, 229–32

R

Railroad-bed trails
    Katy Trail State Park, 47–51
    Lake Mineral Wells State Trailway,
        257–60
Railroad excursions, 107
Ray Roberts Greenbelt, 175–78
Ray Roberts Lake State Park
    Isle du Bois Unit, Lost Pines Trail, 179–82
    Johnson Branch Unit,
        Johnson Branch Trail, 183–86
Red Bird Airport, Duncanville, 22–25
Red Bird Mall, 25
Red Oak Trail, 213
Reunion Tower, 33
Reverchon Park, 48, 51, 69–72
Richardson, Breckenridge Park Trail,
    147–50
Riparian Wetland, Arbor Hills Loop,
    138–41
River(s), hikes along, xvi
River Legacy Trail, 116–19
Rivercrest Park, 56–59
Robert E. Lee Park, 48, 69–72
Rock climbing, 252–56
Rockledge Park, 112–15

Rocky Creek Park, 88–91
Rocky Point Trail, 120–23
Rodeos, 279
Rogers Street Bridge, 244
Rogers Wildlife Rehab and Farm Sanctuary,
    223, 275
Rowlett Creek Nature Trail, 56–59
Runners, hikes for, xvi–xvii

S

Sabine River, 268–71
Safety, 8–11
Samuell Farm Trail, 276–79
Sansom Park Trail, 124–27
Scenic hikes, xviii
Science centers, 116–19
Sculptures
    Downtown Dallas Urban Trail, 32, 33
    Fair Park Loop, 39–42
    museums for, 77
    North Irving, 55
    Williams Square, 29
Seagoville, Post Oak Trail, 272–75
Shady Spring camping area, 218
Shawnee Trail, 32
Shopping, 282–83
    Allen Premium Outlet Mall, 150
    Firewheel Town Center, 38, 59, 63
    Golden Triangle Mall, 178
    Grapevine Mills Mall, 194
    North East Mall, 95
    Red Bird Mall, 25
    Southwest Center Mall, 25
    Trader's Village, 205
    Vista Ridge Mall, 154
    West Village, 72
Sister Grove Loop, 187–90
Skinny Dip Cove, 91
Snakes, 10
South of Dallas, 196–248
Southfork Ranch, 141, 166
Southlake Park, 192
Southwest Center Mall, 25
Speedways, 111
Spillway Hiking Trail, 215

Spring Creek Park Nature Trail, 60–63
Steep hikes, xviii
Sundance Square, 99, 103
Swimming, Benbrook Lake, 88–91

T

TADRA Point, 145
Talala–Duck Pond Loop, 202–5
Texas Discovery Gardens, 42
Texas Motor Speedway, 111
Texas Pioneer Homestead, 279
Texas School Book Depository, 34
Texas State Fair Grounds, 39–42
Texas Tourist Camp Complex, 146
Thanks-Giving Square, 33
Ticks, 9
Trader's Village, 205
Trail etiquette, 13–14
Trees, historic and interesting
    Campion Trail, 29
    Oakmont Park, 135
    Post Oak Trail, 272–75
Trinity River, 99
    Audubon Trail, 64–68
    L. B. Houston Nature Trail, 52–55
    Lavon Lake, 163–66
    River Legacy Trail, 116–19
    Trinity River Trail
        Northside, 128–31
        Oakmont Park, 132–35
Turtle Creek Leisure Trail, 69–72
Twin Coves Park, 113

U

University of Texas planetarium, 46
Upland Forest, Arbor Hills Loop, 138–41
Urban hikes, xviii–xix

V

Victory Park, 50–51
Vietnam Memorial, 39–42
Visitor's Overlook: Joe Pool Lake Dam
    Trail, 233–36
Vista Ridge Mall, 154

W

Walnut Creek Trail, 237–40
Walnut Grove Trail, 191–94
Water, 5–6
Waxahachie Creek, 198–201
Waxahachie Creek Hike and Bike Trail,
    241–44
Weather, 4–5
Weatherford, Lake Mineral Wells
        State Trailway, 257–60
West of Fort Worth, 250–64
West Plano, Arbor Hills Loop, 138–41
West Village, shopping in, 72
Wetland Trail, 67–68
Wheelchair-accessible hikes, xix
Whispering Meadow Trail, 215
Whistle Stop Café, 146
White Rock Lake Trail, 73–77
Wildflower hikes, xix
Wildlife hikes, xix
Williams Square, 29, 55
Wills Point, 271
Wilmer, Cottonwood Creek Trail, 220–23
Windmill Hill Preserve Trail, 245–48
Winfrey Point, 76

Z

Zoos
    children's, 42
    Fort Worth Zoo, 131, 135
    Fossil Rim Wildlife Center, 219, 228

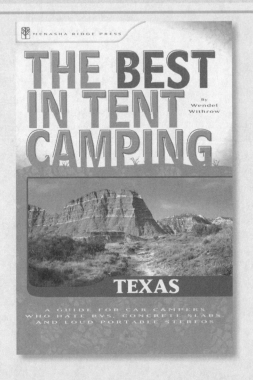
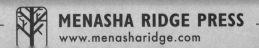

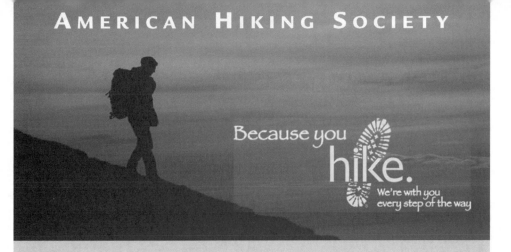
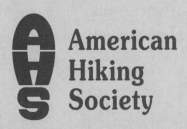

DEAR CUSTOMERS AND FRIENDS,

SUPPORTING YOUR INTEREST IN OUTDOOR ADVENTURE, travel, and an active lifestyle is central to our operations, from the authors we choose to the locations we detail to the way we design our books. Menasha Ridge Press was incorporated in 1982 by a group of veteran outdoorsmen and professional outfitters. For many years now, we've specialized in creating books that benefit the outdoors enthusiast.

Almost immediately, Menasha Ridge Press earned a reputation for revolutionizing outdoors- and travel-guidebook publishing. For such activities as canoeing, kayaking, hiking, backpacking, and mountain biking, we established new standards of quality that transformed the whole genre, resulting in outdoor-recreation guides of great sophistication and solid content. Menasha Ridge continues to be outdoor publishing's greatest innovator.

The folks at Menasha Ridge Press are as at home on a white-water river or mountain trail as they are editing a manuscript. The books we build for you are the best they can be, because we're responding to your needs. Plus, we use and depend on them ourselves.

We look forward to seeing you on the river or the trail. If you'd like to contact us directly, join in at www.trekalong.com or visit us at www.menasharidge.com. We thank you for your interest in our books and the natural world around us all.

SAFE TRAVELS,

Bob Sehlinger

BOB SEHLINGER
PUBLISHER